WHAT ABOUT THE BOY?

WHAT ABOUT

A Father's Pledge
to His Disabled Son

THE BOY?

STEPHEN GALLUP

LESTRYGONIAN BOOKS

SAN DIEGO

ISBN-13 978-0-615-43153-6

Library of Congress Control Number 2011900815

Printed in the United States of America

Book Design by GKS Creative

AUTHOR'S NOTE

This is a work of nonfiction that accurately depicts events and conversations as they occurred. The names of some participants have been changed in order to protect their privacy.

1. SOMEONE TO LOVE

Ku-dun-ku-dun-ku-dun-ku-dun…

"It sounds like a gallop," the Labor and Delivery nurse joked, making a pun on our name.

Judy and I laughed. The fetal monitor strapped onto her belly amplified a signal that did sound like the hollow clatter of hooves. The concussions of that tiny heartbeat reverberated in the narrow room at San Diego's Kaiser Foundation Hospital, making our baby's presence real.

We were already calling him Joseph, although there'd been no prenatal tests that might have established the gender. Judy swore she just knew it was a boy. Besides, folk wisdom held that males had slower fetal heart rates, and 134 beats a minute was fairly slow. Still, either sex would be perfectly all right. Did we want a boy or a girl? For nine months our stock answer had been a resounding "You bet!"

"As long as the baby is healthy …" Everyone says that.

Judy's labor proceeded slowly—or else the hands of our clock were spinning at an improbable rate. Surely *that* much time hadn't passed! But the nurse who'd joked about our name had gone home. A new shift of doctors and nurses checked in with us periodically but gave most of their attention to our neighbors, some of whom were not coping well. One desperate voice in the next room kept insisting, *"¡No puedo! ¡No puedo!"* I can't! I can't!—its owner deaf to the urgent advice offered in two languages. Judy just concentrated on the breathing techniques that had been taught in our La Maze course, and, like all anxious dads-to-be, I tried to help by providing cups of crushed ice and deliberately panting through the contractions with her, face-to-face: *"Hee! Hee!"* A pause, and then a long, drawn-out *"Hoooo."* Another pause and we repeated. For more hours still.

Three-fifteen; this was a.m. Judy had been flat on her back for seventeen hours. The nurses praised her control, obviously meaning what they said. But enough was enough. She needed help. And so an anesthesiologist appeared to give a series of epidural injections (three, since the first two didn't work). The woman offered a little pleasant chatter while waiting to see if her drug would ever take hold. It turned out she was familiar with our home turf in Virginia, which we'd left two years earlier to move Out West. The three of us reminisced about the Blue Ridge Mountains, until we noticed that Judy was no longer suffering.

In the quiet minutes that followed, Judy and I looked at each other and shrugged. The plan had been to have a "natural" childbirth. But this one compromise wasn't so bad. Modern medical science would complement nature. We felt perfectly at ease when they popped an oxygen mask over her mouth and nose shortly thereafter. I recalled tales of babies who in more benighted days had been damaged by birth asphyxia and knew mine at least would be OK. The heart monitor continued feeding out spools of paper with a graphic representation of the galloping hooves, which we took as assurance that all was still well. The IV, now with its piggyback bottles of other drugs—all this high-tech stuff, I knew, would protect us.

"What? Are you folks still here?" The morning shift was back on duty. I could hear someone being briefed on the activity in each of the labor rooms. The Hispanic lady next door had been whisked away for a C-section. I gathered that we were next in the queue.

A handsome, balding doctor strode into the room with a plan. "It's high time we got that baby out," he announced. "I recommend proceeding right away with caesarian delivery."

"Please, no," Judy said weakly.

He raised an eyebrow at me. "We wanted to do this the traditional way," I explained.

"Yes, but you haven't succeeded. Your wife has made very little progress. And now she's exhausted."

"I can still do it," Judy interjected, miffed at being excluded from the conversation.

He shook his head. "The baby might be too large to be delivered normally." He looked us both up and down: a short mom and a skinny dad, people unlikely to produce a giant.

"OK. Let's give it a try," he decided reluctantly. "But just once! *Then* we're doing a section." Attendants appeared and wheeled my wife's bed into the delivery room. I followed her inside, where the pace of events rapidly entered high gear as four or five green-clad specialists donned surgical masks and briskly attended to their appointed tasks.

The wall clock showed 8:35. This day—March 5, 1985—we would gain a new family member, the first of the next generation.

The doctor produced a device that resembled a bathroom plunger and explained that he would make one attempt at a suction delivery. "Set the dial at Six," he told someone. "I *won't* go any higher than that." He glanced at us and friendly crow's feet appeared above his mask. "Well, what do you want, a boy or a girl?" As if all we had to do was place our order now, and he'd bring forth the appropriate gender. Long past the stage of glib replies, we just shook our heads and babbled.

Then Judy's last contraction began. She gripped the rails on the table, bent her head forward, and knotted every muscle in a supreme effort. I kept up a steady patter of encouragement in her ear until I saw the doctor holding my son. Then I collapsed on her shoulder, saying, "God bless you, Judy!" She just smiled weakly at the ceiling.

Joseph was in a tray, having his cord cut. A nurse named Esther called me over, and I gazed at him in awe. Childbirth films we'd seen had hinted that this could be a moving experience. They were right. The baby before me was perfectly formed, with no bruises or blemishes to show for the long ordeal just past. I couldn't believe how beautiful he was. The moment felt unreal. My child radiated an almost other-worldly presence.

"Well, pick him up," she suggested, in the amused tone of a pastor prodding stunned newlyweds to kiss. I did, nervously. She'd popped a little knitted stocking hat on his head, and together we wrapped a blanket around him. I sat down with him beside Judy, where she could watch.

"Hi, Joe," I whispered. That's all I could say, and I said it many times. He lay in my arms quietly, yawning, and running through a menu of facial expressions. Was he going to cry? Sneeze? Smile? He couldn't seem to decide. I thought he was very alert, cutting his little blue eyes back and forth to take in the scenery, and startling when a telephone rang. The doctor, bothered by a string of mucus suddenly dangling from my nose, asked Esther to give me a tissue.

EVENTUALLY, satisfied that wife and son were in good hands, I left to relay the tidings to our somewhat elderly parents, mine in Virginia and hers in Florida.

We slept through the rest of that day, then began the process of get-ting acquainted with our son.

"Look at the way he keeps sizing us up," Judy said. "That shrewd ex-pression reminds me of your father!"

"You're right! It's like he's saying, *Don't think you can pull any fast ones on ME, buster. I wasn't born yesterday.*"

"Except," she laughed happily, "In Joseph's case, he *was*!"

Her recovery from the multiple epidurals was slow, and so we re-mained in the hospital longer than we might have otherwise. Staying close to professionals seemed a good thing. Feeding and burping and diapering him—this was new stuff! Judy and I criticized each other's clumsy maneuvers, especially when he cried or spit up. Occasionally, he would turn very dark in the face, his tiny chin quivering as he gathered air before emitting a pitiful little wail. We looked to the experts around us for guidance.

The nurses frowned and said he had "an irritable cry." The term seemed to have special meaning.

Worse, however, was the vomiting. I fed him and burped him (or tried to), and then invariably, soundlessly, prodigiously, everything came up once again, all over me, the blanket, everything. Judy fared no better. Surely, we should blame this on our lack of experience.

Or, maybe not.

"I'm afraid the little guy will have to stay with us just a while longer," the nurse now said. Checkout time had finally arrived, but instead of bringing us our child, this lady was prancing nervously in the doorway of Judy's room. Because of the problems we'd all observed, she said, the doctors wanted to start him on a course of antibiotics and run some tests. "Your baby isn't critically ill," she assured us, turning sideways and flexing a knee as if anxious to get away. "But he *is* sick. Letting him stay here until we have all these little things sorted out will just give him the best possible start for when you do take him home."

That sounded reasonable. Looking back, I suppose her body language meant that she feared hysterics, but we latched on to the "best possible start" aspect of her message. Of course we wanted him to get a good start. Lacking confidence in our own ability to provide that, we almost welcomed this news.

They'd already moved him to the hospital's Special Care Nursery. Judy and I scrubbed, donned sterile gowns, and went to see him there. We found it a quiet place. The bassinet next to his contained an unmoving bit of life the size of a kitten.

A nurse saw me gaping, and smiled disarmingly. "That's little Gary. He's been with us a few weeks now."

Should we be upset? The staff maintained such an upbeat demeanor that we suppressed our fears. What he had, they didn't know. Possibly it was a bacterial infection. After a day of being fed intravenously he seemed better. That indicated he was probably responding to the medication, which would mean we simply had this hypothetical infection to beat.

Judy and I fell into a routine of visiting him for several hours every day. His color was good. His vital signs were all good. Everyone around us kept smiling! I thought he was too lethargic. He almost never opened his eyes. A passing nurse suggested that this meant he'd have a "laid-back" personality, but when I asked a passing doctor, he admitted that they were a little concerned.

As the days passed, new concerns were aired. The doctors found a heart murmur, and other minor surprises, and they began to casually discuss a range of potential maladies that might account for what they observed. One doctor mentioned cystic fibrosis, and several worried about something called Hirschsprung's disease. Everything was all very speculative. If the patient *did* have this or that condition, it would be manifested in such-and-such a way. So far, all tests were negative.

They did a spinal tap to check for meningitis, and found a trace of blood. To rule out the possibility of internal bleeding, they asked us to authorize a brain scan.

THE YOUNG PEDIATRICIAN in charge of Joseph's case still hadn't quite lost her smile. She apologized for the clutter in her office and began the conference by summarizing other, less alarming issues, in the tradition of delivering the good news first. But we knew what was coming. She had already told Judy that afternoon.

And Judy had told me over dinner at a little restaurant across the street.

I'd absorbed it then numbly, mechanically chewing the tasteless food and thinking distractedly that her voice was too loud. Joseph was missing brain tissue. I imagined that other diners were turning in their seats to look at us. Or maybe they really were looking at us. I must have had more pertinent thoughts, must have said something. But this is all I remember.

Then somebody playfully waved splayed fingers in front of my face. I flinched, blinked, focused on a dapper little man with a white goatee, saw him lose his silly grin and quickly steer his wife past me and into the restaurant. Judy was in there at the cash register, paying our bill. I was standing in the parking lot, utterly unmoored.

Now the pediatrician directed our attention to a set of films clipped onto light panels: cross sectional views of our little boy's head.

"We call these structures the temporal horns," she explained. "The light-colored area represents brain tissue. This black area is just fluid. It tells us brain growth did not occur there."

I tried to compare the black regions with the overall mass of the brain. More than a decade earlier, I'd planned on attending medical school. My rigorous pre-med training had not included anything like this, however. The main thing I'd taken away from all that study was a very high, perhaps excessive, regard for the elite corps who made medicine their life work. I understood that medical professionals accomplished great things, and that runaway emotions could be an obstacle in the process. So I suppressed my own feelings and concentrated on showing this doctor that I would be a reliable ally in implementing whatever treatment she proposed.

"What functions is this part of the brain responsible for?" I asked.

She gestured impatiently. "Who can say, really, *what* the various parts of the brain do?"

"Surely you have some idea."

She hesitated. "Memory and association." After a pause she went on. "I know this is upsetting for you both. Please try to overcome that emotion. There's always an initial shock for parents when they discover that their new baby isn't perfect."

Well, of course, no one's *perfect*, I thought. That was evidently what she wanted me to think. "But this is a pretty serious departure from the norm,—*isn't it?*"

"In terms of physical structure, yes. But I'm absolutely *not* going to prognosticate, because I can't predict the future. A need for occupational therapy may be identified at some point. But for now, the main thing is to watch out for self-fulfilling prophesies. Don't expect the worst." She smiled and stood.

I still had questions. "What caused this?"

"We don't know. There may have been some infection during the last trimester of the pregnancy. I do know that's when the growth should have occurred. However, there's no record or evidence of that."

Judy and I found ourselves outside her office almost before realizing that the conference had ended.

Joseph still lay quietly in his bassinet, appearing smaller and more vulnerable than ever. Just days earlier I'd been happier than at any other time in my life. Even strangers saw the glow. They grinned back at me as I passed them on the street. Now, abruptly, I wanted to shelter him from them all. How could this child hope to meet the world's expectations? Feeling inadequate to the task of protecting him, I bent over and spoke softly into his ear.

"You sweet little boy. Your mom and I love you very, very much."

"I'm glad you haven't changed the way you feel about him," Judy ventured.

"*Of course not!* Nothing that woman says is going to make me not love my kid!"

I thought that sounded good and brave, even as I said it. But at home, we just slumped into chairs and stared at each other bleakly.

"What *is* 'occupational therapy,' anyway?" I demanded. "Something like basket-weaving?"

I had trained for medicine, Judy for special education. So this was very close to her field. But she didn't want to talk about it. Her palm was against her face, her eyes unfocused. She nodded.

"So—although he looks like a regular baby now—."

"Time is going to pass, and he's going to fall further and further behind other kids his age. I guess."

There was a long silence.

After a while I stood and trudged out to the mailbox. I returned bearing a thick handful of congratulatory cards sent in response to the birth announcement. We looked through them absent-mindedly.

I took a deep breath. "Look," I said. "Like she said, we don't want to add our own weight to making this come true. Right now, he's a beautiful baby. Nobody else has to know any more than that."

Judy looked at me wonderingly. "You don't want to tell our families?"

"I don't know how they would react. I want everybody to treat him the same way they'd treat any baby."

As if on cue, the phone rang.

Neither of us moved.

"You answer," Judy said wearily. "I don't want to talk. I don't care who it is."

I picked up the receiver to an exuberant rush of words from her sister Pat, in Virginia. "So! You're a *family* now! *Congratulations*! Are you guys getting any sleep?"

I cleared my throat. "Actually, Pat, the family isn't all here just yet. Joseph's still in the hospital."

"*Still in the hospital*? What on earth are they keeping him for?"

"Well, there's been some concern over his spitting up. They wanted to check that out. And they thought he might have an infection or something. So he's on this ten-day course of antibiotics and he has to stay until that's finished."

So far, I hadn't said anything untrue. Pat pressed for more details. I mentioned sonograms and biopsies of his digestive tract, assuring her that those results were normal, as indeed they were. I steered well away from the real issue.

"It must be a big disappointment for you to have to wait." Pat paused for me to reply and then, sounding less satisfied by the moment, she added "May I speak with Judy?"

Judy had been resolutely shaking her head every time I glanced her way, so I said, "I'm sorry, Pat. Judy's lying down."

"You sound tired."

I *was* tired, come to think of it. I thanked Pat for calling and promised to let her know when we brought Joseph home.

"Your parents ought to be calling," Judy grumbled after I put down the phone.

"They're probably waiting for us to call. Anyway, it's just as well that they aren't, isn't it?"

"You're always making excuses for them. Even now."

Unwilling to respond, I bid Judy good night and found my way upstairs to bed, where I fell asleep grappling with two knotty questions. *How the heck did we get into this jam? And how do we get out of it?* Getting out of it felt akin to evading responsibility for some misdeed, perhaps because until now most of my problems had come as a result of my own errors. Getting out of it would then mean finding a way around whatever righteous authority meant to hold us to account—for what?

An image came to mind, a lovely child in a bright, flowery sunsuit, toddling in the grass beside a blanket on which her happy parents lounged. I'd noted that idyllic scene in passing one Sunday about a year earlier, as Judy and I strolled through San Diego's Mission Bay Park. Five minutes later I'd sat Judy down on a low stone wall and broached the subject. *Maybe it's time we had a baby. Whatd'ya think?*

Initially, she'd been frightened. But the idea took hold in her as easily as it had in me. We'd moved West to start our lives anew. We now had a new home, new jobs. Why not also make someone new to love?

What was wrong with that?

I'D ASSUMED that Judy would follow me upstairs, but learned the next day that she had stayed up most of the night, praying and bargaining. We weren't particularly religious. She was a lapsed Catholic.

A few of the things I'd heard in various Protestant churches over the years had resonated with me. But these days, neither of us ever went to church.

Judy said she'd resorted to opening the Bible at random in hopes of discovering some divine explanation of our crisis.

She landed on a passage from Matthew: "Judge not, that ye be not judged." She derived comfort from seeing this as a reminder that we had no real verdict yet.

Needing comfort myself, I tried it too. I opened to I Kings. "And God gave Solomon wisdom and understanding exceeding much, and largeness of heart, even as the sand that is on the seashore."

This sounded good. But there was room for different interpretations. If such a blessing were coming to Joseph, that would be splendid. *I* on the other hand was not seeking largeness of heart, or even wisdom. I only wanted my boy to be OK.

ON OUR NEXT VISIT, no one on the hospital staff had anything in particular to say to us. We took turns holding Joseph and talking to him. I could see that Judy felt increasingly unnerved by the IV line and needle inserted into his scalp. On the other hand, he was now finally getting, and keeping, some milk. I thought he looked more alert. We studied his chart. There was a notation that chromosome testing had been performed, so I sought out the nearest doctor to ask about that.

He was examining another child. "It was just a routine check," he said, without looking up.

"Well, did you find anything unusual this time?"

"Not as far as I know. Your regular pediatrician will discuss it with you if you'd like."

Our regular pediatrician was not present.

I stayed on after Judy went home for the evening. We'd found a rocking chair in the corner, which I put to use. I liked holding his little body. Having recently memorized the lyrics for "You Are My Sunshine," I tried to sing to him, but got choked up. *"You'll never know, dear, how much I love you—."* Would he ever know? Would he be able to know anything? *"Please don't take my sunshine away—."*

Judy was asleep when I arrived home. As I sorted through another batch of cards congratulating us on the birth, the phone rang again. This time it was her oldest sister Barbara, calling from Maryland. She asked the same questions Pat had asked the night before. I gave the same evasive answers.

"Steve," she said. "Would you like David to do something? He works at NIH, you know. He knows people."

"Thanks for the offer, Barb, but I don't think anything else could be done, really."

But Barbara had her own idea about what might be done, and the next day her husband David called Judy from his office at the National Institutes of Health. He told her he had a prominent neonatal specialist standing by on another line. Would she like to talk to him about Joseph?

Now there was no way out. Judy had to reveal our news in the presence of a family member. The doctor listened carefully and asked a few questions. Of course, since he didn't have the films, he could only speak in generalities. The upshot of the conversation was that he suggested she talk to Dr. Allen Merritt, a colleague of his at University Hospital in San Diego. "Tell him I referred you," he said.

David remained on the line after the doctor had disconnected. "Follow through on this," he urged. "Call that guy. They said he's Number One in that field on the West Coast, so he's bound to be able to help. And tell him who referred you so you'll get his attention." David suggested other names to mention as well, just to be sure. He explained that because his agency funded activities at hospitals across the country, medical people were anxious to stay on good terms with it.

"I know it's tough being out there by yourselves at a time like this,"

David concluded. "But remember that we're thinking about you."

Judy thanked him, broke the connection, and immediately dialed the number she'd been given.

The effect of dropping the magic names impressed her. Dr. Merritt was not in his office, but Judy's call was forwarded to him in another building.

This man had a take-charge manner that she found very soothing. "There are two issues," he said. "The first is diagnostic uncertainty. They ran a test on your son and got a result that they didn't expect. Now they aren't sure what it means. The second problem is simply failure to communicate that to you clearly. Your doctor was a student of mine. Would you mind if I discuss this case with her?"

That evening we met with an entirely different reception. Dr. Merritt's former student greeted us at the door, along with a young man I'd noticed on other nights. They promised to spend as much time talking about the situation as we required. Which was good, because several questions had formed in our minds.

"You said that portions of his brain did not develop during the last trimester of pregnancy," I began.

They nodded pleasantly.

"Well, we're talking about a period that ended just *last week*! Isn't it possible that the development process is still going on?"

The man answered. "No. Once a nerve cell is lost, it can never be regenerated."

"*Lost?* But you guys said this was brain tissue that never formed in the first place."

He sighed. "We don't really know if it didn't form, or if it *did* form and subsequently atrophied. But I should point out that CT-scanning is a fairly recent technological development, especially with babies. We haven't done scans on that many people. For all we know, there may be lots of people walking around on the streets who have brains just like Joseph's." They nodded at each other, as if this were an insight that had just occurred to them. He continued, "So in other words, he may still turn out to be perfectly all right."

"I have faith that he will!" I declared stoutly—noting that this drew a pitying look from Joseph's doctor. "But since there *is* apparently a problem," I went on, "we need to know what to do about it."

More smiles. "Take him home and love him."

"Oh, we will! But what *else* can we do? Let's bring Dr. Merritt in on this."

The smiles were increasingly indulgent. I could see that they found my comments naïve. "Dr. Merritt is not affiliated with this hospital," the man said. "But it's not like you're getting a different level of care from us. I know him. I'm actually his next-door neighbor."

"Are you really?" the other exclaimed pleasantly. "Why, I didn't know that!"

What does this have to do with anything? I almost asked, but instead said, "I just want to make sure Joseph has every chance. And to get it I'll take him anywhere he should go."

I paused, trying to organize my thoughts. Perhaps something in my rudimentary pre-med education might be relevant. I groped and came up with phrases like "cellular differentiation," which refers to the process in which embryonic cells become specialized for one function. This was what we'd want to promote, I thought. But time was probably of the essence. The chances of a good outcome to any intervention would surely be better now than in the future. So I implored them, "Do you know of any sort of program or procedure—even something in an experimental stage—that could stimulate the growth of more brain tissue?"

They shook their heads gravely.

"Nothing at all? Listen, you don't have to *endorse* it. I'm just asking for some leads."

Instead of answering, they had their own question. "Whom do you know at NIH?"

"It's my brother-in-law," Judy blurted. "He works there, in personnel."

"*Oh—*." They sat back in their seats, their interest in us visibly evaporating. They'd been misled. *These people don't have clout, after all!* "So he's not a physician?"

Clearly, that made a difference. There were no further consultations in the four days that Joseph remained in the hospital. He still had to complete the course of antibiotics, and a few of his organs had not yet been sufficiently probed and studied. Nothing else unusual was found, however. On a Monday night, two weeks after that unforgettable all-night labor, they let us take him home.

Judy brought in baby clothes, and I brought a camera. "*Finally*, I'm getting him out of that anonymous hospital white!" she muttered. No doctors were in sight. She dressed him nervously, as if someone might come along and stop us at any moment. Once clad in a tiny T-shirt with a dancing Teddy bear design, however, he seemed more like our own baby. Next was a powder blue cap and gown. A jolly nurse with a Southern accent snapped our photo: two worn-looking adults clutching a tiny, all-blue bundle. "You'd never know he was a boy," she joked. Then we gathered up our blankets and possessions and walked down to the car, for the moment just like any other brand-new family.

2. A GROWING CHILD

"Of course," my dad used to say, "There are two sides to every issue."

He'd be sitting back, long legs crossed, at his accustomed place by the kitchen table, holding forth with a benign smile to the assembled family.

"There's *my* side, and —" He'd pause dramatically, "there's the *wrong* side."

"Oh, Braxton!" my mother would sigh with patient exasperation. But he continued beaming at my sisters and me, unperturbed, as she rose from the table and busied herself irritably at the sink. The joke was that while he perceived the arrogance of this claim, he also tended to believe it. He believed it not because of any illusions regarding his own brilliance but rather because he'd found that the majority of those who claimed expertise in any subject were faking it. If, for example, in some debate I cited the credentials of a renowned PhD who held views Dad wasn't ready to accept, he would snort and remind me, "That clown puts on his pants one leg at a time, same as anybody."

More often than not, proving such people wrong was child's play, and the stories he recited from his long life provided evidence.

Dad gave due, even lavish, credit to the few geniuses he'd met along the way. As for the rest, he believed that one of the worst mistakes you could make would be to allow some ignoramus in a lofty position to determine your course.

IN THE YEARS since Joseph's birth, there have been people who said that the information given to Judy and me at the hospital should have convinced us that our son was a lost cause.

Perhaps Dad's instruction had something to do with my failure to accept that. But Judy found her own reasons to share my view. Maybe we were just in denial. But regardless, we meant to raise up this kid, and by golly he was going to be fine! Things *had* to work out that way.

I've heard it said that Nature makes babies adorable to encourage adults to care for them. If that's true, She must have known our son would need more than his share of attention. He came graced with clear, healthy skin, soft blond hair, and blue eyes framed by extravagantly long lashes.

We marveled at the realization that here was a new human being so small you could enclose his foot in one hand, so delicate that his nails were like tissue. We took turns holding this tiny bundle and looked at each other in wonder. He'd come to this world simply because we wanted him here. And now he counted on us for everything. How could we possibly let him down?

Our optimism did not exist in a vacuum.

Encouragement came from Ferrell, a young occupational therapist assigned to visit our home every month with ideas for infant stimulation. Despite having read the usual parenting books, Judy and I felt way out of our depth. We knew there were developmental milestones to watch for, but didn't know how to help our baby attain them. We welcomed her guidance.

"You know," Ferrell began, "some kids I see actually have had *half* of their brains surgically removed, and the remaining half learns to compensate. Joseph has a *lot* more brain tissue than *they* do! There's no telling how adaptable someone this young can be. And look! When I hold a toy this way, he's actually starting to reach across the midline of his body with one hand. That's an incredibly good sign. You'll see! Try to encourage him to do more of that."

So regardless of the early scare, there might still be a very satisfactory conclusion! I imagined a future time in which the only worry might be whether it would be wise to tell an outwardly normal Joseph that in infancy he'd had an abnormal brain scan.

To help move things in that direction, we gladly made adjustments in our lives. Judy, for example, decided that a return to her job was unthinkable. She didn't even *know* this little guy yet, and already her boss was on the phone, saying, in effect, that her time was up.

She resigned.

At six weeks, Joseph could grab our fingers. He certainly kicked and lunged vigorously enough when distressed. His way of crying for a minute and then pausing (as if to listen) seemed to indicate that he expected someone to come to his assistance. If he were capable of that kind of reasoning, I felt all must be well. On the other hand, he showed little outward response to us or to the toys we offered him.

We diligently filled in the daily squares on a baby calendar that my mother had sent, with cute stickers and notations to commemorate the slightest event and accomplishment. The blank pages stretching into the future—pages that would soon trace the record of when he first rolled over and crawled and stood alone—seemed a new form of wealth.

At Ferrell's suggestion we moved colorful objects back and forth in front of Joseph's face to snag his attention.

In the bath, Judy placed his hands alternately into containers of cool and warm water. "Cold!" She shouted exuberantly. "And this is hot! *Hot water*!"

STILL, beneath all the frenetic activity, two grim words thundered continuously in my mind—*Temporal lobes*. What, if anything, would small temporal lobes mean for him?

The neurologist we saw, a Dr. Mulligan, picked up Ferrell's theme, saying we had every reason to be upbeat about Joseph's prospects. He had no recommendations to offer, but he wanted to see us again because—he hesitated and fumbled for words. "Because, say, three years from now I might see another child like Joseph and following his progress now will help me know what to expect."

Ideally, I thought, doctors should have more in mind than merely "following his progress." But my main reaction to all this was humble gratitude that they were saying nothing worse. Apparently, he needed no intervention!

Dr. Riker, Joseph's primary physician, sounded the same note when we saw him for the usual checkups and immunizations.

"*All* parents are anxious about their kids," he said expansively. "Even when there's nothing unusual in the medical history. And they *go on* worrying until the kid grows up and moves away and starts his first job. You've got to recognize that worrying is part of being a parent. In your case, you've had cause to worry overtime. But try to control it. A high level of tension in the house won't help anybody."

At two months Joseph was pushing himself up on his elbows. He kicked his legs independently of each other, which Ferrell said was another good sign.

But. He was also becoming an *extremely* irritable child. This, we promptly heard, was "colic." Some babies had it, and there was little to do except endure the two or three months needed to outgrow this phase, the doctors and nurses said. They had ready answers like that for every question, never even pausing first to look thoughtful.

Soon he was crying all day, every day, and most of every night.

Compared to Judy, I was lucky. Going to the office gave me a break. In those days I worked for a large aerospace contractor, developing proposals for launching government satellites into orbit. Illustrators worked around me, producing technical line drawings and even spectacular oil renderings of space vehicles set against a starry black sky. Managers and engineers visited continuously, bringing rough text for me to organize and rewrite and then more rough text to replace their previous attempts. Many iterations later, we'd have an impressive multi-volume pitch, just hours in advance of the customer's deadline. The pressure was intense, but at times I needed the distraction.

I phoned home often during the day to get updates on the latest appointment—ever hopeful that there might be real news this time—or just to see how Judy was coping. I remember once she sounded especially demoralized. She spoke in a monotone, giving one-word answers. A frantic shrieking in the background almost drowned her out.

"Is this not a good time to call?" I finally asked.

"It's *never* a good time," she muttered bitterly.

"Wait. Is something *wrong*?"

"Just go do your job. Goodbye."

Putting down the phone, I rubbed my eyes and stared blankly at the papers on my desk. Avoiding tension was more easily recommended than done.

IN A BLACK-AND-WHILE PHOTO from her childhood, Judy stands between her older sisters, Barbara and Pat. Flanked by the larger girls, she seems frail, with eyes too big for her thin face. And yet, while all three girls smile for the camera, only her face is bright and open to the world. The others' smiles are merely dutiful.

Looking at that photo now, I see the same unguarded eyes and smile on another occasion. It was late summer of 1974, the day when Judy and I first knew we had become an item.

We'd reached the end of a leisurely drive along the Blue Ridge Parkway. The highlight so far had been a romantic little picnic in a mountain meadow. Passing motorists tooted their horns at us, and we waved back gaily. But beneath the day's playfulness, recognition of this new relationship prompted nervous thoughts of the future. I knew by then that I would not be a physician. She'd begun to reconsider her career in special education. Neither of us had a Plan B.

At the last stop before turning back to Charlottesville, where I was in graduate school, we found ourselves face to face, clasping both our hands. We leaned away from each other at arms' length, and then, as a game, began spinning in place. Behind her, the scenery blurred. Only her smiling face remained in focus. It was like that moment in *The West Side Story* when Tony and Maria spot each other across the dance floor and all else in their troubled lives becomes irrelevant.

Now, with the unexplained changes taking place in our home, any expectations and hopes for our son, and ourselves, were fading into that blur. But this time, all that remained clear was a growing sense of confusion and horror. No! We could not accept this. We *had* to find a solution!

MY SISTER LYNN phoned occasionally to see how we were holding up in our new role as parents.

I still hadn't confided what we'd heard in the hospital with anyone. In recent years, I've gathered that many families alarmed about their babies' development also seek at first to keep the matter private. Silence is apparently a coping mechanism. Judy's brother-in-law, David, knew how things stood, of course, but evidently he was waiting for us to share the news when we saw fit.

Anyway, what could be the connection between crying and a structural abnormality that might later affect Joseph's memory and association? They were separate issues, right?

Lynn jokingly attributed the crying to cantankerous Gallup genes. "We *are* a pretty ornery bunch, you know," she kidded. I didn't laugh. *Temporal lobes*, I was still thinking. My family wondered at my grim mood, which must have been more than new-parent jitters. "Why worry now?" they all said. "Sure, he spent some extra time in the hospital, but it turned out OK."

Maybe it would yet. But at the moment there remained the business of this *crying*. In later years, it was my fortune to handle two more babies; I've had opportunity to learn that all children can be difficult at times. However, Joseph was something altogether different.

"Well, my advice to you is to invest in some ear plugs," my father finally said, speaking long-distance from Virginia.

Could that be the right approach? Although a continent now separated us, Dad still towered in my imagination as the one dependable source of insight when I could see nothing beyond my own limits.

He was white-haired, had been for as long as I could remember, and was tall enough that the bald patch on top hardly mattered. All my life, he had been striding confidently ahead, leading the way for a family that gratefully followed. And it wasn't just us. Everyone we knew looked up to him, spoke his name with affectionate respect, and sought his opinions.

If an obstacle warranted frontal assault, that's what Dad employed. Once, long ago, when the fast-talking owner of a hobby shop would not let Lynn exchange a defective paint-by-number kit, Dad was in that store like a shot, and out again moments later, holding up the replacement with a satisfied smile. ("He tried that same line, about going back to the manufacturer, that he fed you, but I interrupted and asked, 'Don't you stand behind what you sell?'") Another time, Dad let me cope with a neighborhood bully on my own, until the boy's father joined the fray. Hearing about that, Dad showed up briefly with a few private words, nose-to-nose, with the other gentleman, after which both father and son eagerly and permanently kept their distance.

More often, however, Dad approached challenges with deliberation, taking the brilliant 19th-century violinist Paganini as his role model. Contemporary reports suggested that Paganini practiced *mentally*— either that, or he communed with the devil, which some suspected. They knew only (from spying on him) that the man approached his craft by lying in bed, then leaping up at intervals to seize his instrument and execute new musical passages of groundbreaking complexity. This mysterious quietude, from which genius sometimes flowed, fascinated Dad. It was, he insisted, the place to take your problems.

If you didn't know how to proceed, any action you took would be premature. Or as Dad liked to phrase it, "When in doubt, do nothing." He said that again now.

I was certainly in doubt, but I didn't want to ignore Joseph. If my boy needed something, I wanted him to know he could count on us for it. He was still spitting up his milk. In fact, he did this so frequently and copiously that no one could hold him and expect to keep clean clothes.

NORMAL LIFE STILL BECKONED. The members of a bicycle club we belonged to kept urging me to bring Joseph out for one of their early-morning breakfast rides. "Tell Judy to bring him in the car," one suggested. "We'll meet at a restaurant and pass him around the table."

That sounded like fun, but Joseph was no better in public settings than at home. We'd already tried. I'd carried him out of enough restaurants and similar settings to predict how that would go.

In any event, given the constant spitting up and our inability to stay abreast of the laundry requirement, weekend jaunts for any such purpose just did not seem realistic.

I also gave up my membership in a health club. There was no longer time for regular workouts, and if I stubbornly tried to *make* time, the physical exertion, in my sleep-starved condition, produced crippling headaches.

Work remained more than just an escape for me. As the family's sole wage-earner now, I took my job more seriously than ever and certainly tried to avoid letting this personal situation affect my performance there. No such rule protected home life from the job, however. The projects routinely obliged me to put in very long hours, leaving Judy to cope with things by herself. Many nights I arrived on the doorstep after a fourteen-hour day to find her wide-eyed with terror and at the extreme limits of endurance. "Here! Take this kid," she would hiss, thrusting him into my arms before I could even loosen my tie.

Despite the hour, a long night still stretched ahead of us, during which we took turns holding his thrashing body and walking with him around the house. He seemed less unhappy when I carried him up and down the stairs, and less unhappy still when I did so *rapidly*. Sometimes he stopped crying altogether and looked about in amazement as the scenery hurtled past us. But I was good for only a few minutes of this, after which I had to pause for breath. (Who needed a health club, anyway?) And then we were back where we'd started.

Finally I'd stand holding him beside the crib, rotating back and forth through a gentle arc and mentally calling forth peace, serenity, tranquility. Yes. Crying still reverberated in my head, but the source had stopped. Joseph was relaxing against me. Then, inexplicably, he would jerk to wakefulness and begin howling with renewed energy.

Nearby, somebody slammed a window violently.

"*This is not right!*" I declared through clenched teeth. "Sure, babies cry, but they aren't supposed to cry like this!"

Casting about frantically for help, Judy called on her parents. They had retired to Florida and over the last decade had made it clear to everyone in the family that further travel for them was out of the question. Her father's Army career had taken them around the world, with too many misadventures along the way. He'd survived Pearl Harbor, for example, had seen brutal combat in the Pacific that he would never discuss. Then, with three baby girls in the house and a ten-year-old boy, he'd volunteered for more action in Korea because he believed that was his duty. The family had moved to a base in Japan to be near him, and while there the son had contracted polio and then, in the midst of a catastrophic typhoon, had died. The Army brought her father out of combat for a funeral that saved his life, because his entire company had been killed before he could return.

His name was Joseph, too. He had no other sons, and I had wanted to name our son in his honor.

The elder Joseph decided they should come to our aid. We welcomed the visit. But all their experience with children had not prepared them with answers for this one.

One night while they were with us, and many other nights as well, we loaded our shrieking boy into the car for a panicky trip to the hospital's urgent care clinic, convinced that something had to be drastically wrong. His medical file there was already quite thick. The nurses tried to prevent me from reading it, but I did so anyway whenever a chance presented itself. Joseph's objective, it said, was "to achieve the normal developmental milestones." The prognosis was "guarded." Perhaps we were the only ones who did read this. The doctors on duty just frowned at all the papers and test reports. Audiology. Ophthalmology. "What's his story?" they said. "Just summarize it real quick."

Judy always did so, with a rush of words that was not only quick but thorough, starting with his Apgar scores, and the doctors would nod tolerantly while they looked into his ears and throat. Then came the verdict. "Well, he doesn't have a fever. There's no sign of infection. Looks like you have a healthy baby here."

One kindly old physician did express the concern that we might feel foolish. Although we'd made an unnecessary trip in the middle of the night, it *was* better to be safe than sorry. Another time, a doctor prescribed an antibiotic "just in case" there was some malady he hadn't detected, but no doubt mostly to placate us. We took home a bottle of murky pink solution.

"These medicines have side-effects," Judy grumbled. "They kill off the intestinal bacteria. Do we know what this is supposed to do for him? Did you get that straight?"

"No—."

We worried about the matter overnight and then returned to the hospital. The doctor now on duty shrugged and said we could give Joseph the medicine or throw it away. He didn't think the issue was important. We threw it away.

"HE'S GROWING WELL," Dr. Riker said on regularly scheduled visits. "Whatever it is you've been doing, keep it up."

What Judy had been doing consisted of holding him almost constantly and nursing him on demand—not that nursing ever went smoothly. His sucking reflex was poor. He tended to drift in and out of sleep while eating, so that one scheduled feeding ran into the next. Yes, he was gaining weight, but he looked puffy. Anyone paying attention ought to perceive that this was still a very distressed little boy. Something was troubling him. Eating did provide his only solace. So Judy fed him, gave him her undivided attention all day long, and played soothing lullaby tapes that helped her own rattled nerves if not his.

Joseph was in no danger from us. But the point arrived, early one morning, when she dialed the number for a child abuse hotline. "What do parents do?" she asked anxiously. "*What do they do*, when their babies keep on crying and crying and crying?"

The counselor on the other end thought we might be dealing with some kind of medical problem and should see a doctor.

I HAVE READ ARTICLES in which physicians lament the "unreasonable expectations" of parents. They say we've become "programmed to expect a 100 percent normal baby" and we want to blame the doctor when anything goes wrong. These articles warn that fear of litigation is driving doctors out of business.

The argument made is that patients need to understand the concept of risk. There are no guarantees, and the correct response to disappointment is to accept it philosophically, rather than looking for someone to sue.

Other literature makes light of the human desire to identify causes for misfortune. People like to think that things happen for a reason. Personally, I find that urge very understandable. The fact that we don't know why a child is born with problems does not mean we shouldn't search for explanations. How else can we hope to treat him effectively or to avoid a recurrence with the next baby?

Judy and I were not blaming the doctors for Joseph's condition. We were not thinking of lawsuits. We were, however, becoming extremely frustrated with their evasiveness. At some point, Judy phoned the woman who had taught our Lamaze class, just to see what she might suggest. We remembered her as a down-to-earth expert, somebody sure to give us straight answers. She did. If we were having difficulties with the hospital or the doctors, she said, we needed to understand that her sympathies had to lie with the professionals, not with us. She was pleasant about it, but said she did not want to be called again.

JUDY'S SISTER BARBARA had given us a subscription to a monthly publication called *Growing Child*. Each issue targeted the present age level and consisted of defining a normal baby's abilities at that stage and suggesting games that the parents might profitably attempt with him. We took it as a benchmark for gauging Joseph's progress.

The first few months brought no surprises. Like the typical child described, Joseph sometimes babbled and pivoted on his tummy. Other differences could be chalked up to individuality. But then some alarming discrepancies began to appear.

At five months, Baby likes to:
- Roll over
- Sit with support

Joseph was nowhere near either of those "milestones"—at five months or for several months thereafter. And the challenges continued to escalate. Each issue, there were fewer items on *Growing Child's* list that he could manage.

At nine months, Baby likes to:
- Pull himself up
- Creep on the floor
- Play interaction games like pat-a-cake

We certainly had experienced some interaction with him by this time. His crying was an effort to communicate—*Right?* Sometimes we even thought he wanted to imitate our speech. I didn't much care about his disinterest in pat-a-cake. But in terms of mobility he was at *zero*.

With the approach of each scheduled evaluation, hope still swelled that perhaps *this time* some specialist would get to the bottom of the trouble and prescribe a course of action. It seemed a reasonable expectation. During the pregnancy I had suggested that ongoing advances in medical science might enable Joseph's generation to live into the 22nd century. We were asking for something far less dramatic than that! But we seemed caught in an invisible revolving door. The file grew ever thicker, but no one put it to any use, such as diagnosing his problem.

No one had confirmed that there really *was* a problem.

Then, with his first birthday approaching, Judy took him back for a follow-up exam with the neonatal specialist who had first told us about that brain scan.

I missed that event, but heard enough about it to feel as if I'd been there. Judy walked into the examination room with a baby she hoped might still, somehow, be OK. She stood, carefully holding him on the scroll of slippery paper that stretched across the padded table. The doctor entered, uttered brisk pleasantries, and set about trying to get Joseph up on all fours. Failing in that, she moved a penlight in front of his eyes and then tried unsuccessfully to interest him in a toy. I'm sure Judy was talking nervously throughout the process, until the doctor stepped back and presented a jaw-dropping list of major deficits that stopped her cold. Chief among them was the lack of motor development, "Which may mean something, in view of what we know about the temporal lobes." She flashed her sterile smile, making no effort to square this explanation with her earlier statement: Presumably, as far as anyone knew, abnormal temporal lobes might impair motor functions as well as memory and association.

To explore mobility further, she recommended an appointment with the physical therapy department downstairs.

Next, although the vision specialists had already seen him many times, she wanted still another ophthalmologist to look at his eyes, because he was not attentive.

Furthermore, his lack of focus suggested to her that he might be having "subclinical seizures" (episodes so mild or brief that we were overlooking them).

Still more appointments were in order to investigate that.

The doctor left the room and was replaced moments later by a psycho-social nurse, who wanted to know how Judy was reacting to this news. She found Judy in tears.

"Dr. Bunker would be very sorry to think you got the impression that she doesn't care," the nurse said, almost chidingly, after letting Judy rant for a few minutes. "I know that she cares very much indeed."

Collecting herself, Judy gradually became more coherent. "I know I'm blaming this doctor because she's the bearer of bad tidings. Probably I should be more upset with all the rest of them. They're always so upbeat! They *tell* us, 'Don't worry!' That's what they've been saying for a year! If Joseph really is in such bad shape, why do they do that? They keep telling us to go to another appointment, and then another appointment, and then another one." She waved the new slips of paper she'd just been given. "I guess the drill is just to keep us busy. Meanwhile, nothing gets accomplished. I'm sick of this."

Suddenly, Judy really was sick. At home, she went to bed for a few days, letting me take Joseph to the next appointment solo. I carried him back to that all-too-familiar hospital and found my way to a sign reading Physical Medicine.

We were shown to a large padded area, and in due course a young therapist arrived and introduced herself as Michelle. Like her colleagues, she was not familiar with Joseph's chart, and this time I remained silent, letting her arrive at her own conclusions.

Michelle stretched herself out casually beside Joseph on the mat and began getting acquainted with him. After a few moments she began to look puzzled.

"His muscle tone seems OK, a little tight maybe, but nothing—. Motorically, well—. This is interesting." She hesitated and looked at me. "Has anyone suggested that he might have autism?"

"No."

"Hmm. Well, I don't know, of course. It would take a lot of testing to find out for sure. But certain things about him suggest that to me. Look at him right now, for example."

Joseph was on his back, gazing in the general direction of the ceiling. For once, he was not crying and in fact his face glowed with a beatific smile. Based on that, I thought he looked great.

"Now that smile is not appropriate. He's not interacting with us socially. It's almost like he's in a world of his own. Does he usually relate to you more than this?"

"I can't say that he does."

"Does he seem to get—um, excited—about rhythmic, repetitive things? Noises?"

I tried to be helpful, to think of an example. "Well, he looks at the pendulum of the clock when I show it to him."

Michelle nodded. All this evidently made a lot of sense to her. But she looked worried. "*Can you handle this*?" she asked. "I don't want to come down too heavy on you. Is this too much for you right now?"

I told her I could handle *anything* approaching a real diagnosis. Besides, I had only a sketchy idea of what the word *autism* meant. "What is the fate of an autistic child?" I asked.

"It depends on how soon the condition is detected. They *can be* intelligent in certain ways," she added distractedly. She seemed to be looking for something positive to say. "They're often very attractive, like Joseph is. Just look at those gorgeous blue eyes!"

"I want to find out one way or the other as soon as possible."

She said there was a doctor in the health maintenance organization—a psychologist, she thought—who specialized in this sort of thing. His name escaped her at the moment, but she would find out and report back to me. Then we could arrange an appointment with *him*.

"Sounds great," I said. "How soon can I talk to you again?"

This was late on a Friday afternoon. She agreed to see us again Monday.

I drove home feeling more optimistic than usual. At last we might be on the track of something! But when I told Judy, she was crushed. Literally. Already seated, she sank deeper into the chair as if a heavy weight had been laid upon her.

"No," she murmured hopelessly. "Oh no, no, no. Not autism."

"Is it that bad?"

"Steve, autistic people live in a world of their own. They wind up in institutions. It's incurable! Almost always."

"*Almost* always? *Some* people get over it, then?"

She sighed heavily. "In college I read about a father who worked with his son, for years, and finally pulled him out of it. The parents—um—sort of crossed over into their son's world, and did everything he did. And eventually they got his attention."

We could feel the tentacles of a grim, dry despondency gathering around us—and then the phone rang. A panic situation had developed at the office. The customer wanted to see a new presentation, and I was the only one in my department with the right security clearance to prepare it. My presence there was mandatory. Automatically, I agreed to come in, then after hanging up realized that I probably should not. However, I didn't know what to do for my family in this state, and Judy seemed indifferent. Joseph was much calmer than usual, so I encouraged her to put him to bed and to try to sleep, herself.

And so she and I got through that bleak evening separately, I by immersion in the busy-ness of office work (while simultaneously cooking up desperate schemes for somehow crossing over into Joseph's world) and Judy by sinking into and (with divine help, she thought) finding her way out of a desperate mental state. But I didn't hear about that until much later.

This was 1986, two years before the film *Rainman* introduced autism to the general public, more than a decade before organized parent-activists began demanding media attention for a crisis they said was wrecking an entire generation. I truly did not understand the implications of what Michelle had suggested. Judy, however, had taught developmentally disabled students when we lived in Virginia. She understood. Years passed before she told me what almost happened that night. Had I known the agony she was experiencing, I'd have stayed home.

3. "YOU CAN SAVE A LIFE"

The next morning, all three of us paid a visit to the public library to see what it had on the subject of autism. We came away with arm-loads of books, old and new, which we tried to study for the rest of the weekend. Most were intolerably grim. "Placement" of the afflicted family member was inevitable, they said. Divorce was not uncommon for the parents. The only one I could bear to read was the story of an unmanageable child whose behavior supposedly resulted from a rigid and unloving home environment. The situation described was so un-like our own that it became merely an interesting tale.

Autism did seem to be a heavy cross to bear, but I wasn't sure its characteristics dovetailed with what we were seeing.

Monday morning found Joseph and me on the mat once again with Michelle, who had changed her approach completely. Now Joseph was simply one more patient undergoing physical therapy. She showed me various exercises to do with him.

Finally I said, "About the question we were discussing Friday—."

"Yes?"

"Well, we've been reading up on autism since then."

"Have you really? I'm surprised."

"And—I don't know, but it seems to me that it's not exactly the same condition that Joseph has. Unless there are lots of different varieties of autism."

"There are. But look, I did not tell you he *was* autistic. Only a doctor could do that."

"OK. Well, what about the guy you mentioned Friday?"

"I can't refer you to him. Only your primary care physician can make referrals. That's how you came to me. You'll be referred to another doctor if it's appropriate."

"I think a determination of some sort is *very* appropriate. How can we treat him if we don't know what's wrong with him?"

"Listen," she said anxiously. "Please don't tell your doctor what I said! I could get in real trouble for saying he was autistic, because like I told you, I'm not qualified to make that diagnosis."

Michelle paused then and looked with surprise at a speaker on the wall, where she was being paged. (I hadn't noticed.) She excused herself for a moment and then returned to say that the psycho-social nurse wanted to meet with me upstairs. So we ended our session early, and I proceeded to the office of a lady who had just been talking with Judy—or, more accurately, listening to Judy—on the phone. Unfortunately for Michelle, the cat was already out of the bag.

"Your wife tells me you feel that you have been getting different stories from different people within our organization," the nurse began. "I'd like to help if possible. How would you like it if we arranged a conference with all the different doctors who have examined Joseph over the last year? Would it make you happier if you could interview *all* of them in one room at the same time? I can set that up for you."

I remember squinting at her while digesting this unexpected new idea. "You guys don't have to jump through hoops for us," I finally said. "A meeting like that doesn't sound like a real productive use of people's time."

"Well again, from talking with your wife, it sounds like you're not happy. I'm trying to find a way to address that."

"OK. Here's how to make me happy: *Fix my kid!*" The vehemence behind those three words startled me, but I pressed on. "Somebody needs to find out what's wrong with him. And fix it!"

If this were a conflict between us, I felt that the righteousness of that demand should be so effective as to give me an unfair advantage. There could be no defense against a parent asking medical people to help his kid! But why did there need to be any disagreement at all?

Her face did hint that she felt bullied. This *was* a conflict. "You've got to recognize that a large part of the problem is in yourselves," she said soothingly.

"No! I don't buy that. I am not the patient!"

She sighed and said nothing, so I continued.

"We keep waiting for somebody around here to start talking about *treatment*. Nobody ever does. If you guys don't know what to do about this, I think the time has come for you to refer us out to somebody else." I mentioned as an example Dr. Merritt, the eminent physician Judy had called when Joseph was still in the newborn ICU.

"That won't happen. I'm being blunt but you have to understand this. Your policy does not cover providers outside Kaiser Permanente. And furthermore, there's no need to see them, I assure you. Anything they offer is available right here, within our organization. So again, did you want to schedule that meeting?"

I exhaled heavily and shook my head. "I want results. Not meetings."

She selected a few printed brochures from a shelf. "Well then, if you really want to go outside our HMO, you can always contact Regional Center. In fact, I recommend it."

She placed the literature on the desk in front of me. The Regional Center was a state-funded organization, she said, which meant it was free to us. Families with "delayed" children went there to see counselors, nutritionists—. I made an exasperated noise at this point. "They'll provide an independent doctor, too," she continued quickly. "That will give you the second opinion you want. There's even a respite-care service. That's free babysitting. Respite care will allow you and your wife to get out of the house and do something just for yourselves."

Totally confused, I carried Joseph to the car, looking at the brochures doubtfully. I wondered about this nurse. Did she feel satisfied with the conversation we'd just had? Was it possible that she thought she had provided something of value? If not, what kind of person would choose a job like that? Now, Michelle, on the other hand, had freely offered help—at least until someone had told her she could not.

Apparently, the medical world had done everything it intended to do for Joseph. I felt uncomfortable at the idea of progressing from there into what was basically a community service—possibly Joseph's first step toward becoming a ward of the state. I had no intention of accepting that scenario. My boy *was* going to recover from whatever it was that afflicted him. I didn't know what route recovery would take, but surely there was an expert somewhere with an interest in this stuff— some pioneer putting leading-edge brain research to practical use. We just had to find him.

"I THINK WE'LL ALL BE A LOT SMARTER when he gets older," Dr. Riker told me a few days later. "I do expect his delays to continue, based on what I've seen with other babies. And I suspect that, down the road, some sort of program for him will be advisable. But I don't recommend anything at present."

"Nothing? So you're saying we don't need a psychologist?"

"What? For you, or for him?"

"For him!"

Dr. Riker knew I was referring to Michelle. "The person who made that comment was out of line. We don't diagnose autism until much later—age three at the earliest. No, just be patient and enjoy the little guy."

DESPITE OUR ANGUISH, time seemed to speed past at a totally unfair rate—that is, in view of any changes we might have been seeing.

At 14 months, Toddler likes to:

- Eat finger foods
- Participate in dressing and undressing
- Hand objects to mother and father
- Stack blocks

Joseph could do none of those things, and he certainly was no toddler. He frequently choked on food. He was still mastering the art of rolling over, although his preferred position was flat on his back. He liked to turn his head repeatedly from side to side. We didn't know why he did that, but the habit looked awful and we tried to discourage it. He persisted, however, wearing a wide patch of hair from the back of his head. The "colic," if that's what it was, had not even diminished. He still cried bitterly much of the time, thrashed around uncontrollably, and vomited at unpredictable moments.

As soon as his teeth came in, he had begun grinding them audibly and by now had actually worn the front teeth down to mere nubs. When held, he was likely to stiffen, arch his back, and rake us with his nails (or bite us). Judy learned to switch to a "football hold" to keep from dropping him at such times.

What did he need? What could we do?

Ferrell kept tossing ideas our way. For example, "finger-thumb prehension"—the ability to pick up cheerios from his highchair tray—appeared to be a key test of development. She didn't say how to help him pass the test, however. The question arose that perhaps he couldn't see the cheerios clearly, and Judy hit upon the idea of covering the white tray with a brightly-colored vinyl mat. With better contrast, he definitely saw the cheerios, but generally he just swept them onto the floor.

ANOTHER THING FAMILIES in this situation tend to do, besides withholding the dreadful secret from everyone they know, is to look at themselves for plausible explanations. In our recent appointments, the medical people had begun warning us away from that line of inquiry. Incredibly, they seemed content with the notion that there was *no* cause for our child's failure to develop, other than the luck of the draw. Parents often needlessly blamed themselves (or each other), they said. And doing that was never helpful.

But this was still not a question of blame. We simply needed to make sense of what was happening. If we understood it, maybe somebody would know what to do about it.

We began with the obvious. Neither of us used tobacco or consumed alcohol beyond the infrequent beer. During her pregnancy, Judy had avoided even aspirin in hopes of safeguarding her baby. But life brings unplanned turns, regardless. Shortly before taking maternity leave from her job, she'd slipped on a wet floor at her office. The fall had been gentle, but might have hurt Joseph. Another time, she'd given our cat a flea dip. Possibly, her skin had absorbed some poison in the shampoo. And speaking of poison, her office had been upstairs from a factory that used strong-smelling industrial solvents. She'd always been sensitive to odors. Even a coworker's perfume could give her headaches.

But surely other pregnant women experienced the same, or worse, with no ill effects.

On our own, we couldn't begin to pursue these questions. Further pondering brought forth nothing better than scenarios in which Joseph's affliction might be construed as poetic justice for ourselves. For example, looking back on her previous career as a special-ed teacher, Judy recalled all the students she had not helped.

She had gone into that profession expecting to improve the lives of disabled youngsters. Instead of being improved, clueless eighth-grade girls in her classes became pregnant. The boys imitated TV violence by brandishing knives. When she addressed these matters, she only antagonized parents (who were in denial) and administrators (who had no interest in whatever zany goings-on transpired in special-ed). Eventually, she admitted defeat and quit. She then tried taking disability claims for the Social Security Administration, but even there felt helpless when exposed to people's misfortunes. She simply could not keep an emotional distance from her clients and reacted to their suffering as if it were her own. Her heart went out to claimants, such as a woman who had abruptly gone blind, and she sought to find help for them in ways that went beyond the constraints of her job, whereas succeeding in that job depended on how many claims she could close out each week. Her most recent position, in a corporate accounting department, provided the insulation from human misery that she needed to work effectively. There, it was all numbers. She had no contact with the public. But she nursed a sense that she'd run away from her calling. Now perhaps that calling had turned up again in the form of her child.

For my part, I had supported environmental causes and endangered species over the years but had shrugged off the needs of people. *You can help save a child's life*, the magazine ads used to read, adding for effect the photo of an innocent waif in some impoverished land. For only twenty dollars a month, I could sponsor someone like this. *Or you can turn the page.*

I'd always turned the page.

Well, we couldn't turn the page and leave *this* child behind. This time, job changes were not an option. Nor did we seek an escape— only a remedy. This was our boy and our responsibility, and he had no other advocates.

Gradually, the necessity of sharing our news became inescapable. Having kept our parents in the dark this long, we didn't know where to begin the story of what they were missing. To test the waters, Judy broached the unavoidable subject to her close friend Anita.

"Steve isn't handling it too well," she said. (I don't know what led her to that opinion. Personally, I thought I coped, but it's true that I seldom smiled.) "He just can't accept the idea that Joseph—might have a lasting problem." There, she had put it into words.

"What do you expect *me* to do about it?" Anita asked crossly.

"Nothing!" Judy stared questioningly at her friend. She had just wanted a listener.

She turned to others, and within a short time became a one-topic conversationalist, scarcely noticing the transition until seeing the reaction it drew. Once a month, Judy traditionally met with four or five friends at a restaurant for an evening of networking and chatter about families, jobs, and so on. She'd tried to keep this one diversion, which was far more important to her now than before Joseph's birth. But it suddenly turned out that the attraction was no longer mutual.

As one evening drew to a close, she realized she'd monopolized the conversation with a litany of our concerns, theories, and hopes. "I probably shouldn't go on and on about this," she apologized.

Her friend Lois mustered a brittle smile. "Oh well. If it makes you feel better."

Anita and Lois both had babies within a few months of Joseph's age. Their children were developing normally, however. Perhaps the fact that ours was not made them uncomfortable. Our new openness about it certainly did. They saw Judy less often.

Next stop was Lew Fry, the Methodist pastor who had christened Joseph. Judy stood in the church office holding Joseph and sobbing out our story.

"Steve wants him to go to the University of *Virginia*," she wailed. "That's where he went, and his father and his grandfather. What he wants is so, so—*different* from this!"

Lew frowned thoughtfully. Social isolation, he said, did not improve our ability to cope. He suggested involvement with others in the congregation. Possibly an older person would welcome this opportunity to be a surrogate grandparent, for example. He promised to put an announcement in the church bulletin and to sound out members who might be interested.

This led to a call one evening from a lady who told Judy her son had cerebral palsy. He was now in his twenties and lived elsewhere in a sheltered environment. "I want to be honest with you about this," she said. "Having a handicapped child has been the worst thing that's ever happened to me. It was even worse than losing my husband to cancer."

Now, with her son finally out of the house, she was trying to pick up the pieces of her life. She'd called us this once because Lew asked her to, but no way was she going to involve herself anew in a situation like ours. It was just too painful.

"I wanted to tell her, 'Gee, thanks a bunch for all the encouragement,'" Judy told me. We wanted honesty, and here at least we'd gotten it. But we could not believe that there would be no guidance beyond this.

For lack of anything better to do, we turned back to the brochures describing the Regional Center and made an appointment. The intake process there involved yet another pediatric exam, which brought nothing new to light. Joseph was bigger now, but functionally had progressed very little. The pediatrician handed Judy a typed summary of his medical record and moved to end the meeting.

"There's *got* to be something we can do for him!" Judy insisted.

The pediatrician said, "Oh, there are programs out there for children like yours. But they're controversial. I'm not about to recommend any of them."

"How are we supposed to make intelligent decisions if we don't know our options?" Judy demanded.

"Talk to other parents," was all the good doctor would suggest.

4. NOT A DOCTOR?

When Judy and I met, and throughout the early phase of our marriage, friends saw me as an outdoorsy guy who liked to hike in the mountains and who enjoyed live Irish music. Beneath that wholesome exterior, however, I was a mess. All my life, I had expected to become a doctor. But as I moved through my mid- and late twenties, I fretted more and more about how that cherished plan had been derailed. Amusements helped keep the sense of frustration at a manageable level, but I just couldn't stop picking at the old emotional scab.

My grandfather had been a physician, in the quaint old days of house calls. My dad remembered him being called out at all hours to deliver babies and set broken bones, and he also remembered that payment for these errands was never a sure thing.

Accordingly, Dad found a more stable line of work. He chose chemistry as a major simply because employers in his day wanted chemists, and with that he built a career in a series of large corporations. To me, however, providing professional care to patients seemed a great thing.

Unfortunately, a lot of others in my generation had the same idea.

Nowadays I'm hearing that medicine has lost some of its appeal. Ambitious young folks see that greater financial rewards, and perhaps greater prestige, can be obtained in fields that don't require medicine's long, arduous apprenticeship. Arguably, increasing government involvement makes it less attractive still. The numbers of applicants to medical school are trending downward.

But in my time, the pool of qualified applicants drastically outnumbered the spaces available. The odds against being admitted were so terrible, in fact, that the director of admissions at one school warned me that final selection criteria were essentially arbitrary. Still, in my senior year of college I did at least get invited for interviews at my favorite medical schools. Progressing that far in the process is considered significant, so if any one thing kept me out, it likely was what I said. For long years afterwards, I replayed the exchanges that occurred, mentally substituting answers that might have had a better effect.

The interview that stands out most clearly in my memory involved sitting at a long table facing several faculty members. Each held a pad for jotting down his impressions, although nothing was written in my presence. I remember a youthful chap with an open face and a down-home Southern accent, and a grey-haired gentleman with kind eyes. Most of the talking was done by a chunky middle-aged guy whose earthy small talk had startled me before we got under way.

"Bicycles!" He'd snorted, when I said biking was my favorite exercise. "Riding a bike is just working your legs off to give your ass a ride."

He put on a totally different persona at the table. Rubbing his palms together, he frowned and spoke slowly:

Let's say you're a family doctor, with your own clinic. And a teenage girl comes in late one afternoon just before you close, without the knowledge of her parents. And let's say you know the parents very well. They are your good friends, and you've known this girl all the time she was growing up. And now she confides to you that she is pregnant and wants a secret abortion. What do you do?

The personal relationships in this scenario provided an opportunity to show some understanding of professional ethics, or so I thought.

"Knowing the parents doesn't matter a whole lot in this situation, does it?" I began. "Maybe I could predict whether they'd be supportive. But the Hippocratic Oath would prevent me from going to them without her permission."

Over on the right-hand end of the table, the older one said, "I think you'll find as a doctor that the Hippocratic Oath won't be much of a guide in making decisions. It's not the point of reference it once was."

"No?" I must have looked astonished.

"It's more of a formality than anything else," the younger one explained helpfully. "When I graduated from med school, the Oath wasn't part of the main ceremony. I think it was being administered in some room in the basement, for those who wanted to go take it. A lot of us missed that because we were shaking people's hands and having our pictures taken."

"Oh," I said flatly, having lost the thread of what I'd intended to say.

"Back to the girl who wants that abortion—." The man in front of me prompted.

This was early in 1973. Roe v. Wade had been decided by the Supreme Court just two months earlier and was still being discussed in the news every day. And so I blurted, almost without thinking, "Well, it *is* legal now." Everyone sitting across from me audibly gasped.

"It's legal. So you would just do it?"

"I wouldn't *do* it," I said uncomfortably, meaning that I never expected to perform abortions myself. "We're getting ahead of ourselves, I think. Of course, there would have to be a lot of counseling, over a period of time. This is a major decision!"

"But the bottom line then is that it's legal, and so it's OK if that's what she wants?"

"Well, ideally, she would decide in the end that she *didn't* want to."

"*Ideally*, son, she wouldn't be pregnant."

"She's coming to me because she trusts me," I explained. "If she is convinced that she cannot carry the child, and her doctor turns her away, what is she going to do? We don't *know* what she would do. She might go find a quack. She might try to abort herself, possibly at the cost of her own life. If that happened, I would have failed her."

In trying to remember the details of that day, I can almost see my inquisitors pushing back from the table and consulting wordlessly among themselves. *Do we end this now? Fred, do you want to carry on a bit more?* That's no doubt my imagination intruding, but cues of some sort must have been passing among them. I recall a moment when their focus was not on me. Fool that I was, I used the opportunity to glance surreptitiously at their notepads, hoping they'd recorded something favorable.

Well then, let's say instead that you have a very elderly patient who is in a coma and is on life support. He is not expected ever to regain consciousness. Would you keep him on life support indefinitely, or would you pull the plug?

Oh, why did I not perceive by this point that these questions were designed to gauge my belief in the sanctity of life? Why did I not react to the disapproving body language inspired by my first response? Again, I began by equivocating. Surely, I said, state laws and hospital policy and family wishes would be the most important factors in determining what to do. But my interviewers wouldn't let me off the hook. "Everyone is counting on you to make a decision," the younger one said. "I can tell you from experience that the family won't be thinking clearly. That's their dad lying there. They will just look at you and say, 'Doctor, what do *you* recommend?'"

Thus pressed, I sighed and said that, if it were up to me, I would recommend pulling the plug. They frowned again.

"You've said the patient has no chance of recovering," I argued, belatedly sensing danger. "That's a given in this scenario, right?"

"There are very few 'givens,'" the older physician said. "Patients surprise *me* all the time." This drew affirmative rumblings up and down the table.

"Well, I'd have a different answer if he had a chance. But if you're just hoping that he wakes up one day, without doing anything to make that happen, and meanwhile he's running up a huge bill that somebody's going to have to pay, and he's tying up hospital resources that might be needed by someone else—I just don't know that I would be in favor of that."

My delivery probably sounded clumsier than represented here, but the arguments I offered were essentially the same as those I'd make today. I would not try to block the girl from having an abortion if I perceived that she was determined to get one, would still advise against prolonging life by extraordinary means—assuming there truly was no reasonable hope of recovery. But I might have made my points in a way that showed more sensitivity to the issues.

When it was over, my interviewers took turns shaking my hand and wishing me well. And in due course gave my seat in that class to another applicant.

Yes, I'd known admission was a long shot. Nevertheless, I had absorbed stories from the popular culture in which the underdog with a personal resolution to succeed always beats the odds, and had not prepared for the possibility of actual rejection.

On one level, the sudden change in career plans meant I now confronted a job market with a college transcript full of highly specialized and irrelevant courses, like histology and embryology.

I might have reapplied the following year, as a physician friend of my parents suggested. However, he warned, youth was another of the acceptance criteria. In those days, being even one year older than my competition would count against me.

No, I decided, the sting of being passed over was too great to bear twice. Better to pick a totally different career path. So I returned to school, earned a graduate degree in English, flirted with the idea of becoming a professor, and eventually found work as a technical writer. That at least made some use of my background in the sciences. And then, with the passage of time, I slowly became obsessed with remorse, not just for having blown the interview, or having invested so much of myself in the study of difficult subjects I would never need, but for missing the chance to prove to myself that I could handle the rigors of med school, and be a good doctor.

Maybe their strategy in that interview was to challenge *anything* I said. I think now that those guys would have expressed dismay, regardless of the answers I gave. Their real strategy was probably to see me take a stand and defend it. But I do think I handled their challenges poorly. I hadn't prepared adequately. My dad, who'd interviewed hundreds of job applicants in his day, advised me only to go in there with a firm handshake. "Just look them in the eye and give straight answers," he'd said. Nowadays, there are websites where med school applicants share their interview experiences. In every way, kids are infinitely more savvy now.

But if they truly didn't like my answers, which also seems likely, I have to wonder what criteria they used for right and wrong.

AT LEAST, Joseph's life was not in jeopardy. In another society, in another era, a child like Joseph would not have survived this long, but in fact he and all of us were physically safe. Financially, we were reasonably secure, too, as long as I kept my job and avoided new expenditures. I knew some people had worse problems.

But we had precious little room for complacency when we glimpsed other families. Mercifully, our exposure to normal children was minimal; we really didn't know how thoroughly charming little kids and child rearing could be. But we knew we had a problem.

And I was ready to debate right and wrong with anyone who felt medicine ought not to grapple with it.

If I wasn't good enough to be a doctor, then I sure as hell expected doctors to be good enough to do more with this issue than they had thus far.

In my experience, their profession had performed reasonably well prior to Joseph's birth, not that my family had ever presented major crises. They hadn't always diagnosed everything correctly the first time, hadn't always begun with the right course of treatment. But there *had* always been a good-faith effort to resolve matters. So I could not understand the way Joseph's providers had avoided treating him for a year. And now one of them had mentioned the option of venturing into some alternative that was too controversial even to name, let alone endorse.

Yes, my dear, there are people who can help you with your unwanted pregnancy. But I'm not about to tell you who they are.

I had little curiosity about the alternatives, but Judy was already heading full-speed in that direction. One evening she floored me by saying she had taken Joseph to a psychic. "I just went in there and said I had to find out what Joseph is thinking and experiencing. And the psychic told me he is in pain! She said there's an almost constant pain that wraps around the top of his head."

"What does she think is causing it?" I asked automatically.

"She said in a previous life Joseph had a lot of people depending on him. He always had to be the strong one for them. This time around he chose to be helpless. So we need to help him understand that it's safe, and he won't be put in that situation again."

"He's in pain? And we have to somehow tell him not to be in pain? *Come on*, Judy! We can do better than this! What did you pay for that wonderful advice?"

Judy gave me a disappointed look and said no more. But she had barely started. Now she was reading a book describing something called iridology. It claimed that a practitioner could read the state of one's health from markings in the iris.

She studied Joseph's eyes carefully and thought she saw concentric rings in the irises. Three rings indicated a very significant level of stress, according to the book. She counted *five* rings.

She took him to a practicing iridologist who confirmed the rings were there. Yes, the man said, this was a very sensitive, highly stressed child. "He'll be the kind of adult who cries at sad movies," he predicted. He offered a selection of medicinal herbs in capsule form, and Judy bought everything he suggested.

Years later, I found the draft of a letter she wrote to her sister Pat during this period. They'd had trouble getting along in the past (at one point, Judy had even cut off all contact for a year or more). However, recently the two had grown close, with frequent calls in which their parents, my parents, and I were all fair game for discussion. This letter held a lot of personal insights about their family background, but part of it bears on the situation.

> [The iridologist] said they would read Joseph for free but felt they could learn more about him from my eyes (since much is inherited). It was very interesting. After looking at my eyes he recommended some things for my liver and adrenals and nerves (I have three nerve rings myself. Five equals a full-blown nervous breakdown in an adult.)
>
> He asked if I ever had a blow to the head and I remembered getting hit with a rock (by the kid next door to us in our apartment in Italy). I was six years old, and following that I had blackout spells every so often—remember? He said I was very stressed as a child, with more than the usual number of fears.
>
> Also he said both Steve and I need to be treated for stress if Joseph is to be helped, because Joseph is almost totally telepathic, very sensitive and greatly affected by those around him.
>
> I am now taking an herb called valerian and it is great for calming me down. Joseph is less cranky, seems to sleep better. Steve is very resistant. He took his valerian and licorice root one time and slept almost all Saturday. Then said he felt numb and didn't even want to take a reduced dosage. Frankly, he is completely stressed. He has been driving me crazy for months. He is a bigger problem than Joseph. When he found out what I paid for the reading and the herbs for all three of us (most were for me) he hit the ceiling. …

Yeah, I probably did hit the ceiling. But what I meant to express wasn't anger with her so much as it was frustration at the thought of her spending the day on such a patently useless errand, and spending more than I earned in that day on jars of dried grass that I knew would catch dust for the next several years, until somebody cleaning out the pantry found the decomposing stuff and finally tossed it.

THE FOLLOWING WEEK brought another appointment with the ophthalmologist. Judy asked him about stress rings. The doctor was puzzled. "No. I don't see any unusual structures in his eyes." He'd never heard of such a thing as iridology, and didn't want to hear about it, either.

"Your son's vision is basically OK. There's some astigmatism and nearsightedness, but certainly nothing to be alarmed about. The problem is that he just doesn't seem to pay attention. In that, he's like a younger baby." He sighed and took a seat. "Visual development typically goes hand-in-hand with physical activity. So as he becomes more mobile, theoretically he'll be more alert."

That was assuming he did become more mobile.

A SOCIAL WORKER from Regional Center visited periodically. The woman sized up our situation and entered notes in her folder. Then she left, and that was all until next time.

"Why do they pay people to do that?" Judy wondered. "The government thinks they've got a program, but what does Joseph have to show for it? *This* isn't making him better! They're just putting notes about him into a filing cabinet somewhere."

"Well, they're building up a database," I suggested.

"So what? What does it tell them? Who's looking at it, even? What is anybody going to do with the information?"

Continuing with her research, she read about allergic reactions. One researcher claimed that various substances in food, water, or air could produce symptoms similar to Joseph's. By administering or withholding these allergens, the author had been able to turn the symptoms on or off. Was something like that at work here? If so, was it dairy products? Airborne dust? Some chemical? A combination of factors? The variables seemed endless. Identifying the culprit(s) would be a complex task, and Judy looked for a professional who could go about it properly. To her dismay, no one agreed that the effort was justified.

"Your son has an immature nervous system," Dr. Riker said patiently. "Extraordinary measures aren't going to change that. But just the same, you might as well look into regular physical therapy at this point." He described another state-funded organization called Crippled Children's Services, which he said existed for patients whose disabilities might involve long-term financial hardship for their families.

If I HAVEN'T UNDERSTOOD the guiding criteria used by medical people, I should at least explain my own at this point. In that 1973 admissions interview, I'd argued against artificially prolonging the life of an elderly patient in a vegetative state. My own father had often said that when his time came, he hoped to be allowed to go in peace; so when the interviewers compelled me to take a stand, I chose the preference he'd expressed.

On the other hand, extraordinary efforts aimed at improving the quality of a child's life did seem justified, and not just because this was my child. Why? Why should the question even be asked? I sensed then, and later formulated the conviction that wellness and potential are every child's birthright. And I'm quite sure that society is served when children have it.

Still, since this notion is not universally shared, I have spent some time wondering how I arrived at it. Reaching back, I recall the story of Helen Keller, told in *The Miracle Worker*—specifically, the moment when the deaf and blind child first connected the sensation of water on her skin with the word for water, signed into her palm. Prior to that breakthrough, she had been living in a state of virtual idiocy because of the barriers sealing her off from the world. That one event opened the way for interaction with others. As she later wrote, "It was as if I had come back to life after being dead."

Joseph did not have Helen Keller's disability, but the effect on him was similar. If he was capable of thought, which I had no reason to doubt, then the problem was impaired ability to make sense of things and express himself. He too would want to participate in life. And finding a way to help him *had* to be the responsibility of anyone presuming to act in his interests.

ARRIVING FOR THEIR FIRST APPOINTMENT at CCS, Judy carried our son through a sad gauntlet of older children strapped into wheelchairs, leg braces, and stretchers, all lined up at a curb and waiting to be loaded onto buses. Once inside the building, she met a young occupational therapist named Jan, who rolled her eyes comically when Judy repeated what the doctor had said. "They make us sound so *grim*," she complained. "'Long-term hardship,' indeed! Gimme a break. Anyway, we changed our name long ago. It's '*California* Children's Services.' Same acronym—just not so depressing."

Then she looked at Joseph. "Yes, he's behind schedule on his motor development, but he could make a lot of progress with improved muscle tone. Right now it seems a little exaggerated."

She was referring to a rigidity in some of his joints that we had noticed. If placed on his tummy and lifted by the hips, he did not assume a four-point creeping posture but rather came up stiffly, with his legs straight out behind him.

Jan began the session by trying to interest Joseph in various toys. He took note of marbles that she rolled noisily down a track, but he didn't want to touch anything.

"He doesn't seem to fit into any obvious category," Jan mused.

"Have you seen kids like this before?"

"Oh, sure!"

"How long does it usually take them to learn to crawl?"

"That varies with the child, you know. I wouldn't want to make any predictions at this point."

"Do these kids eventually get well, or what?"

Jan's answers became increasingly vague. Finally, when Judy refused to give up, she confessed that CCS never actually "cured" anybody. The object was to help patients compensate for their disabilities, rather than to overcome them. Another part of her role was evidently to help the family adjust. She gave Judy a reprint of a magazine article describing the classical "grief process" that parents of a disabled child pass through on their way to acceptance.

An arrangement evolved in which Jan performed occupational therapy with Joseph for an hour, every Tuesday, and a physical therapist named Jean worked with him again on Thursday.

In the evenings I always wanted to know how the sessions had gone. At first Judy was noncommittal, but then—.

"It doesn't look good," she said. "Joseph has started protesting so violently they can't do anything. Today Jean was trying to put him on his hands and knees and he just shook his head and screamed, and yelled, 'No!'"

"He *said* 'No'?"

"*He yelled it.* Plain as day. You could have heard him anywhere in the building."

"Well, that's kind of interesting." I hadn't heard a lot of recognizable words from him.

"Come to therapy with us and you'll hear him say, 'No.'"

BY THIS POINT, Judy had begun locking herself out of the car at inconvenient times. She'd taken to phoning her parents and sisters on the East Coast with blow-by-blow accounts of the unfolding crisis. "The physical therapist said they're not sure, but he might have cerebral palsy," she told her sister Barbara. "Yes," Barbara said knowingly. "Dave and I have been telling each other it sounded like that. But at least that's not a progressive illness. I mean, you know, it doesn't get worse."

I said nothing about Judy's phone bills and little mishaps. After all, I committed blunders of my own, such as the time I put a casserole dish full of leftovers into the kitchen cabinet instead of the refrigerator. And compared to her, I was lucky. I had distractions at the office. The Space Shuttle *Challenger* had recently exploded during launch. That calamity, distressing enough in its own right, had driven all elements of the space program into crisis mode. Where I worked, an entire product line—an upper-stage rocket designed to be launched from the Shuttle—was abruptly terminated, and people were scrambling to find new assignments.

Joseph never strayed from my mind during that turmoil, but Judy remained the one who cared for him all day, receiving only rare smiles and virtually no speech for her trouble. (Sometimes, unprompted, he'd utter a recognizable word, but no amount of coaxing led to any sort of exchange.) She assumed the main burden, too, of finding help, however erratic that search was becoming.

The suggestion that he might be in pain remained before us. Why else would he cry so much of the time? Every day, she gently traced fingertips over his head, noting the high crown. The molding his skull had undergone during birth was still apparent, even now, well into his second year of life.

"I wonder if we should take him to a chiropractor," she mused.

"A *chiropractor*? For *him*?" I'd never once heard of babies going to chiropractors. "First a psychic, then someone selling snake oil, now this. You're going crazy, honey. You know that, don't you?"

"Well look at his head! You're telling me this is normal?"

"Hey, I don't know if *anything* we're looking at is normal. But surely, if chiropractors had something to offer here, we would have been advised by now to see one."

"Oh, so you still think mainstream doctors have answers for this? Who's crazy now?"

5. THE PARTING OF THE WAYS

Because the physical therapy still wasn't going well, I took time off from work and sat in on a session. Jan was placing Joseph in a sitting position on a mat and encouraging him to twist so that he could use his right hand to pick up a toy that was on his left side. First he cried and resisted her efforts to guide him through the motions. Then he arched his spine and fell backward. He began rolling his head from side to side and making the repetitive siren noise that always pierced me like an ice pick.

Jan pulled him back up into sitting, and he screamed furiously. "Well, now he's tantruming," she observed in a matter-of-fact tone. "Look, Joseph. The toy is over here."

"Should Judy and I work him past the point of crying, the way you do?" I asked doubtfully.

Jan frowned. "Well, it's a little different for *me* to do this, because I'm an outsider. But you *could*, depending on how fast you want him to progress."

Naturally wanting him to progress at a perceptible rate, I began putting Joseph through a similar routine that night. Immediately, I had a fight on my hands.

Within a few days, when mere vocal protest hadn't worked, he began biting.

He began thrashing violently in his car seat as soon as Judy parked outside the building where the therapy sessions were held. When she picked him up he would hit her in the face, scratch her, and struggle with such force that she nearly dropped him.

I gave up the unproductive evening sessions, and Judy talked to a counselor at Regional Center. Behavior modification was suggested. "Take him to the clinic every day, even when he doesn't have an appointment," she was advised. "Just walk him around there for a few minutes and then leave. If you desensitize him in that way, he won't react when he sees the building."

"That sounds a little dishonest," I muttered when Judy told me the new plan.

"It *is* dishonest!" She agreed. "Joseph's trying to make sense of his world, and now we'll be confusing him. I hate it!"

We frowned at each other. "When he resists," I finally said, "Of course we don't like it. But that's a form of communication. He's trying to tell us something. That in itself is worth a lot. I'm not saying he's *right*. I'm not saying the therapy should *stop*, but—."

"I know. We need to respect him. But give me a better idea."

I could always find fault with the ideas I heard, but as a source of them I was bone-dry. "Well, I'm going to give this a try," Judy decided. She gave everything a try.

On their first bogus trip to therapy she found an old, out-of-tune piano in the corridor, and she entertained Joseph by picking out familiar melodies on it. While loitering there, she told me that night, she met a woman carrying a very small, fragile-looking child.

"My daughter's therapy just got cancelled," the woman announced mournfully. "She hasn't responded, so the doctor who referred us said we have to stop."

A long discussion ensued. The mother said she'd made arrangements to have a therapist carry on with treatments at their home. "We can't afford private sessions," she said. "But we can't just do *nothing*!"

All this made a big impression on Judy, who saw our own future in the other family's situation. Joseph wasn't responding, either. How soon would they cancel *us*?

She told me how the other mother continually wiped her eyes with a palm, ranting. "I know, I know: If it hasn't helped so far, why is more of it going to help? I just think we need to continue with this until something better comes along. They don't know what's wrong with her, is the problem. But if we could just—get somebody's *attention*, maybe get her case written up in a medical journal or something, then maybe she could get included in a study."

"Even being part of a study is no guarantee of treatment," Judy warned. "You might be in the control group."

"Yeah. Maybe I'll have a better idea tomorrow."

ONE AFTERNOON Judy called to say she had locked herself out of the car yet again. They happened to be at a chiropractor's office. She added that as long as I had to come unlock the car, I might as well stick around to hear what this doctor had to say.

This was too convenient, I now see. Surely, she locked herself out on purpose, because she knew there would be no other way of getting me into the chiropractor's office.

It worked. I arrived, grumpily, to hear a young woman who wanted to be called by her first name—Dr. Lori—saying in effect that the psychic had been correct. Joseph was indeed in pain. "This is the most severely distorted head I have ever seen," she added. "You say Joseph was delivered with suction? Well, it looks like that pulled up the back of his skull. The plates of the skull are actually overlapping! I wish you had come sooner. This is going to take quite a few treatments!"

Dumbfounded, I just stared at the floor. If this were true, why had nobody else noticed? Of course, if the method by which Joseph had been delivered had caused the problem, I could imagine why the employees of our health plan might have avoided telling us.

IN THE DELIVERY ROOM the doctor had said, "Set the dial at Six. I won't go any higher than that!" And hoping to avoid caesarian delivery, I had stupidly thought, *Go ahead! Set the suction as high as you need to. Let's finish this.*

IN THAT LONG-AGO INTERVIEW, I'd been told, "The family won't be thinking clearly. They will say, 'Doctor, what do *you* recommend?'" But Judy and I had told our doctor what we wanted: natural childbirth (or something as close to it as possible, given that she was already loaded up with meds). Had we influenced him to make the wrong choice? If we'd gone along with the C-section, would that have saved Joseph from all this misery and apparent disability?

AT ANY RATE, for about a month Judy took Joseph in for a chiropractic adjustment almost every day. These were brief sessions, in which Dr. Lori thumped him a few times at strategic points, using a spring-loaded device about the size of a pencil. After a few treatments Joseph did cry less often and slept more easily at night. I conceded that Judy must have been right, and that I'd been way too conservative. Prepared to learn, I took him in for his appointment one Saturday and watched carefully.

"His nervous system is completely shut down," Dr. Lori explained. She was demonstrating a way of massaging his back that might encourage circulation of the cerebrospinal fluid. "Still, he's making progress."

"What does that mean?"

"It means he's beginning to hold his adjustments. You can go down to three appointments a week."

"When do you think he'll start to crawl?"

She looked thoughtful. "Crawling is something he has to *learn*. It's hard to predict when that'll happen." However, my focus on achieving this overdue milestone may have made an impression. When Judy took Joseph in for his next appointment, she said, "There's a book I want you to find. It's called *Teach Your Baby to Read*."

Judy was puzzled. "Well, I'm sure the idea of teaching babies to read is very nice, but what does that have to do with us? We're still trying to get ours to *move*."

"Just get the book. You'll see."

Two days later Judy and Joseph returned for the next appointment. "Have you read that book I told you about?" the chiropractor wanted to know.

"No. Not yet."

"Don't wait around! You can probably find it at the public library. The author's name is Doman." She wrote the title and author on a slip of paper.

And still another appointment day arrived. "Well?" she demanded. "Have you gotten that book *yet*?"

Judy sighed. "OK. I'll go by the library and get it today."

That was a Friday. By Sunday night Judy and I had both read Glenn Doman's book from cover to cover. It wasn't just a how-to book. On the contrary, the author wanted mainly to explain what he'd learned while treating brain-injured children. Neurological growth was not the static and predestined fact everyone supposed it to be. It could be slowed or even stopped, but it could also be restarted and accelerated. Teaching very small children to recognize printed words was one technique for accomplishing this.

Mr. Doman headed a place in Philadelphia called the Institutes for the Achievement of Human Potential. He cited cases of brain-injured children who learned not only to read but to do all the other things necessary for full participation in life.

I closed his book gently and gripped it in both hands. This sounded like the very thing we'd been looking for. Here was *one* therapist, at least, who believed in making a difference.

Philadelphia was a long way from San Diego, but we would bridge that distance. For starters, I called the Institutes as soon as their switchboard opened Monday morning. A woman answered and I launched into an urgent monologue about our son's problem and the book we'd just read. When I let her speak, she gave the impression she handled calls like this all the time. No one was available to talk with me, but she promised to send a package of information in that day's mail.

Unable to wait for its arrival, we plunged ahead with Joseph's introduction to the written word. Following the instructions in the book, we bought sheets of poster board, which we cut into strips, six inches high. Using a bold, red marker, we began printing, starting with the obvious—*Joseph, Mommy, Daddy*—and progressing through every word that was part of his experience.

He directed a brief, suspicious glance at the cards when we presented them, but at least he looked. That was encouragement enough for us to continue.

SESSIONS WITH DR. LORI continued as well. In fact, hardly a day went by when Judy wasn't loading Joseph into the car and rushing off to see some specialist. Often, there were two or even three appointments in one day. On a typical Monday he might have an audiology exam and a chiropractic adjustment. Early Tuesday morning brought a home teacher who'd replaced Ferrell. That would be followed by occupational therapy, and then I would take time off from my job to meet Judy and Joseph at some doctor's office for yet another unproductive consultation.

And so it went. We felt like detectives, hot on the trail of the answer to Joseph's problem as we ran down one lead after another. And, like maverick TV detectives, we felt stonewalled by the authorities.

"Did you see the way that pediatrician looked when you said we'd gone to a chiropractor?" I asked Judy. "I thought she was going to barf right there on the floor!"

Judy laughed in agreement. "But she didn't actually say anything against it."

"I guess they have to respect each other's turf. So, looks like we're expected to listen to what they say, and also to read between the lines for other meanings."

I said this feeling a complicated mixture of anger and sadness. These people likely had nothing of value to tell us, verbally or otherwise. *Did* the small temporal lobes of Joseph's brain represent a handicap? Or were the experts I'd trusted using that peculiarity as a convenient explanation for anything they didn't understand? Why did they show no professional curiosity? If this chiropractor was right about the plates of his skull, did that mean the doctors knew something about him that they wanted to hide from us? Or were they just hiding the fact that they felt as confused and helpless as we did? They sure didn't like being asked for anything more than the next appointment slip!

I still had doubts about Dr. Lori, too, despite Joseph's initial improvement under her care and the sage advice to read Doman's book. Although her waiting room held a folder of testimonials written by other patients, they didn't inspire confidence. One joker praised her ability to twist his head around without actually twisting it *off*. No one seemed to have been cured of serious problems, or even to have had any.

Worse, she was offering discounts if Judy and I—and even our friends—would become patients. More appointments would bring economies of scale. She insisted that we could all benefit. I resisted any discussion that moved the focus off Joseph.

Even more disturbing: her sessions with him now included some New Age foolishness called crystal therapy. She explained that certain crystals vibrate at a pitch that harmonizes with good health. Bringing them into close proximity with his body was supposed to change the flow of energy in his spine. Yes, my views were evolving. But that notion remained too far-out to take seriously. I knew we had to move on.

A large envelope arrived from Philadelphia. It contained a brochure that profiled several truly outstanding children—musicians, gymnasts, all-round *geniuses*, apparently—and concluded with a promise. "There is nothing they can do that is not available to all babies at birth … Those children, together with *yours*, are the one, last, best, bright hope for tomorrow."

Although it sounded great, the phrasing did not completely mesh with my expectations. For example, why stipulate "at birth" when the kids seen at the Institutes would not be newborns? If the writer thought that distinction was worth making, then what potential applied in Joseph's case?

Still, no other promises looked as good. Of course, no other resources were promising anything. There was a letter assuring us that the primary work of the Institutes was with "hurt kids." Many parents of normal children also applied the Institutes' methods to achieve exciting results, it said, but the real focus was on accomplishing the same thing with families like ours. Finally, there was a list of reading materials to help us understand the methods and lifestyle involved in such an endeavor.

This time there was no delay. Judy and I searched the public library yet again and brought home several more books, most notably *What to Do About Your Brain-Injured Child*, also by Glenn Doman. The subtitle covered all the bases. *Or Your Brain-damaged, Mentally Retarded, Mentally Deficient, Cerebral-palsied, Spastic, Flaccid, Rigid, Epileptic, Autistic, Athetoid, Hyperactive Child.*

Here was literature of a totally different stripe from any we'd read previously. Avoiding professional jargon, Doman addressed himself to the people out in the trenches, the parents. He wrote confidently of TOTAL WELLNESS for kids whom the doctors saw as hopeless. He dismissed as "unmedical" the practice of compensating for neurological disabilities—using leg braces, for example—without addressing their cause. The cause was always in the brain, and despite assumptions to the contrary, the brain could be changed, reprogrammed, *made to grow*!

Growth was accomplished by providing specific stimulation and opportunity, with enormous "intensity, frequency, and duration." A hurt kid absolutely needed this if he was going to recover, and the sooner one started providing it, the better.

"Aha! They do *patterning* at the Institutes," Judy said. "I read something about that in college. So *these* are the people who invented it!"

We scrutinized the diagrams and accompanying text. Patterning was a practice in which three adults simultaneously manipulated a child's arms, legs, and head while he lay prone on a table. Many hours of repetition told the child's brain, by sensory input, *This is how it feels to crawl.* The people most suitable to take responsibility for this project—indeed, the only people, according to Doman—were the child's parents.

In short, instead of passively waiting for medical professionals to do their job, we had the option of becoming educated enough to do it for them.

We read a discussion of patterning that had originally appeared in the *Journal of the American Medical Association*, in 1960. Twenty-six years earlier.

"How come nobody around here seems to know about this?" I demanded.

"Well, I've asked about it," Judy said. "More than once! Jan just brushed aside my questions. She told me nobody does that anymore. Said it's been proven not to work."

She asked again.

Jan was appalled to learn that we had actually been in touch with the Institutes. "That approach is all *wrong*," she insisted.

"Have you read any of the Institutes' books?"

"No—. I don't *have* to! I know they make big claims that aren't founded."

"Have you ever seen any children who had been patterned?"

She hesitated. "Well, yes. There was one boy."

"Did he learn to crawl?" Judy felt like an attorney cross-examining an uncooperative witness.

"Oh, he finally got to where he could scoot along on his stomach.

Like a lizard. But look. We don't know that patterning was responsible, even for that."

"I don't see the harm in trying it," Judy said. She thought for a moment. Jan, she knew, was very athletic and had a special enthusiasm for rock-climbing. She must have taken chances at some point. "Jan, have you ever tried to do something that you weren't sure would work?"

Jan said no more.

GLENN DOMAN'S BOOK summarized how the small team of specialists that evolved into the Institutes had begun by faithfully employing the accepted therapies of the time. They couldn't avoid noticing, however, that the children they treated never improved. In 1950 they'd stopped to evaluate the results achieved thus far, and what they saw was so discouraging that they wondered if they had any business treating patients at all.

They changed course after raising a simple question that apparently no one had considered before. *What are the factors necessary for a child to develop?* Since the authorities of the day had little to say on this subject, Doman wrote, "We decided to go to the source, the infants themselves." From observation of normal children, they gradually identified four essential stages of mobility, though which everyone apparently passed—first, moving arms and legs without mobility, then crawling on one's belly, then creeping on all fours, and finally walking.

A child like Joseph, who at fifteen months remained stuck at stage one, needed specific help if he was going to advance. And Doman's book was about providing that help.

ON THURSDAY Judy and Joseph were back at CCS for an appointment with Jean, the physical therapist. As usual, I heard all about it that night. This time she didn't need to bring up the subject of patterning. News of our potential defection had spread through the clinic. "Judy, families who go that route end up driving away all their friends and alienating their relatives," Jean warned.

"Joseph needs us more than our friends and relatives do," Judy retorted.

"It drives people away because it's hard," Jean said earnestly. "Believe me, that kind of program is too hard on everybody. It's *not* a good idea!"

Jean was wasting her breath. Judy said, "Just having a disabled child is already hard on us. It's no picnic for him either, I'm sure. If we're going to improve things, we need to move him toward wellness."

There it was again—that pained expression we encountered at any mention of wellness. After all their attempts to educate us, we were still being unreasonable. Jean said, "*These children* do everything in slow motion. Nothing's going to change that. Nobody can promise to speed up their development!"

"That's exactly what they *have* promised."

"You need to understand something here, Judy. If you insist on starting a patterning program, we won't let you continue as a client with us. Think about that. Promise you'll talk it over with me some more before you do anything rash."

JUDY MET with the neurologist who had seemed so confident a year earlier. She described Joseph's resistance to therapy. "I feel if we could just get past his irritability, we could stimulate him more effectively," she suggested.

The doctor mentioned Melaril, "a mild sedative" that could help. Judy demurred. How could she *stimulate* him if he were sedated? Finally, the doctor asked that we both return to his office that evening. He wanted his colleague, Dr. Green, to talk with us.

It happened to be one of the nights when I had to work late at the office. In fact, by the time Judy called, I knew that it would be a very late night. But I could slip out without dire consequences. My boss agreed to cover for me, and I drove to the clinic.

Dr. Mulligan ushered us into his office, where we found an older gentleman in a brown suit, thumbing casually through Joseph's chart. He glanced up as we took our seats and asked why we'd come.

"Are you familiar with Joseph's history?" I asked, privately irritated that here was one more professional who hadn't taken the time to prepare himself for us.

"No."

"Would you like me to summarize it for you?"

"Well, yes. If you can."

Heaven help families who can't spell out their situation for these people, I thought. I began retelling the story, in what I hoped was a sensible, professional tone. I really wanted them to take our problem seriously.

Dr. Green asked about Joseph's personality. I said he'd always been extremely irritable, seemingly in distress. Judy interrupted to amplify that with voluble descriptions of how he arched his back and slung his head from side to side.

Dr. Green had a friendly mustache, high forehead, and kind, Jewish eyes, which were filled with sympathy. "Well, to begin with, you needn't feel that you have been singled out as the victims of some rare calamity," he said.

"No indeed," Dr. Mulligan put in from behind his desk. "The incidence of this sort of thing is—*several* per thousand."

"Of the people affected, how many recover?"

The doctors glanced at each other. Then Dr. Mulligan spoke in a gentler tone. "We can't say for sure what the future holds for Joseph. But looking purely at the odds, the chances are that he will have intellectual and language deficits, and quite possibly other problems as well. Such children often have difficult births, as he did, and he's continuing to fit that pattern."

There was a long pause. I looked at Joseph, asleep in his stroller.

Dr. Green said, "The important thing I want you both to understand is that this is *not your fault.* A lot of parents make the mistake of blaming each other, or even blaming themselves. And they worry that there may be something they haven't tried yet that's going to help their child. That's the wrong approach. You shouldn't see Joseph's progress as being critical—to *you*—because if he fails to accomplish something, what happens then? Where does that leave you? Just looking at Joseph there—looking at the way you have him dressed, for example—it's easy to see that you love him very much. He certainly looks healthy and well-nourished. I know you've done everything you can for him."

They let us talk about all the avenues Judy had, in fact, been pursuing. "I read a book about iridology," she said. "Are you familiar with that subject?"

They weren't. She told them about the stress rings in his eyes. She went on to describe the therapy at CCS, Joseph's resistance to it, the behavior mod. She spoke of the suggestion that he might be autistic, and that truncated line of inquiry. She mentioned a nutritionist she'd seen, and her unsuccessful efforts to have Joseph tested for allergies. "I even took him to a *dentist*," she said, "because he has worn his teeth down so badly by grinding them. I thought he must be in pain. But the dentist told me that the nerve in a tooth will 'retreat' in a case like that, so it shouldn't cause any discomfort. So then I tried a chiropractor."

The doctors had listened patiently. Finally, as she launched into the subject of overlapping skull bones, Dr. Green said, "I recommend that you pick just one source for the answers you're seeking. Find someone you trust. Settle on an authority whom you think has something to offer your son. That would be a lot less stressful for you than constantly trying new ideas and new services. The way you're going, I'm afraid you might wear yourselves out."

"Doctor," I said. "Since she brought this up, *does* taking Joseph to a chiropractor have merit?"

Another uncomfortable pause. Dr. Green leaned forward, elbows on knees, and said, simply, "Anything has merit if it gives you hope."

"That's true," Dr. Mulligan added quickly. "But you should stay *far away* from anybody who preaches Doman-Delacato stimulation methods." I was startled, since we hadn't gotten around to that topic yet. Evidently Judy had mentioned patterning in their earlier meeting.

"Oh, right," Dr. Green conceded. "That approach ruins lives."

"What I'd *rather* have you do," Dr. Mulligan continued, "would be to see a counselor."

I bristled. "I keep trying to tell people that Judy and I aren't the ones who need help. *Joseph* needs help!"

"The advantage of getting counseling is that you could acquire 'tools'—for coping—while you make sure Joseph gets the care he needs. You have to look after yourselves, too. I have to say that both of you look quite *wrung out*."

Joseph stirred and awoke from his nap. As always, he promptly began shrieking. We concluded the meeting.

The doctors had delivered their intended message, but to me, matters felt unfinished. "I'm sorry we didn't have time to talk more," I said regretfully as we stood.

Dr. Green clapped me on the shoulder. "I daresay you're just beginning to talk."

Judy and I parted in the parking lot. She took Joseph home for a late dinner and I returned to my office, where I dodged my boss's questions. What would be the point of telling him? Right now any more pity, from any quarter, I thought, would make me physically ill. The doctors had set up a whole current of pity, trying to commiserate with me over my long working hours for example. That's what they'd done instead of considering Joseph's needs. Granted, stress reduction for us was a good thing. But what about the boy—the patient? Why expend so much energy addressing our stress, when the *cause* of that stress was being ignored? OK, so his odds were not good. He was counting on us to find a plan for beating those odds.

I sat at my desk and steamed. Skip the pity. Skip the assurances that we were not at fault. I took no comfort in the news that others were also afflicted. Doman's program ruins lives? These turkeys don't know ruined life when it's staring them in the face. *Anything has merit if it gives you hope*, remember? Screw them, we're going to see Doman.

6. TWO NEW PATHS

Joseph was sitting placidly on the floor (for once, at least, not crying!) during our one session with the family counselor Dr. Green had recommended. Her advice—to "take each day as it comes, and avoid worrying so much about the future"—did not strike us as an option.

He was crying, and doing little else, when Judy's younger sister Debbie visited from Florida over the Fourth of July. It was Debbie's first trip to California, and we tried to be good hosts. Instead, we found ourselves betraying our addled state by making wrong turns on familiar roads and snapping at each other over trivia. "I have never seen Judy like this," Debbie told me several times in an awed voice. "She's like a different person."

The doctor at Regional Center had suggested comparing notes with other families, and we did. Judy had found a local support group for families with disabled children. We attended meetings in which less-experienced parents vented frustrations and the old hands offered perspective.

One mother confessed to using up an entire box of tissue at every medical evaluation.

"You're still in the 'Kleenex stage,'" a lady named Peggy observed knowingly. "It's natural. I used to take a box of tissue with me to every appointment! I'd start out by telling the doctor, 'Sorry, but I'm going to have to cry. Please don't let it bother you.' Then when my daughter was four, I finally got to where I didn't do that so much."

Following Peggy's lead did not look like a great option, either.

DEBBIE FOLLOWED UP on her visit with a letter. "You need to go back to work," she advised Judy. "Get out and think about something different. Hire a nurse to look after Joseph during the day. Even if that takes all or most of your salary, it'll still be worth it, because the burden you have is just too much."

Now that we'd shared our secret, Judy grumbled about the fact that no one, in either of our families, was stepping forward to help us. I generally defended them, pointing out that they had lives of their own, thousands of miles away, and adding that we didn't have a clear idea of how they might help, even if it occurred to them to offer. But in Judy's mind this letter indicted the whole clan.

In her view, my own family scored even lower. By now, my parents had seen Joseph twice and granted that something was definitely troubling the little fellow. But I guess they found it inconceivable that their only grandchild would have a lasting problem. They felt sure I would call some day to announce that all was well. Until I did, they still recommended patience.

Debbie's advice notwithstanding, there was no way we were going to turn Joseph over to a stranger. The few "trained" respite workers who'd been provided by Regional Center had proven to be far more interested in our television set and the contents of our refrigerator than in our son.

No, the thing that would help us would also be the thing that helped him. And we were beginning to understand what that was.

Mobility was his most obvious problem. According to the Institutes' books we were reading, the first and most basic requirement was to keep Joseph in a prone position, so he would at least have opportunity to learn how to move. He still preferred lying on his back, where he

WHAT ABOUT THE BOY?   71

tirelessly rolled his head from side to side. If we placed him on his stomach, he flipped over again as soon as we released him. Our reading contained references to something called an antiroll device, which children at the Institutes wore to prevent this kind of nonproductive behavior. We had no idea of what such a thing should look like but began experimenting with designs.

We read about the advantages of encouraging an immobile child to inch his way down a smooth inclined plane. The slope would make forward motion easier and in turn might inspire crawling on a level surface, too. I set to work constructing one right away. Clearly, I needed to meet the people who generated such common-sense ideas.

THEN THE DAY ARRIVED that Judy had been half-expecting since her chance encounter with the mother at CCS.

After a routine therapy session marked by Joseph's usual protests and resistance, Jan invited her into a room where she found Dr. Mulligan and two other physicians waiting. Rising to the occasion with newfound confidence, she placed Joseph on the examination table and gave Dr. Mulligan a cheery greeting. "Looks like you've picked up some sunshine!"

He seemed embarrassed by this overture. "I took some friends out on my boat yesterday," he murmured. Then, with his colleagues crowding around impatiently, he went on. "Our purpose in asking you to meet with us today is to agree on a point for terminating Joseph's therapy here."

One of the others hastened to add that there was no need for alarm— they would recommend allowing him to continue until his second birthday, still a good six months away.

"Is he going to be well on his second birthday?" Judy demanded.

They didn't seem to think so.

"Why would you want to cancel him, then?"

"We don't have a qualifying diagnosis," Dr. Mulligan explained. One of the others moved Joseph's arms and legs and said, "He's not spastic," as if that settled everything.

"Well, I'm *glad* he's not 'spastic.' But obviously he does have a problem. We're still waiting for somebody to tell us exactly what it is." Judy looked back and forth at their blank faces. "Jan told me once that he moves like someone who's brain-damaged."

"I did *not* say he was brain-damaged!" Jan cried out defensively for the record, no doubt fearing the sort of reprimand Michelle may have received.

"That's not necessarily so," Dr. Mulligan said blandly, "Although the abnormal CT-scan *is* probably related to his lack of development thus far. But there's no evidence that there was any trauma, either before or after birth. This is just the way he grew. It just happened. Granted, he *is* slow." He paused significantly. "The word *retarded* means 'slow'—."

Judy interrupted him hotly. "I used to be a special-ed teacher. Believe me, I know what 'retarded' means!"

"—but physical therapy, unfortunately, is not a treatment for retardation."

AS WE CIRCULATED among families with disabled children, we heard references to a local osteopath, Viola Frymann, who specialized in treating children with disabilities. One mother assured us that she'd given up on other medical providers altogether and relied on Dr. Frymann for everything, from sniffles on up. We hesitated to pursue this course, however, because of the expense. As long as we used providers within our health maintenance organization, there were no medical bills. But the chiropractor had not been covered. We'd handed over $1,000 to her before discontinuing treatments. The Institutes would certainly not be covered! I tried not to think about the outlay we might be making in the months—or years—ahead.

We began our exposure to this new wing of medicine by attending an evening lecture that Dr. Frymann gave periodically. She turned out to be a spare-framed, elderly woman with a prominent forehead and a precise, deliberate way of speaking.

She began by saying, "Most people bring their children to our Center because someone has suggested that it might be a good idea, but they have no clear understanding of what goes on here. Typically, we see parents who have been dealing for some time with conventional physicians, where the pressing urge was to find a diagnosis—a label that describes the problem that their child presents. That label may eventually be 'cerebral palsy,' or 'mental retardation,' or 'learning disabled,' or some sophisticated-sounding name of a syndrome, which simply means that a doctor has made himself famous by describing a set of conditions that occur together and affixing his name to them.

"And once you have gotten this label, this diagnosis, there is a tendency to feel that you have accomplished something. But as you think about it, you realize that you haven't traveled much farther than where you were to begin with.

"We are more concerned with what is *behind* that label—that is, the state of the child himself. We are looking at a human being, rather than a case of this, that, or the other."

Then the proceedings became really interesting.

She exhibited a tiny skull that had belonged to a newborn baby and pointed to the opening at its base, through which the spinal cord passed.

"This hole should be symmetrical," she declared. "If a baby has a history of excessive vomiting or 'spitting up,' that is the first indication that there has been compression in this area. Deformation of the baby's skull, caused by trauma at the time of birth, results in irritation of the vagus nerve. And you have a child who is unable to suck or swallow properly or who can't keep his food down. Also, when you have any sort of structural deformation, you find a baby who is nervous or tense—one who cries excessively and has trouble sleeping."

Judy and I stared at each other in amazement. She'd just described Joseph! Were his symptoms *that* typical, and *that* easily explained?

"Fortunately," she said, "the body has the most extraordinary capacity for righting itself. Your own inherent forces within the body take care of most injuries most of the time. The function of our discipline is to encourage the body to do what it wants to do on its own."

A mother in the audience spoke up. "My son is two years old," she said. "And he's functioning at a ten-month level. We've been seeing pediatricians and neurologists and all, and they keep saying not to worry, that he'll catch up on his own. Is that reasonable?"

Dr. Frymann said, "I can't comment on your child specifically without having seen him. But if he is two years old and already more than a year behind schedule, the idea of 'catching up' is rather like running after a train. Isn't it? Catching up with other children might not be as appropriate a goal as simply addressing whatever it is that has happened to him."

Another woman said, "Is patterning an appropriate response when a child is behind schedule like that?"

"Yes," Dr. Frymann said. "In many cases, patterning does help. I have been to the Institutes in Philadelphia. I've seen the kind of work they do there and the results they're getting. Patterning definitely can be useful."

The first mother said, "But what do I say to those doctors who tell me to do nothing? They say anything I do will be a waste of time!"

Dr. Frymann shrugged. "I wouldn't talk to them," she advised. "I don't believe in trying to persuade someone who has a mind block about something. That's a *real* waste of time."

EVIDENTLY, then, two options remained for Joseph—repair of what Dr. Frymann called his structural mechanism and stimulation to accelerate his development.

We meant to pursue both.

I scheduled an initial evaluation for him with Dr. Frymann, and together Judy and I hastened to complete the Institutes' application. Mainly, it asked us to evaluate our child's "competence" in six areas—visual, auditory, tactile, mobility, language, and manual—and to certify that we had both read *What to Do About Your Brain-Injured Child.*

This was the beginning of an extensive correspondence. The staff asked for his medical records, but their main interest appeared to be in seeing him through our eyes. *We* were the real experts on our son, they suggested, not the specialists we'd relied on thus far. Also, they wanted to clarify what would be expected of us. After Joseph's program was prescribed, we would have to perform it with him *all day, every day.* So that we realized what that meant, we were instructed to visit a family currently doing an Institutes program. The nearest one, apparently, was 100 miles away, across the desert, in Mexico.

IF WE WERE GOING all the way to Philadelphia, we would certainly make a day-trip to Mexico, too. But for the moment Judy turned back to the mothers she already knew in the support group.

Peggy said that she'd written to the Institutes once. She hadn't applied, however, because her husband was opposed. He believed the doctors who'd said their child could not be helped and thought it was outrageous to cross the continent for some unrealistic pie-in-the-sky.

However, another parent mentioned knowing a family that actually patterned their child. When Judy pounced on that news with a demand for their phone number, the other backpedaled, saying, "I don't know if it would be wise to start you down that road. Jennifer is pretty gung-ho."

"*You're* not starting us down any road," Judy protested. "*We'll* make the decisions about what to do."

At length, the phone number was grudgingly produced and that night Judy dialed it.

"Patterning works," Jennifer told her. "I don't care what anybody else says. I've seen the difference with my own eyes. If *you* want to start, you can have the patterning board we used."

We wasted no time in driving to their house. Once the initial greetings had subsided, their two-year-old son Lucas padded into the living room to look us over. He sat on the floor, tilted his head back, and regarded us from the bottoms of his eyes. Jennifer explained that the odd posture was necessary because of limited vision that was part of Down syndrome.

They had patterned for several months, Jennifer said, until he began creeping. Then they'd stopped. "We decided that it wasn't worth continuing the program if everything else was going to fall apart," she explained. "I had to think about the rest of my family."

Her husband Mike added, "Lucas is *always* going to have Down syndrome. No program is going to change that. I figure this is the way God wants him to be."

Judy and I let that go by. Chromosomes notwithstanding, we didn't believe God wanted anyone to have a permanent disability. But we hadn't come to argue.

They brought the patterning board out of a closet. It was a flat plank, two feet wide and almost four feet long, with ample padding under a brown vinyl cover.

Lucas grinned with recognition when they set the patterning board on the living room floor. He promptly flopped himself down upon it.

"Do you want to be patterned one last time, Lucas?" Jennifer asked. "All right! Let's demonstrate how it's done."

Three of us knelt around the board, one on each side and another at the head.

"OK, with one hand the person where I am takes him by the wrist, like so," she said. "Press your fingertips on the back of his little hand, so the palm flattens out against the vinyl, up here beside his face. Now, watch. See how I drag it back, all the way down to his hip."

As she wiped her son's hand across the surface, she used her other hand to push his knee forward. "This is what happens on one side," she repeated. "Over on your side of the table, Judy, you're doing exactly the opposite of what I'm doing. When his left hand comes back and his left leg moves up, his right hand goes forward. The right leg straightens out."

Judy and Jennifer moved Lucas through a couple of cycles while I waited at his head. Thanks to the illustrations in Doman's book, I had the general idea of what I was supposed to do, but felt reluctant to take hold of her son in such a familiar way. Jennifer looked at me.

"You, meanwhile, have to hold his head gently between your palms. Put your fingertips along his jaw line. Now turn his head from side to side, so he's always looking at whichever hand is forward."

More cycles continued as Judy and I clumsily tried to coordinate our movements with Jennifer's. "You think this is tricky?" she said. "We're lucky these are *little* kids! It takes five people to pattern the older ones."

I couldn't imagine doing this with a larger team. "What did you and your husband do about getting a third person to help?" I asked.

"You'll have to recruit volunteers. Get as many as you can. Believe me, doing a home program is no cakewalk! Nobody can handle this alone."

This family's program had not been directed by the Institutes, although it incorporated techniques that had been developed there. Jennifer described another practice called "masking," which had been mentioned in some of the books we read. She showed us a small plastic bag designed to fit over a child's mouth and nose, with an elastic string that went around his head. A straw in the end permitted limited amounts of air to enter, but the level of carbon dioxide accumulated inside the bag while it was being worn. The advantage of repeated short maskings was that the child learned to inhale more deeply, with the long-term result of enhanced oxygen flow to the brain. She told us how to obtain masks of our own.

"Good luck!" she said warmly as we left. "The board is yours. If you want to repay us, just pass it on to somebody else when you've finished.

There's always going to be another brain-injured child who needs help."

The patterning board fit nicely on top of a desk in our living room. We adjusted the height with phone books until we could work over it comfortably. All we needed now was that elusive third pair of hands.

Like our families, our best friends were all on the East Coast. Local friends had drifted out of our lives over the past year. I hated the thought of knocking on doors in our condominium complex, calling strangers away from their dinner tables and TV sets, and asking them for help.

Until we could get started, we tried at least to keep Joseph prone on the floor in his new antiroll device. By now, Judy had come up with a very effective design that used half of a Styrofoam swim ring sewn into a fabric tube across the back of a vest.

He *did not* appreciate being forced to lie on his tummy. His first response, upon discovering he could no longer roll over, was furious indignation. Finding that tears did not change matters, he then typically resorted to sleeping. We, in turn, spread a blanket over him where he lay, and placed a toy just out of reach to motivate some effort whenever he again opened his eyes.

Dear Neighbor,

You may have seen us walking around the neighborhood. We need your help. Our son Joseph is a beautiful boy with blond hair, blue eyes, and a brain injury. Because of the brain injury, he is just starting to crawl at one and half years old. His physical therapy program calls for three people to move his arms, legs, and head in a crawling pattern for five minutes, four times a day. This input trains an undamaged part of his brain. Since we, his parents, are only two people, we need your help. If you have five minutes you could give us once or twice a week, you could help immeasurably in Joseph's development. We can't pay you, but the reward is great.

If you can help us by coming to pattern at our unit (even once), please call.

Patterning is not difficult and it can be fun! Bring your children with you and let them play while you help for five minutes. Don't be shy, please call. That's why we wrote this letter. We need you.

Judy, Steve, and Joseph Gallup

NANCY SEDLMAYER, NAN O'HARA, AND CAROLYN NELSON were the first neighbors to respond to our plea, and the germ of Joseph's growing volunteer corps. They readily accepted our explanation of what was needed. In patterning our child they would be reproducing movements that normal kids make. Hopefully, repetition would awaken dormant instincts and bridge the injury in his brain. That was all the theory most people needed. Newcomers listened as they stood beside the patterning table, stroking his hair gently, blinking back a sympathetic tear, and said, "Just tell me what to do."

Judy predicted (accurately, I feared) that the regimen we had in mind would soon involve "a cast of thousands." So far, we were terribly unprepared for coordinating their efforts. Many times in these early days Nan would call in the morning to ask, "Is your schedule full today? Will you need me?" The fact was that we had not thought ahead far enough even to *have* a schedule. So far, *nobody* was lined up; we merely hoped to find people as we went along.

Everyone remained unreasonably tolerant of our rattled state, even when it resulted in too many helpers showing up at one time.

One neighbor never stepped forward herself or even spoke with us, but did take our letter to her church. It was read from the pulpit, and that afternoon our phone began ringing anew. A retired teacher named Marge became a regular thanks to this publicity, and she brought in her friend Nell. Both of them claimed the role of honorary grandparent.

"I can't get over how lovable little kids are at this age," Nell gloated. "I could just eat 'em up!"

Because Marge and Nell came together, they made a complete team with Judy. This simplified the schedule enormously, especially when they lingered to do extra sessions.

"Now, it's going to *cost* you if we stay over," Marge warned teasingly. Then she and Nell would make good on the threat by fixing coffee for themselves while Judy urged Joseph to practice crawling. They added their encouragement as she coaxed him down his new ten-foot inclined plane.

I had constructed something that resembled the illustration in Doman's book: a smooth plank, about two feet wide, with railings. One end remained on the floor and we propped the other on whatever object would create a slope steep enough to prompt movement.

At first, Joseph hated all this handling. Early patterning sessions were accomplished over a steady roar of deep-throated protests, although this tapered off as he began to make sense of the routine. Patternings always lasted a predictable five minutes and required nothing of him but patience. He soon learned not only to accept the imposition, but to know within five or ten seconds when the time was almost over.

When placed on the inclined plane, he tried to find some way of escape, other than the obvious route before him. He raised himself up on his arms and peered down over the railing. Then he directed a wounded expression at the adults, apparently thinking everyone was being terribly hard-hearted about asking this of him. However, a peeled banana at the bottom of the ramp changed his focus. He kicked his chubby, unused baby legs and moved an inch, and then another.

Joseph was crawling!

THEN JUDY BROUGHT HOME another tale from CCS, where she was continuing to keep the appointments until they kicked us out, just in case standard therapy might still help. She hated to give up on anything.

This time, she'd gotten into a fight with Jan.

"She had him up on a rocking horse and he was crying," she told me. "Maybe what he objects to there is the way they take him from one task to another without any transition. Or maybe he felt insecure, because she was holding him by the hips. He *did* bounce on it for what I thought was a good while. But he was so miserable, so I suggested we stop. But Jan didn't want to. And I said, 'Joseph, do you want *down*?' And he turned toward me and held his arms out! And Jan—." Judy stopped and just breathed for a moment. The memory was stirring up her emotions anew. "Jan put his hands back on the bars and snapped, '*No!*' Well, you should have seen his face. It just turned red, he was so upset. So I said, 'We are stopping now.' And I took him off."

I nodded at Judy with admiration. Joseph could have no better champion than this.

"I put Joseph on his tummy and patted his back to calm him down, and I told Jan we were going to have to come to an understanding. No therapy is worth destroying his trust in me. He'd responded appropriately to my question, which was a big deal, I thought, and it was wrong of her to ignore that."

"My bet is that parents aren't really supposed to get involved in the therapy," I suggested.

"Yeah, but we're involved, aren't we. And that was the *other* part of it. I know Jan was biting her tongue, but things smoothed over and to change the subject I told her he crawls down an incline at home now. She didn't believe it. She got out this big foam wedge and I put him at the top. And he crawled right down, toward some bells at the other end! He did that twice. All the other therapists in the place came over to watch."

We'd been sitting at the kitchen table as she told me this, but now I had to stand and pace around the room. The scenario she described was too exciting. Maybe it was premature to call this a breakthrough, but then maybe not. For the very first time, we had what felt like momentum.

"Jan looked very surprised," Judy went on. "She agreed that he's definitely crawling now. She seemed puzzled. She said, 'It's late. He's sixteen months old. But he has a normal crawl pattern, and he's exploring like a normal child.' I'm so proud of him. What do we credit this to? We started patterning, and now he can crawl. *He wasn't even close to doing this before!*"

7. "THIS LITTLE BOY IS IN PAIN"

Finally the day came for our first appointment with Dr. Frymann. She worked in a cramped, old cottage in La Jolla just a block from the scenic Cove (a setting, I gathered, that she deemed to be more important to the well-being of her little patients than the modern clinic she might have had elsewhere). Her receptionist showed interest in our planned trip to the Institutes, but for a surprising reason.

"Doctor Frymann has *lectured* at the Institutes," she said with great pride. "She knows all about their approach. With her, you may not have to go to Philadelphia after all!"

The first phase of the appointment was an interview in which Judy recounted Joseph's history. Meanwhile, I had to wait with him in a tiny room called the "chapel," surrounded by shelves of worn, old books with titles like *What Would Jesus Do?* and *Love Is the Healer* and *Peace with God*. Scanning them, I felt more removed by the minute from the crisp, businesslike world of modern medicine.

Next, Judy joined me there while the doctor and one of her students examined Joseph for themselves. We could hear his irritated protests and the high-pitched gargling noise to which he resorted when particularly stressed.

Finally we were invited into the examination room to hear the findings.

The doctor began bluntly. "This little boy is in pain," she said. "This little boy has a head that's in *constant* pain. It was subject to tremendous compression, for hour after hour, in the course of being born. It is still compressed. And the first thing that needs to be done about that is to treat him structurally so that he can be more at peace within himself."

She laced her fingers together forcefully to illustrate her point. "There's very, very little movement between the bones of his skull. There is some movement, yes, or he wouldn't be alive at all. But it's very restricted. *That's* why he arches and throws his head back. It's so compressed back here, the only slightest degree of relief is when the head comes back."

"I figured he was doing that to get relief of some sort," Judy said faintly.

"And you'll also notice that his breathing is extremely slight. It's very, very shallow."

"I was just beginning to get an idea about that." Judy interjected. I, meanwhile, merely listened, sensing that this was by far the most important information anyone had yet given us, determined not to miss anything.

"And he cries," the doctor went on, "Which is a way of generating breath. And many times when we have these children who have breathing problems, they will cry until the tears come. Because when you cry, you *have* to take a deep breath. Crying is the only thing he can do to motivate adequate breathing."

I thought back to the times as a baby when he had cried for a moment and then (so I'd thought) listened for someone to come. Maybe he hadn't been listening! Maybe he'd been unable to breathe!

Judy leaned forward in her seat. Doctor," she said earnestly, "Are you saying that his head can be reshaped? And then he won't have all these problems?"

"I am saying that I believe one *cannot* at this point estimate accurately the potential of his development. But once that structural mechanism begins to function more effectively, then—."

Judy was increasingly agitated. Her questions came so rapidly that she was interrupting almost everything the doctor said. "Hasn't his head had time to expand since he was born?" she asked.

"It *can't* expand."

"The chiropractor who worked on his head said that she'd fixed the overlapping—"

"I'm not talking about overlapping. I'm talking about—"

"So it's all locked together? Does this look like it was due to the suction delivery?"

"It wasn't just the suction. It was the whole birth process. How many *hours* was he in that birth canal?"

"Doctor," I finally said, "it seems to me that long labors are fairly common. Does this problem occur very often?"

"Yes," she said. "What percentage of newborn babies do you think have some degree of problem related to birth?"

"I don't know, but how many have the degree that we're looking at here?"

"The degree that we're looking at here is probably 10 to 15 percent."

I felt my jaw drop. Surely *that* many kids weren't in this kind of distress!

"So what caused it was long labor?" Judy went on.

"Yes. And that was *probably* associated with some degree of brain damage, too, you see."

Again I spoke up. "The CAT-scan showed a lack of brain tissue that supposedly dates back before birth."

"That may be," said the doctor. "That may be. But the thing that is accessible, the thing we can do something about, is the body's structure. And the brain will benefit from an improved structural mechanism. Remember that the central nervous system has a tremendous capacity for adaptation. So if he is given the opportunity, at this point in life, *then* one will begin to see the potential for his neurological growth."

"Did the chiropractor help him at all?" Judy was looking very discouraged.

Dr. Frymann had no idea. "I didn't see him before the chiropractor," she said simply. "So I can't evaluate what she did."

Continuing, she said the time had come for us to stop running around aimlessly and to make decisions, the first of which concerned the therapy at CCS.

"Oh, that therapy is traumatic for both of us," said Judy. "And they're planning to discontinue it. The only reason we haven't gone ahead and stopped is we haven't gotten to the Institutes yet, and we don't have anybody else to give us guidelines on child development. Anyway," she added, "we don't have to pay for CCS. It's free."

"And that's about what it's worth, too." This blunt statement stopped us cold. Finally given silence in which she could elaborate, Dr. Frymann added reasonably, "If it isn't answering his needs, then it isn't really worth your while. Is it?"

With that, she dismissed us to talk things over and pick a course of action. The result was that we cancelled CCS, redoubled our efforts with patterning, and signed Joseph up for a series of Dr. Frymann's treatments, which unfortunately could not begin until several weeks off in the future. Our appointment in Philadelphia would occur first. Actually, she questioned the value of our going there at all while Joseph was in such bad shape; she doubted whether he was ready to benefit from a neurological stimulation program. But hopefully the two separate approaches would complement each other.

I looked at Joseph with new compassion. Dr. Frymann had said he probably did not even know what it was like to be comfortable. The poor kid! And all these people, ourselves included, had been so oblivious to his needs. How lonely he must feel! One day as he was sitting in his highchair I said, apropos of nothing that was going on at the moment, "Joseph, you are my son. I love you so much."

For a split-second he looked directly at me with an expression of profound relief and gratitude. As if he'd been worried about that. Then the connection was broken. But we'd had that exchange. I had communicated that much to him.

THE SUMMER HAD BROUGHT a reorganization at my job. I now had a new boss named Terry, a hard-driven athletic guy with a sharp, hungry face. He was new to the company but already had a much better grasp of its politics than I ever would. In getting acquainted with me, he showed some polite interest in my home situation. I still did not feel comfortable talking about it there, but Carolyn, his bubbly secretary, was one of Joseph's new volunteers. She'd probably given Terry more details about it than he wanted—certainly more than I would have.

Terry mentioned that he had a retarded brother. "You know mothers," he said, in an affectionately disparaging tone. "Ours was always convinced that somebody at the hospital dropped him on his head when he was a baby."

"She may be closer to the truth than you think," I suggested. "At least, *something* caused his problem."

"Nah!" He grimaced, already bored with the subject. "Some people are just born that way."

Quite a few people were apparently born that way! Suddenly, it seemed that coworkers all around me had family members with poorly diagnosed disabilities. As word spread, thanks to Carolyn, they stopped me to talk about uncles, brothers, and grown children, each of whom had been a subject of anguish and sacrifice for many years. "If only we'd known about this 'Institutes' place when he was little," they lamented. "If we had done what you're doing, the outcome might have been better."

Word of mouth also led us to yet another household that had implemented a home program. We met a short, energetic woman named Dotte who was investing virtually all her energies into her disabled five-year-old daughter.

The three rooms she rented in a bad part of town contained almost no furniture. Instead, they were cluttered with stacks of large-print reading materials fashioned after the instructions in Glenn Doman's book. An overhead horizontal ladder, similar to what one might find on a public playground, filled the living room. She said her daughter Lizzie spent up to an hour every day brachiating—swinging from one rung to another—to improve her eye-hand coordination and her breathing capacity.

All this activity was directed by advisors at the Institutes, with whom Dotte consulted by phone. Actually traveling there was not possible, given her lack of funds. The father had disappeared from their lives as soon as Lizzie's disability became apparent, leaving them to Welfare and occasional checks from the grandparents.

"When I compare Lizzie today with where she was a year ago, it's worth the effort," Dotte said confidently. "I hear about other things you can do, too. There's a German doctor who comes to this country every year and gives kids injections of fetal brain cells. It's supposed to restart brain growth. It's not legal," she added quickly when she saw my interest. "If you ever do that, *do not* tell your regular doctors about it! There'd be no end of trouble. In case you don't know yet, they will give you *enough* trouble just for doing this." She gestured at the room behind her.

"I've looked at every option anyone has ever mentioned," she continued as she walked us to the door. "My conclusion is that the Institutes is on the leading edge. I can do only one thing for my kid, and I believe this is the right choice."

ABOUT THIS TIME, Judy received a letter from Betty, our former next-door neighbor back in Virginia. She and her husband had had a baby a few months earlier, and Judy had tried to share the excitement with them long-distance. They'd sounded oddly subdued when she called. Finally, when we found time to send a gift, Betty wrote with the real story. Their son David had Down syndrome.

"We won't really know the extent of David's problems for several years," the letter said. "Evidently, his growth and development will be slower than 'normal' until he reaches his potential. There aren't a lot of physical problems, but unfortunately that does not mean his mental will be better. We just don't know."

We just don't know. That line sounded familiar. If the passive dread it carried was wrong in our situation, why not in theirs as well?

Our former neighbors had bought and completely refurbished a rundown old house on a shoestring budget. They'd put in an oversized garden every spring. They gave voice lessons and organized ambitious musical productions at the community theatre. They threw themselves into multiple jobs at the same time, and they thrived and made friends in the process. Just watching their intensity used to make me tired. But if anybody was cut out for running a home therapy program, they were. Judy and I both wrote replies as soon as possible, telling our friends about the Institutes and our hopes for Joseph. We said this might be the answer for David, as well.

THE LAST HURDLE in our preparations for Philadelphia was the required interview with the Institutes family that had been selected for us. Jennifer didn't count, because her efforts had been directed by another organization, one that had learned about patterning second-hand. Dotte didn't qualify, either; although her program looked intensive to us, it was not *the* Intensive Program, for which we had applied.

We couldn't avoid that trip to Mexico. Although the border was only 18 miles away, we'd never had cause to drive across it. In my life I'd walked across maybe three times.

Frankly, we'd been reluctant to go. Until someone called from Philadelphia to say our appointment would be cancelled if we didn't see that family very soon. So we faced up to it. We could dwell on the stereotypes that had Mexico as the point of no return for stolen cars, a semilawless realm where our auto insurance would lapse. Or we could look forward to this rare opportunity to visit with a Mexican family in their home. Either way, Joseph was leading us into new adventures.

We drove east over the mountains, passed through the desert, and crossed the border at Mexicali. Immediately, we had to stop at a traffic light. Kids, who'd been waiting for people just like us to appear, leaped from opposite sides of the car and began cleaning the windshield while another stood at my window to claim payment.

Here was an unexpected dilemma. Giving them money would only encourage their begging. But if I ignored them, I would again be turning the page on third-world poverty, one of the defects of my prior life that I might be atoning for now.

Once past that gauntlet, we proceeded along a thoroughfare that was about three lanes wide but with no markings on the pavement. The traffic pattern varied between two and four lanes. *Well OK*, I told myself. *I can handle this.* For protection, I tailgated a retired school bus with the words "El Viking" painted across the back in slanted letters.

"What are these street signs that say 'Alto'?" Judy wondered, counting on my rudimentary grasp of the language.

"Stop signs. You can tell by the shape and color."

"Well, be sure you stop completely. We sure don't want any mix-ups with the police—Whoa, this is our turn! Turn right here!"

I swerved to the right but cut back immediately at the blast of a horn. I hadn't thought there was room for another vehicle on my right, but one was there. Its occupant gave me a hard look in passing.

"Like I said, can we at least *try* to stay out of trouble?" Judy grouched. She tended to become a bit overbearing when she felt out of her depth.

Soon we were checking house numbers. We found the one we sought on a stucco wall and reversed into a parking place at the curb.

Immediately, a gate in the wall opened and a sturdy man in a khaki shirt strode out to greet us with a powerful handshake.

"Mr. and Mrs. Gallup? Welcome! I am Manuel. This is my wife, Silvia." He indicated the smiling lady who had followed him. "We've been watching for you. Did you have a pleasant trip? And this is little—is it Joseph? He is so beautiful. Hello, Joseph. *Buenos dias*! Does he understand espanish?"

They led us across their courtyard, and past an overhead ladder just like Dotte's. As soon as he was on the floor in their large, dimly-lit parlor, Joseph rolled onto his back. Somehow, Judy and I had forgotten to bring his antiroll device. We grimaced at each other, hating the fact that there was nothing we could do to keep him prone today.

Silvia ushered a thin adolescent girl into the room. She walked with a shuffle and sat next to me on the sofa.

"This is Angie," her mother announced gently.

"*Hola, Angie,*" I ventured, hoping to connect. If exchanges with Joseph still weren't possible, perhaps I'd be able to communicate with *this* disabled child. "*Mí hermana se llama Angie, tambien.*"

The girl smiled, not exactly at me, but didn't speak. Then she noticed Joseph and became more animated. She pointed to him and grabbed her mother's sleeve.

"Yes, I see the baby." Silvia responded. "Angie is thirteen years old," Silvia told us. "She was a normal baby for the first nine months. Then she started having violent seizures. We took her all over Mexico trying to find help. Nothing worked. We didn't learn about the Institutes until four years ago."

Manuel joined us, and together they continued telling Angie's story. They had known that time was running out for her. If they didn't find a solution soon, they probably never would. When they did finally discover the Institutes they were told that different countries were assigned a quota of seats in each incoming class. Of about thirty places in a given class, roughly twenty would go to families from the United States and only one or two to Mexicans. This might have meant a wait of more years before they could begin the treatment that was their last hope. Fortunately, they had a post office box across the border in California, and they applied as Americans.

"We've been on the program for two years now," Silvia told us. "When we started, she was like a wild animal. No one could reach her. Now she helps around the house. She washes dishes. She takes care of herself. And of course she can read."

"She knows all the U.S. Presidents," Manuel said very proudly.

"In a little while we'll show you her intelligence materials."

Their enthusiasm was a bit overwhelming, but I sure liked what we were hearing. Would we do as well? Maybe we could do even better. I'd never thought of Joseph as being like a wild animal. OK, maybe he was, when he lunged in our arms so that we nearly dropped him. But he didn't have seizures. He was much younger than Angie. If they'd gotten this far in two years, surely we could, too.

Two older sisters came in with coffee and a tray of snacks, and they lingered to coo over Joseph. Already, Judy and I felt completely relaxed with these fine people. In opening their door to us they were revealing intimate details of their greatest struggle. And they seemed to be coping with it extraordinarily well. We had only to get comfortable and absorb the information they were now eagerly presenting.

Manuel produced an envelope of photos they'd taken at the Institutes. What a place! The lecture hall looked like the United Nations. The parents in the audience sat behind placards that identified them by name and city of origin. Those who did not understand English wore earphones, which they plugged into their tables, and listened to simultaneous translations.

"Lectures are so important because the parents are the ones who have to do the program," Silvia told us. "The staff will evaluate your child and tell you what he needs. But they want you to understand everything, because you're the ones who have to do it when you get back home."

"And they make *sure* you'll understand," Manuel added. "They are really strict about those lectures. A bell rings, and you have to be in your seats and ready."

"One time I didn't return from the restroom before the bell stopped," Silvia said. "I had to spend the next hour in the translators' room, because they wouldn't let me disrupt the lesson by walking in."

"I'm not sure I like that part," I said. "It sounds awfully regimented."

"It's how they make sure you get your money's worth," Silvia explained. "They go at a fast pace, and nobody is allowed to interrupt."

"They repeat themselves some, too, don't they? I mean, we've read their books, and we've heard a tape series they sold us through the mail, and doggone, I keep hearing some of the same anecdotes. Don't get me wrong. They're *interesting*. But enough is enough. Have you felt that?"

Manuel shrugged expansively. "Sure. Sometimes we have wondered, 'Do they think we are *donkeys*?' But they have a reason for repeating themselves. They believe that what they have to tell you is the truth about what kids need. After all these years, the rest of the world still refuses to understand. You have to *know* it and believe it deep down, or you won't last long enough to succeed."

"You'll receive certificates at the end of the week," Silvia added. "They will want you to understand that you've been given important information."

Manuel crossed the room and returned with their most recent certificates, which he showed proudly. "We got these on our last trip. This says that we are human developmentalists on the Intermediate Level. We have reached the point where we can even diagnose some of a brain-injured child's problems and choose the therapy. After our sixth trip to the Institutes we will be certified at the Advanced Level."

"It's so hard to go back there each time," Silvia continued. "It's so expensive! They know that not everybody can return again and again, and so they try to make us independent of them as soon as possible."

A timer began beeping and she turned her attention to Angie. She placed a long, tubular bag made of stiff, clear plastic over the girl's mouth and nose and held it there while monitoring her watch.

"This is part of her respiratory therapy," she explained. Further progress for Angie hinged on eliminating her seizures and her dependence on anticonvulsant medications. To achieve that milestone, she needed a superior respiratory system. As we watched, her breathing became noticeably deeper, and then deeper still. The bag clouded with condensation, and after another moment Silvia removed it. "We call that 'masking,'" she said. "The people at the Institutes will explain how it works."

"We've already started doing that," Judy bragged, "although we don't have the same kind of mask."

Silvia frowned. "The Institutes won't approve. They like to see the child first, to make sure he can tolerate it. And they want to give you the instructions on how and why it's done."

This warning led into a discussion of the relationship between families and the Institutes staff. "They are very, very strict," Manuel said. "When they give you Joseph's program, they will expect you to do it all, and to do it their way. They know it's hard, but you still have to do it. If you don't, believe me, they'll tell you goodbye."

Well, why *wouldn't* we do it? Judy and I were ready to work hard. We couldn't wait to start.

Hours passed quickly, and before long we were staying for dinner. It so happened that our hosts were planning their next trip to the Institutes in just one week. When we learned that they would take an early-morning flight out of San Diego, we urged them to come the night before and stay over with us. We were glad to simplify their departure somewhat and to save them the expense of leaving their car at the airport.

In a letter, Glenn Doman had predicted that we would establish meaningful ties with other families on program, and that was already proving to be the case. That night Judy and I drove home under the desert's brilliant canopy of stars, wondering why we had dreaded this trip. It seemed that we had been unaccountably slow to embrace several of the ideas coming out of Philadelphia. No more! It had become abundantly clear that the Institutes represented optimism, and an inside track to real answers. On the other hand, every time we went back to standard caregivers, and the families who relied on them, we encountered ugly limitations—and a willingness to settle for that. One course offered growth, the other stagnation. One meant acceptance into a loosely knit society of people determined to win; the other meant subsisting on an inferior footing with respect to the rest of the world, being pitied and avoided.

Shortly before we left for Philadelphia, Joseph developed a scary illness that came on quite suddenly. His temperature soared and he began shivering violently. He gave Judy an indifferent, glassy-eyed stare. What was it now? Seizures? Yet another anxious run to the pediatrician ensued, but this turned out to be nothing more than a routine infection. Afterwards, they were waiting for a prescription in the hospital pharmacy when a young mother carrying a newborn took an adjacent seat.

"You might not want to sit close to us," Judy warned, smiling. "We have germs here!"

This didn't deter the other, who was eager to compare notes on motherhood. She'd come in to pick up a medication that would help her one-month-old sleep at night, she said. She thought it cried too much. Then she asked the question we'd learned to dread. "And how old is your baby?"

Judy began to explain that Joseph was more than eighteen months old, although he looked younger because he was brain-injured. Now that we had found a way out of the problem, she could talk about it easily with anyone. She was almost gushing, in fact, in her relief that this day had brought no more bad news. She'd scarcely begun, however, when the woman abruptly moved to another chair on the far side of the room.

Judy pondered that reaction. *Communicable disease*? No worries. But *brain injury*? Don't taint my space! As things stood, the world at large meant to reject Joseph. If we could alter that fate, by overcoming his handicap, no sacrifice would be too great.

One Saturday I found myself putting in another long day at the office. My employer was bidding for a critically important contract to launch a series of government satellites into orbit. Various engineers came and went with last-minute changes to the content they'd already given me. As the editor in charge of the proposal, I knew I would be among the last to finish.

Terry had other things on his mind, but he asked about progress with Joseph as we walked between buildings. I said efforts were under way and the momentum growing.

"What happens at home when you're here?" he asked.

"When I'm at work, my wife just has to find extra volunteers to replace me."

He stared ahead for a moment, thinking. "Well, do what you've gotta do."

He said no more about it, but from that point on, I somehow found myself able to stay with forty-hour work weeks most of the time. Some of my coworkers received promotions, headed up new subgroups in Terry's ever-expanding department. But I got evenings and weekends to devote to my son.

In fact, I came to see new advantages in my job. With the resources of a graphic arts department at my disposal, I was able to create an eye-catching poster about Joseph's home program. Copies found their way onto bulletin boards at a private college near our home, and still more volunteers began calling.

Even relatives got into the act. Judy happened to have an aunt and uncle in Philadelphia. She hadn't seen them in years, but they heard about us through her mother, and offered us a room in their house. Our lodging there would be free.

We were just bound to succeed.

8. "YOU'VE GOT A FRIEND IN PENNSYLVANIA"

Like wormy apples, travel plans conceal surprises. Our first trip to Philly meant arriving at the airport for an early-morning departure, only to spend the next several hours on the wrong end of the snorkel that led to the aircraft. While we waited, Judy fed Joseph all the milk and food we'd brought for the day's journey and I paced fretfully, glaring through the glass at the idle plane. A mechanic was supposedly flying in from another city to fix a problem with its landing gear.

At length, the agent announced that this plane would not be going anywhere today, and that Northwest had no others. However, American had empty seats on a flight going to DC, if we would settle for that destination.

Washington sounded fine at this point. I made mental adjustments immediately. We could rent a car and drive north from there. No sweat! Where was this other plane?

Well, that was the catch. The other plane was at the airport's other terminal. It was boarding now. And we first had to locate our checked luggage.

There followed a mad sequence in which Judy did her best to keep up while I cradled Joseph against my chest with one arm, clutched the heaviest suitcase with the other, and sprinted as if life itself depended on making that flight. Sure, we might have waited a day and still arrived on time. But I was done with delays. Pent-up frustration powered our transit to the other gate, and in very short order we dropped, gasping for breath, into our newly assigned seats. As San Diego's terra-cotta rooftops dropped away below us, I muttered through clenched teeth, to no one in particular, "Ha! Take *that*! *Nothing's* going to keep us from getting the help we need."

In the years that followed, most of our trips to the Institutes involved misadventures of one sort or another—air sickness, trouble with rental cars, even a robbery at a restaurant where we were dining. We accepted it all as part of the scenery along the way toward Joseph's recovery.

A bit later in life, when Judy and I were reading the works of Bernie Siegel, we encountered his suggestion that it means something when elevator doors open and traffic lights turn green at one's approach, when glances at the ground reveal coins just waiting to be picked up. Small fortuitous events, according to Siegel, are signals from the Universe that one is on the right course. Conversely, obstacles mean some alteration is needed.

While I've always thought that sounded good, it doesn't address the fact that great accomplishments tend to require perseverance and triumph over adversity. Judy and I saw no other way to the goal we all needed to reach. We simply *had* to get there from here.

In our case, perseverance accomplished a lot. And there were pleasant surprises, too. This time, the change enabled us to spend the night with old friends in Maryland and then enjoy a drive up to Philadelphia the next day past autumn foliage of such jaw-dropping beauty that I wondered why I had ever wanted to move out West.

Memories of our former life felt strong here. Although still 100 miles from the terrain I'd hiked in earlier years, this nevertheless felt like home. Even Interstate 95 seemed just a hop away from the hills where I used to inhale the faint scent of wood smoke and scuff my carefree way through dried autumn leaves. Fall had been one of the two seasons that delighted me. The other was spring, with its succession of colors—first the subtle bits of crocus, poking up bravely into the chilly air, then the bands of forsythia hedges, the random bursts of redbud, and finally the four-petaled dogwood blossoms. I used to imagine that, if one looked at the Eastern states from a high enough vantage point, this sequence would take the form of waves of color—yellow, pink, and white—ahead of a darkening tide of green, each slowly moving northward as the season advanced. Then of course in the fall the green would ebb, trailed by a rich froth of red and gold like that now surrounding us.

Not for the first time, I pondered the course our lives might have taken had we not left Virginia three years earlier. Terry and Myriam, those solid-gold friends who'd expressed delight at putting us up without warning, had been *so* much fun to see again! Had Joseph been born here, would he have been spared whatever it was that hurt him?

As we neared the end of the trip, Judy and I noticed that the cars around us bore blue license plates that promised YOU'VE GOT A FRIEND IN PENNSYLVANIA. We grinned at each other. Driving across the bridge into Philadelphia, I flung back my head and impulsively sang a verse from the old rock opera *Tommy*, by The Who.

There's a man I've found could bring us all joy!
There's a doctor I've found can cure the boy!
There's a man I've found could remove this sorrow,
He lives in this town, let's see him tomorrow.

"We *will* see him tomorrow!" Judy reminded me happily.

Her Aunt Julie and Uncle Jim welcomed us graciously into their home and installed us in a spare bedroom. Until that point, Joseph had been an excellent little traveler. But then he had one of his bad nights. He thrashed about in his little bed and screamed for hours, in spite of every strategy Judy and I devised to calm him. Familiar tapes that we'd brought from home, our own soft singing, even resolutely ignoring him—nothing worked. Occasionally, the volume of his complaints tapered off, and we'd start to breathe more easily. Judy's cousin Rob resumed the snoring that came faintly through the wall. Then Joseph would startle at some invisible irritant and come fully awake, howling with renewed fury. Rob's snoring stopped again, and I buried my face in the pillow in exasperation.

To simplify the equation, so it involved only Joseph and me, I finally carried him downstairs through the dark house, to a family room that was as far as possible from everyone's sleeping quarters. There I reclined on a sofa, holding my squirming little boy, and tried to will both of us to relax. Eventually we did, and that's where we slept.

The next morning Julie and Jim insisted that the night's turmoil had not disturbed them. "Heavens," Julie laughed. "We raised five kids in this house. Don't you think we've gotten used to babies by now?"

Rob was not available for his impressions. I imagined he was catching up on his Zs.

"I thought it was pretty bad," I ventured.

"Listen, with you stop that? It was nothing." Julie was moving ahead with her first item of the day, getting us launched. Her plan was to ride to the Institutes with us to make absolutely sure we didn't lose our way, with Jim following in their car to pick her up again. To me, this arrangement seemed too much of an imposition on them, but she refused to discuss it. This last leg of the journey turned out to be very short and easy.

We arrived at the Institutes promptly at nine o'clock, as they'd admonished us to do. The first thing we saw was a formidable stone wall enclosing the grounds, with very mature evergreen trees overhanging a drive. I turned into the entrance and stopped while Julie stepped out of the car and wished us luck. Then we continued into a circular parking area in front of a three-storied mansion with several gables along the front, a steep slate roof, and ivy-covered walls. I turned off the motor. This was it! The Institutes for the Achievement of Human Potential, a place defined almost as much by the contempt of its detractors as by the inventiveness and hard-headed optimism of its founders, by its professional isolation as by its reach. Every week of the year, families like ours converged on this little fortress.

Inside the door, a lady with dark hair pulled severely back stepped forward, hugging a clipboard. "Welcome to the Institutes," she said formally. "I'm Janet Caputo."

"*Cara's* mother?" Judy gushed. She was referring to a student in the Institutes' International School, a model of accelerated development who got star billing in their brochures.

"Why, yes, I am. I see my little girl's fame has preceded me. This way, please."

She led us to a large, oval dining room. "Would you like a cup of coffee? No? Well, a staff member with be with you very shortly." She handed Judy a blue loose-leaf binder with plenty of sheets of blank notepaper, and photocopied information. Then she excused herself and returned to the front of the building.

I sat, holding Joseph on my lap, and looked at an ornate marble fireplace. Above it hung an oil portrait identified as A. Vinton Clarke, the benefactor who, we'd read, had made it possible for Glenn Doman to acquire this property in the 1950s.

We examined the papers Janet had just given us. One typed alphabetical list was headed INITIAL EVALUATION WEEK, NOV 3, 1986 – FORTE 19. Joseph's name appeared halfway down the first page, with our names and address to the right. Also listed were families from Spain, Canada, Guatemala, Italy, Mexico, and Germany. There was a family with a mile-long name from India. And of course, others represented all parts of the U.S.—Florida, New York, Wyoming, Kentucky.

One of those other families arrived: a bearded guy easily three times the size of his wife, and a boy about five years old who could walk but obviously needed some kind of help. We nodded shyly and they took the next table. I watched surreptitiously as the youngster blundered nervously around the room.

A younger lady appeared at our table. She wore a black blazer and had long, wavy hair. "Hi!" she said brightly. "I'm Rosalind Doman. If you'll come this way, please, I'd like to take Joseph's history." She led us toward a door at the back of the room. "You might want to button up your coats again because we'll be walking to another building."

A flagstone walkway led down a grassy hillside to a newer, white structure, whose angular lines contrasted starkly with the stone edifice behind us. This, we later learned, was the Veras Building, often called the Clinic by staff members. It consisted mainly of a large open room with a high ceiling and several offices arranged in tiers along two outside walls. Rosalind took us into one of these offices and invited us to sit. The wall behind her desk was all glass, and looked out onto a wonderland of autumn color.

She opened a folder that was already bulging with Joseph's medical records and our correspondence. "Now then. This is Joseph." She looked at him carefully for a moment. Hoping to make the right first impression, Judy was already zipping him into his vest with the Styrofoam swim ring. He lay prone on the floor. His arms were stretched out straight in front of him, and he was playing with the fringe on a throw rug.

"That's a very ingenious antiroll device," Rosalind observed. "Did you make it, Mrs. Gallup?"

"Yes. I tried another design first, but that didn't work very well. This was the best thing I could come up with."

"Well, it looks just perfect. As long as it keeps Joseph from rolling onto his back, it does everything it's supposed to do."

"Sometimes I tell Judy that she should have been an engineer," I said.

Rosalind smiled. "Our home programs have a way of bringing out a lot of latent talent in the parents." She watched Joseph for another moment. "Joseph, you say, is now twenty months old."

"That's right."

"And he doesn't yet creep."

"No, although he has gotten up on his hands and knees a couple of times in the last week or so. And he started crawling on his tummy last month. We've been patterning him four times a day for six weeks now."

"That's terrific." She made a notation on a sheet in front of her. She watched Joseph a moment longer, and jotted down something else.

"Now, I'm going to ask you both a lot of questions, first about your pregnancy, Mrs. Gallup, then about the delivery, and finally about Joseph's history up to the present time. This usually takes about an hour, but we'll spend as much time as we need. I want you to be as complete and as accurate in your answers as possible."

And we were off. We covered everything, starting with the earliest days of Judy's pregnancy and continuing through every medical evaluation, every mishap, and every crackpot suggestion we'd heard along the way. Rosalind took copious notes and clucked sympathetically. She probed for more details whenever we skipped the smallest episode in Joseph's story, but for the most part she just let us talk.

"You may know the osteopath we finally settled on for his medical care," I said. "We're told that she has been here."

Rosalind thought for a moment, then brightened. "Oh, yes. I do remember. Dr. Frymann lectured to the staff on the terrible things that can happen to a baby's skull during childbirth. I happened to be pregnant at the time, and it made me pretty nervous."

Judy yelled, "Steve! Will you look at Joseph!"

I turned in my seat to find our little boy up on his hands and knees—and moving! He came forward about ten feet before settling back onto his stomach to think about it.

"This is the first time we've seen him do *that*!" Judy exclaimed.

Rosalind's eyes sparkled happily. "Well, we're getting off to a great start."

Finally, Rosalind closed the folder and sat back in her chair. "You've been very helpful. We're always glad to get folks who have kept such good records." She handed more papers across the desk. "This is a list of all the people you'll be seeing here today. The Chairman wants to meet with you for a few minutes. Then we'll do a neurological evaluation. Let me see," she referred to the sheet again before handing it to Judy. "Susan Aisen wants to see you at three o'clock. She represents our Institute for Intellectual Excellence. We need to squeeze in a physical exam with Dr. Sosin. Ann Ball is scheduled to talk with you in general terms about brain injury. Then my husband Doug will discuss the very special relationship that the Institutes has with families who are on program. And finally, Gretchen Kerr, our director, will present our functional diagnosis of Joseph, based on today's observations."

She escorted us back to the large, open area we'd crossed earlier. It was now filling up with newly arrived families, who were mostly sitting on benches around the perimeter of the room. The voices of their children echoed off the distant ceiling. "Just put your stuff inside one of these benches," Rosalind said, showing us how to raise the cushioned seats. "And make yourselves comfortable!"

For a moment we were left to ourselves. I shuffled through the papers we were accumulating and pondered the lecture schedule for Wednesday and Thursday. I saw topics like "Who Is Brain-Injured?" "Range of Brain Injury," "Physiology vs. Pathology," "How the Brain Grows." Lectures were scheduled for *twelve hours* each day, with ten-minute breaks every hour and two half-hour breaks for meals.

Meanwhile, Judy was looking at the other families with a stricken expression, as many had children far more seriously hurt than Joseph. One very little girl writhed constantly on her back, emitting faint mewing sounds. She gave every indication of being in agony. A teenage girl wandered aimlessly about the room, sweeping her hands through the air and grinning into space as if she saw wondrous things invisible to the rest of us.

An Asian lady in a green blazer approached and shook our hands. "I'm Elaine Lee. If you've finished giving Joseph's history, the Chairman is ready to see you in his study."

"Sure!"

"It's in the other building. Just leave your things here, and I'll show you the way."

Judy hastily zipped Joseph out of his antiroll device in order to put on his jacket, and, right on cue, he began screaming. "Come on honey," she pleaded. "We're going to see Glenn Doman!"

The volume increased even more, and continued as we returned to

Clarke Hall, passed through the dining room, and entered a pleasant old-fashioned parlor.

"Once this kid gets going, he's hard to stop," I said miserably. "I don't know if Mr. Doman wants to try and talk over this commotion or not."

Elaine looked at him thoughtfully. "Maybe not. If it's OK with you, I'll just borrow the little guy from you for a while, so you can talk in peace. But Glenn *will* want to see him, at least." She led us through two intervening rooms and to the door of Glenn Doman's study. Inside, we found him seated at a desk.

Elaine announced us very formally. "Glenn Doman, I'd like to present Mr. and Mrs. Gallup, from San Diego." He smiled genially and stood to shake our hands. The chairman of the Institutes looked like his pictures: beige three-piece suit, a beard that was nearly white, glasses with heavy plastic frames. Although shorter and stockier than I'd anticipated, he wore a tangible aura of command. I remembered reading that this man had been an Army officer in the Second World War. Dr. Frymann had warned us that he still thought of himself as being at war. This time, we were his soldiers.

Elaine explained that she would keep Joseph, who had not stopped howling for even a moment during this exchange. Our boy's eyes were beaded with tears, and his expression said plainly that he was more than fed up with everything he could see. Glenn smiled. "Yes, Joseph. I understand. You're not very happy today, are you? Well, we're going to get you fixed up anyway." Then he turned his attention on us, and suddenly we were alone together. Judy and I found ourselves perched on a sofa, and Glenn took a chair opposite us for what he termed "a little chat."

He began by acknowledging the significant effort we had made in getting to Philadelphia. "But if you think *you're* a long way from home, we get people from behind the Iron Curtain—people who have to wait *years* for permission to leave their countries. We had a family from a remote area of Indonesia. The first part of their journey here was downriver, in a boat. It took them the first day just to reach an airport.

Parents from all over the world beg, borrow, and steal in order to get here, simply because they think their kids are worth it. We tend to agree with them."

He focused on me then and spoke slowly, with emphasis. "Mr. Gallup, I want to promise you—In fact, I give you my word—that we at the Institutes will do everything in our power to make sure your son is one of the *answers* to the world's problems, and not another of its problems."

This was the most wonderful, powerful sentence I had heard from anyone since Joseph's birth. I caught my breath in an audible sob of relief. To my left, Judy glanced at me in concern. I think she often worried that I was about to crack.

"Naturally, you want very badly to see him succeed," Glenn continued. "You wouldn't have come this far if you didn't want very badly to see him succeed. His success is in your best interests.

"Well, you have some company. Now it's in our best interests, too. But may I suggest, Mr. Gallup, that it is also in the best interests of everyone in the state of California. Furthermore, to a certain extent, I believe that it is in the best interests of everyone in the United States— and indeed, the world—that Joseph succeed. Everyone stands to gain if he does, and to lose if he doesn't."

He then turned to Judy and made another promise, just to her. I wish I could say what it was. Perhaps he was offering assurance that the staff would respect and value her son's unique qualities. But for the moment I couldn't process anything further. Had there been a coherent thought it my mind, it would have been gratitude to God that we'd found a place that understood and believed in our dream. Like that time outside the restaurant, when the news sank in that our newborn baby had a problem, for a few beats I missed whatever was happening around me.

Glenn cocked his head and looked at me inquiringly until we had eye contact again. He seemed to relax a little. Although he was doing all the talking, perhaps he had also been making an assessment of our attitude. "Our days are long here," he said. "It's not uncommon for us to still be seeing families well after midnight. If the long hours are hard on you, well, we're sorry about that, but"—again he smiled—"unlike the rest of the world we haven't learned how to solve everyone's problems in an eight-hour day.

"So my advice to you is to relax and enjoy yourselves while you're here. All too often, families are tense when they first arrive at the Institutes, and they don't start to unwind until the end of the week. Don't let that happen. Talk to the other families. Talk to the staff. And take it easy. Rest while you can.

"Before long," and here his eyes twinkled, "we'll be asking you to work very, very, very hard."

Judy started to say something, but Glenn continued. "This booklet I'm giving you explains the advocate system that we follow here. As you may know by now, every kid on program with us has his own staff member who knows that kid and his family intimately. All of us want to get to know you, but your advocate will be your special friend and mentor. We find this arrangement works to everyone's advantage. This way, when you call, nobody has to run down to the basement to look for your kid's chart."

He explained that the advocate described in the booklet would study Joseph's case and get in touch with us during the week. He stood. The interview was over, although we were suddenly boiling with questions, particularly about this advocate. Silvia had emphasized that rapport with one's advocate was vitally important to success. She'd said some staff members made far better advocates than others. But did we have any say in the selection? What if we didn't get along? Who—? "Have a great week!" Glenn repeated, shaking our hands warmly and ushering us out through a side door.

Our round of initial meetings with staff members continued until late that evening when we met Gretchen Kerr, a tall, lean woman with steel-gray hair and a tired smile. Judy and I were worn down as well by that point, having hurried from one office to another almost nonstop all day. All the fight was out of Joseph, who now slept in our laps. Gretchen said, "With the information you've been given, you probably have an idea of what we're going to say about the nature of Joseph's injury."

"Then he *is* brain-injured?" Judy asked.

"He is indeed brain-injured. You've come to the right place."

Confirmation that a child has a brain injury may hardly seem like good news. Still, as Judy and I saw it, knowing that the problem had been identified, by people with a solution, meant that from this point he could only improve.

As in our dealings with physicians back home, I matched Gretchen's studious tone. We were going to be partners in resolving this. "Presumably, the damage is in more than one part of the brain," I said carefully. "Because he has many problems. 'Multiply handicapped' is what they call it back in San Diego."

Gretchen nodded. "Joseph has a moderate, diffuse, bilateral mid-brain injury. 'Diffuse' because, as you say, more than one function is affected. 'Moderate' because he's performing at more than fifty percent of his chronological age." She showed us a chart giving his neurological age as 11.3 months, versus his chronological age of 20 months.

We hunkered over the paper for a few minutes. "They figure the neurological age based on what he can do," Judy told me.

"Right," I said, catching on. "And according to this, if he weren't crawling yet his neurological age—at least in mobility—would have been only five months. And that would have been *less than* fifty percent."

"He started crawling because we started patterning him!"

"So if we hadn't already been patterning him, Joseph's injury would now be classified as severe, instead of moderate!" I glanced up at Gretchen, who seemed to enjoy our enthusiasm.

"Can you say what caused this injury in the first place?" I asked.

"The immediate cause of any brain injury is lack of oxygen to the brain. But as to what brought that condition about, it's often hard to say. In Joseph's case, it may have been the toxemia you say Judy experienced during the last two weeks of her pregnancy. It may have been birth trauma. It may have been something else. Anything is possible. We'll probably never know."

"But what about the abnormal CAT-scan? The doctors said that was a condition that developed over a longer period of time during the pregnancy."

"You're referring to the small temporal lobes. These are a cortical structure. The problems you've observed so far are due to injury in the *mid*brain, a much lower area, developmentally. Joseph is a classic example of a midbrain-injured kid. He is relatively competent on the sensory side—almost up to his age level in some areas, but on the output side he isn't doing so well. Mobility and manual competence are his weakest areas. Now it may be that once we progress past the midbrain injury there will be cortical problems, too. But I wouldn't be alarmed about that now. For one thing it's too early in his development to see any clear manifestation of a cortical injury. For another, the program we'll give you will address the cortex as well as the midbrain."

WE HAD SCARCELY UNPACKED our belongings into our bench the next morning when a handsome blonde lady called us into her office.

"I'm Phyllis Kimmel," she said, unfolding the document that Gretchen had showed us the night before. "I just want to go over Joseph's Developmental Profile with you." We looked again at the chart that would track his progress over the coming years. There were six columns, divided by seven color-coded rows. Phyllis reviewed this with us now. "Joseph has been evaluated in each of the six pathways that we see as being vitally important in human development. These functions are all fully developed in the average six-year-old. The Profile measures seven giant steps under each function. You can see for example that language culminates in speech with complete vocabulary and proper sentence structure. Manual competence culminates in writing, using a dominant hand. And so forth. All kids are somewhere on this scale, no matter how badly they're hurt. The sequence of developmental events is the same. The timetable is what varies.

"We use the Profile to see what levels have been attained, and this blue line drawn across each column shows where Joseph is right now. "We'll update his Profile on each of your revisits and show his new status with a red line. The degree of success will be the difference between this blue line and the red one.

"We also use the Profile to diagnose the area of injury and to define the treatment needed. Glenn will have a lot to tell you about that in the lectures. The rest of us will be here with the kids." She smiled and gestured at her neat attire, beige blazer and skirt. "When you drop Joseph off in the morning, you'll find us wearing entirely different clothes, because we spend the day right down there on the floor with the kids. We work with them and get to know them."

Elaine had us next. In ten minutes she measured Joseph in just about every way imaginable: his weight (25 3/4 pounds), height (80.3 centimeters), head circumference and diameter (side to side and front to back), and chest circumference and depth. Watching her handling him, I was impressed with two things. This woman certainly knew her way around a kid, and she cared about him, too. She handled Joseph with the utmost respect and tenderness. He may have noticed, too, because for once he didn't protest all the manipulation.

9. A STROLL ACROSS THE ROOM

The prospect of two full days of lectures may have worried some of the parents. However, nothing, short of a breakthrough for Joseph, could have pleased me more.

Now, answers we had been pursuing, yearning for, would be presented to us. In a sense, this was the medical education I'd missed the first time around. It was a second chance—and not just for Joseph to become a normal little boy. It was also another chance for me! No, I had no illusion about becoming a doctor at this late date. But now I would be preparing myself for a challenge that felt every bit as formidable as medical school.

As a young applicant, I'd wondered, like a soldier yet to see combat, whether I would be equal to the relentless demands of medical school, the information to be mastered, the sleep deprivation, the critical decisions, the stress. That question remained unanswered. But this time we were going to see what I could do. And what Judy could do, too, of course.

So my spirits were high as we drove back to the Institutes through an early-morning drizzle. Our first order of business there was to check Joseph in with the staff members who would be caring for him all day. We joined a crowd of families entering the Veras Building through its dimly lit back entrance and inched our way to the top of a staircase, where we handed Joseph and his belongings across a table.

When they saw what was happening, some of the kids panicked. One Italian boy in particular cried piteously after his parents as they retreated miserably back down the stairs. Judy and I smiled sympathetically, thinking how doubly hard all this must be on the foreign families. Even the adults were struggling with language issues and all the subtle details that can make another country seem so alien. But their kids quite likely had no idea of why they'd been brought here, or what was coming next.

Separation anxiety wasn't among Joseph's problems, and he didn't object to being taken from us. Feeling strangely empty-handed, Judy and I stepped back outside into the light rain to walk the short distance to the auditorium.

"*That* was a rocky experience!"

We turned to see a couple following us out of the building. Both were tall and long-limbed, like professional tennis players. The man who'd spoken shook his head and tapped a fist on his chest ruefully. "Our rascal was one of the screamers in there."

"Don't feel self-conscious about it. Ours exceeded his crying quota for the whole week, on the first day!"

We recognized the auditorium from Silvia and Manuel's photographs. For each of the fifty-four parents in our group, a white placard was affixed to the front of a table, giving the name and hometown.

Judy and I descended to the very front row, where we finally located our seats. I started to shed my coat but noticed a distinct breeze coming from a vent and decided to keep in on.

A four-toned bell sounded over the PA system, similar to that used in opera houses to summon audiences to their seats after intermission. The rustle of people behind and around us died away abruptly. Glenn Doman had entered from a side door, and before the bell stopped he was standing at the front of the room, hands in pockets, aiming a smile of genuine pleasure at us all.

He began with a short apology for the temperature of the room. "People come here from all over the world every week of the year, having sacrificed a great deal to do so. This room has twice as much air conditioning as is normal for a room this size. Even when it's below zero outside, we are paying money—very hard-to-come-by money, I might add—uh, to cool the room! The room is cold because we have always known that intelligence is operating better in cold than in heat. It's cold here for *you*. My wife Katie tells me that every time I give one of these lectures, my feet are cold for three days. And I often get the sniffles. That doesn't seem important to me, compared to you understanding the precious things we want to tell you about your children. How much each of you knows as a result of this is directly related to your child's chances for success. You are the ones who will implement his program. We want to help you, but in the end what happens is up to *you*."

Then the first lecture began.

"We at the Institutes are in complete disagreement with almost all other professionals regarding the diagnosis, treatment, and objectives of brain-injured children." He recited the list of terms, like autism and cerebral palsy, that made up the lengthy subtitle of his book. "All these labels just add to the confusion surrounding the issue," he said. "Only one is meaningful, just as there's only one condition, and that's 'brain injury.' The other terms refer to symptoms, at best, and are not medically sound diagnoses, any more than fever or sore throat would be a diagnosis for someone who had flu."

With this first point established, he proceeded to define brain injury, proceeding slowly and carefully. "A very large number of events can cause brain injury," he concluded. "But all of them have in common the effect of preventing a sufficient flow of oxygen to the brain. Once the injury has occurred, it will be manifested in a variety of ways, depending on the degree and location of injury."

The bells chimed again, signaling a break. It was hard to believe, but an hour had already passed. Glenn stopped speaking abruptly and signaled for us to leave. When we reassembled ten minutes later he launched into the next phase of his presentation, Range of Brain Injury. Nothing I had heard on the topic had ever made so much sense, or given me so much hope.

"I would like to propose to you a spectrum of conditions," he said, strolling to the far left-hand side of the room. Once there, he turned to face us. "Let's pretend we have an eight-year-old child here who has just died." He took a sideways step and looked at us again. "And let's say that here we have another eight-year-old who happens to be in a profound coma. Now, if you had both of them side by side, I submit to you that it would be difficult to say immediately which one was alive and which was not. We have two children, in two fundamentally different conditions, but they look similar."

He then took another sideways step, moving toward the center of the room. "Likewise, if you put the kid who is in the profound coma next to one in a *moderate* coma, you would find that these two also had a great deal in common."

I could see where he was going. During the break, a large display had been unveiled on the wall behind him. Like Joseph's Developmental Profile, it was a vertical scale, with each gradation represented by a different color. At the bottom was DEATH — NO NEUROLOGICAL ORGANIZATION. Above that were a series of conditions of diminishing pathological intensity, all bracketing alongside the term NEURO-LOGICAL DYSFUNCTION. Several more conditions appeared above these, labeled POOR NEUROLOGICAL ORGANIZATION. At the top of the chart was COMPLETE NEUROLOGICAL ORGANIZA-TION.

Glenn continued to take new positions, moving across the room to illustrate the same progression. "Higher on the scale are those who are able to make sounds but unable to walk or talk, and then those whom the school system calls 'trainable mentally retarded' kids."

By now he was near the center of the room. He glanced back over the ground he had covered. "Here at the Institutes we see kids who make the whole trip. Because these are *not* separate and unrelated conditions. How could they be? *How could they be?*" The idea clearly irritated him.

He was talking to us, but I guessed that he was really addressing all the absent professionals who stubbornly insisted on applying different diagnoses depending on degree of severity.

But Glenn had more ground to cover. He stepped to the right again. "Somewhere along the way across this spectrum, you start to find kids who are not demonstrably brain-injured. Any problems they have are seen as discipline problems or learning problems. The rest of the world doesn't even look for a neurological explanation."

He paused and gave the audience a steady look. "Incidentally, *total wellness* is the only sensible objective for kids at all levels."

He was getting no argument from us.

"OK. Let's talk about wellness," he continued. "Still higher on this scale is the 'average' kid—the one who gets passing grades in school." Glenn's tone of voice made it clear that he did not view average as a satisfactory state. "Then there's the 'above-average' kid—who may still have a reading problem, by the way, in spite of his high IQ. The 'superior' kid is excellent, both physically and intellectually. These two, physical and intellectual excellence, often occur together, it turns out. And finally, at the top of the scale is the ideal kid. What is ideal? Who can say? Frankly, *I* don't believe we have even come close to where we ought to be."

Sitting at the front, Judy and I missed whatever went on among other people in the audience, but I sensed a stirring behind me at this point, as if people were becoming excited. Ah, if only the progression Glenn had just described were as simple as a stroll across the room! He hadn't suggested that it *was*, of course—only that such a progression was possible. The idea certainly had appeal. Proving it would be the best possible use of my time and energy.

Now he was summing up. "The function of the brain is to relate its owner to the environment. The degree to which a brain does that is a function of its neurological organization." He returned to his original position in the center of the room to conclude. "The principles involved in moving up the scale to increased organization are pretty much the same, regardless of where you happen to be. Where you stop along the way is up to you."

Amazingly, another hour had gone by. The bells chimed again, and we left for ten minutes to restore our circulation.

Lectures continued throughout the day, combining theory, inspiration, and occasional doses of humor.

If it were possible to send men to the Moon and bring them safely home again, then it was certainly possible to move a brain-injured child up the spectrum toward wellness. "Of course," Glenn allowed, "there were people who predicted quite confidently that we'd never get to the Moon. And when we did, some tried to say that footage of Neil Armstrong was actually filmed at some desolate location here on Earth, such as, oh, maybe downtown Hoboken."

There were loud guffaws. "No, you'll hear that kind of talk," he warned. "People will try to take your victories away from you. Because they won't accept the fact that they were wrong."

Glancing back, I saw the Italian mother of the little girl who could only writhe and make mewing sounds. She sat with headphones clamped on her head to absorb the translation. Humor did not register with that lady. She stared at Glenn fixedly. Her expression said *I'll be impressed when my daughter improves.*

I was willing to be impressed now. He said, "You can spend your time lamenting those dead brain cells. Or you can be strong enough and determined enough to get busy on the *billions* of cells that your kid has left."

He said we should think of brain injury as a physical barrier separating our child from the rest of the world. The person behind that barrier had boundless intelligence and potential, simply because that was his makeup as a human being. Failure to reach him therefore implied a greater tragedy than one could guess.

"In a comatose patient the barrier is complete," Glenn said. "But it can still be penetrated. The proper treatment for arousal from coma is to use *every* road into the patient's brain. We use bright lights, and loud noises, and rough textures and strong odors, and even pungent tastes, to send the message: 'Come back! Come back! Come back! Come back!'" Glenn advanced almost into my lap and shouted to drive his point home. "'We're *not* going to let you give up on life. *COME! BACK!*'"

The moment had become pretty intense. I shrank into my seat. People around me were crying. He retreated and lowered his voice dramatically.

"By contrast, one of the best ways to destroy someone—even someone who's very healthy—is by sensory deprivation." He suggested that the traditional response to a comatose patient, a quiet, dimly lit hospital room, had more in common with sensory deprivation than with any form of arousal.

"Looking at the spectrum we've talked about," he continued. "The biggest difference you see, going from profound coma to the ideal, is in the degree of consciousness. Ask any schoolteacher to describe her brightest pupils and she'll probably use words like 'alert' and 'aware.' Ask her about the ones who are least bright, and she'll tell you that, somehow, things just don't seem to get through to them. She knows that she's sending out the same message to all the kids in her class. The trouble is that what reaches one brain is different from what reaches the others.

"Well, our purpose with your kids is to make sure more of the message arrives."

WE HAD BEEN WARNED that our last day of the week would be a long one. Before it was over, each family needed to have one-on-one discussions with several different staff members.

It was no surprise to find that we had to begin by waiting. We chatted with Paul and Laura, the couple I'd pegged as tennis players (actually, it turned out that both were airline flight attendants), and Judy got into a long conversation with a mother who, like her, was a former special-education teacher. Several parents were surprised to hear that we were already patterning at home. They asked about the appeal for help that we had mailed to our neighbors. We had a copy, which we passed around, and they took notes. Eventually, we went to the dining room for lunch, still without having seen any staff members. Where was our advocate, anyway?

We ate with a family who held a little red-haired baby. Rather, we thought he was a baby. They said he was almost five years old.

The parents explained that they had won a strenuously contested malpractice suit against the hospital where he'd been born. But thus far mere cash, even lots of it, had done little for their struggle to help him.

"One of the clinics in our town has a library of books about disabilities," the mother told us. "I kept going there, trying to learn something that would help Joshua. "Most of it wasn't worth much. Then one day I found Glenn Doman's book, *What to Do About Your Brain-Injured Child*. And you know what? They wouldn't let me check it out! They actually refused! They said the author was all wrong and I'd be wasting my time."

"So what'd you do?"

"Well, I carried it back to the shelf where I'd found it. And I opened it up and skimmed a few paragraphs. And, you know, it just sounded like it made so much *sense*! So—nobody was looking—." She grinned sheepishly. "I just put it under my sweater and took it home."

Judy and I laughed.

The father chuckled. "We brought the book with us, and on Monday we asked Glenn to autograph it. He thought that was amusing, signing a stolen book!"

"A *rescued* book," I suggested.

The young man who'd been assigned as our advocate never made an appearance. Instead, a lean, no-nonsense woman named Lidwina van Dÿk called us into her office to discuss the physical portion of Joseph's new program, and during the meeting she apparently decided that *she* would claim us instead.

Lidwina began by opening Joseph's file and producing two copies of a printed form on buff-colored paper. "This is what we call a Program Sheet," she said, handing one to us. "On it, each staff member who sees you will be writing down goals and programs for Joseph. These are the objectives that we see for him right now, in order of priority. OK?"

"Sure."

"Joseph's Number One objective is Physical Growth Toward Excellence." As she spoke, she wrote this on her copy of the program sheet, and following her lead, Judy did likewise on ours. "By this," Lidwina continued, "we mean to take him from where he is right now to the next phase in the mobility pathway. The Number One means of achieving that is the Floor Program." She and Judy wrote this as well on their respective copies.

"Now, even though we've said here it's *physical* growth, creeping will address every single problem that he has. Creeping is a treatment for the midbrain, and that's where a big chunk of his problems are. Also, it's creeping that will dramatically affect the intelligence and the neurological age. What we're after, and what you have to be very clear about, is that the objective has to be *total wellness*, and not just mobility. Because otherwise we can get sidetracked into looking at things too narrowly."

Lidwina unfolded Joseph's Profile and turned it around so that we could see it. She pointed to the Functional rating he had been given on visual convergence. "I think you will start to see a lot of change in his vision as a result of creeping. If you watch Joseph lying on the floor on his back—." She demonstrated his way of turning his head back and forth. Judy and I winced. "He does that to stimulate his vision. And he also gets quite keyed into making sounds." She tapped the auditory column of his Profile. "All this stuff is purely random stimulation. It becomes a bad habit. Creeping has a major effect on changing that."

Judy said, "So we could expect that the more he creeps, the more that self-stimulation—the noises and the head shaking—will die out?"

"Yes. He won't have that far-out visual look, and the random noises should be less. Also, with language, the role of creeping is to get words.

Then to get words relating to one another. We can expect couplets, and then for him to draw ideas together. Just through treating the mid-brain, all these pathways will clear up."

Judy and I grinned at each other. If creeping was what it took to achieve that end, we would make sure Joseph crept.

Lidwina gave us a printed sheet headed THE FLOOR AS A WAY OF LIFE and asked Judy to read aloud "The Philosophy of the Floor."

1. Every moment your child spends in the prone position with the opportunity for movement, he is having the best opportunity to become well.
2. Every moment your child is sitting, or lying on his back or rolling over, he is wasting precious moments of his life.

Then she dictated the details of our Initial Floor Program. "First, Joseph must be on the floor all day and all night. He will *sleep* on the floor. Visitors must observe this law. They can give him loving and hugging, but only as a reward after he has crept. Secondly, Joseph must not lie on his back. Furthermore, he may not sit in the 'W' position." She walked around her desk and demonstrated what she meant. It was an awkward-looking posture in which she sat back on her legs with the ankles spread out to either side. "The 'W' position is totally out, and Joseph is to have an anti-sit device to prevent him from ever getting into it." She found an example for us. It was a big, pillow-shaped canvas bag with a zipper across one face. It made a rattling sound. One end was closed with Velcro, and she pulled it open. "There are aluminum cans in here, squashed up. It's *not* a comfort pack, not something he'll want to sit on. It attaches to the seat of his pants with this zipper. So, obviously, you'll have to add zippers to his clothes."

Returning to her desk, she gave Judy a pattern for making our own anti-sit pack. "Mum and Dad are responsible for making this work," she said. "Mum and Dad must become experts at creating a need for Joseph to creep. Remember that Joseph *must* succeed! Create a reward system that is based totally around the creeping he does. For example, when Joseph creeps six meters he gets to be tossed up in the air. When he creeps seven meters, he gets to be tossed in the air *and* to hear his favorite song. Later, when he gets to where he's just a solid creeper, then we follow the same kind of system but work it toward time. For example, if he usually creeps twenty meters in so many minutes, he gets a bigger reward for going faster than that. Because our objective is *distance*.

"Also, you must record daily progress. You'll find we're sticklers for records. This is, first of all, for Mum and Dad. You need to know at the end of the day where he stands, relative to where he needs to be. If he's behind schedule, you need to know that so you can make it up on the next day.

"The ultimate objective," Lidwina continued, "is to do a mile of creeping in one day. You may achieve that by the time for your Revisit. We can adjust our expectations regarding that when you send in your Interim Report, but I certainly expect him to creep half a mile."

"Half a mile?"

"That's eight hundred meters. Also, when you return, be sure to bring the anti-sit device. And absolutely no wheelchairs!"

"Wheelchairs!" Judy and I recoiled. "Of course not!"

"That includes strollers."

"OK. We've already stopped using Joseph's stroller. But—"

"You can carry him on your hip when you must. Just remember. We don't permit wheelchairs or strollers. They do nothing to promote mobility. They're a waste of your child's time, and they're terribly demoralizing for the other families if you bring them here."

And that concluded our instructions for Joseph's Initial Floor Program. "Do we talk to you about the intelligence program?" I asked.

Lidwina smiled. "I'd love to do that, but I've changed departments. I *used* to be in the Institute for Intellectual Excellence. No. One of the 'beige blazers' will see you shortly."

And that was to be our advocate! She was cheerful and chipper, without a trace of frivolity. On her spare frame the simple black and white uniform denoting her affiliation looked especially austere. What I took as a proper British accent lent her a bookish air, but there was something tough as nails not far below the surface. It didn't seem at all inappropriate for her to be specializing in physical development.

There would be at least an hour before our next conference, and the clinical coordinator advised us to take this opportunity to grab an early dinner.

We were beginning to find that the other parents who came to Philadelphia were as interesting as the staff. This time we sat with George and Elizabeta, a family from West Germany. There was a communication problem, since we had only a smattering of each other's languages. But the desire to talk carried us through the frustration of having to say the same things several different ways.

"*Sie ist sehr schön,*" I said of their four-year-old daughter Orly, and she thanked me with a lovely smile. No problem with this child's comprehension!

George asked where we were staying, and we explained that Judy had an aunt in the neighborhood. "You're lucky," he told us, impressed. "We have nobody in this country. I do have a relative in New York City, but all he thinks about is his money. He's a millionaire. I tell him I am *three times* a millionaire, because I have three daughters!" He startled me by producing glossy eight-by-ten portraits of each.

Joseph's intelligence program would be given to us by Teruki Uemura, one of the staff members who'd cared for the kids on the lecture days. We took seats in his office and he began by asking if we had any questions about intelligence in general.

I said, "We have already been showing Joseph word cards, and just for the record I have a list here of the words he's seen. The problem is that he doesn't show a whole lot of interest."

"How big is your print size?"

A detailed discussion ensued. Terry thought our lettering might be too small for Joseph to see it easily. Also, he worried about the number of times we were showing him things. Because we had no way of knowing whether he'd learned the material, we presented some words several dozen times.

"That's far too many exposures. A child learns very quickly, and if we continue to teach the same things over and over he'll be bored. Also, a child may not show 'a whole lot of interest' the way an adult would. You want to show materials to him at high speed, so you won't tax his visual convergence. But since you're unsure, let's start by going back to basics.

"In reading, we're sending bits of discrete information to the brain for future use. We do this using two pathways—visual and auditory. Now, when a child's understanding is very low, we may also use something else—feel or smell or taste. Joseph doesn't need that. However, for now, why not show him objects or pictures along with the word. Later, you can drop these out when all is going well."

He described how we could present Joseph with a word card reading "banana," for example, and then, whisking the card away, we could follow through by giving him the actual fruit. This sounded like fun. Already, I was eager to go home and start, but Terry wasn't through with us yet.

As Lidwina had done with creeping, he outlined a very detailed program. And the goal: "To enjoy reading and receive a Reading Victory at next visit." He explained that a "Victory" would be awarded when Joseph demonstrated an ability to recognize written words. For now, we were to avoid testing him. "Remember that reading is silent," he admonished us. "Just choose an interesting vocabulary, and present it in a distraction-free environment. Give him time to rest between reading sessions. Above all, do not bore him. Finally, have a great time! It's fun."

WE STILL WEREN'T FINISHED. The next order of business was a lesson in patterning, to be given by Dawn Price, RN. She had a very businesslike approach, which she used to check the giddy excitement that had been building in us all week.

"Patterning is the clearest example of what we call 'closed-brain surgery,'" she said. "Now if you'll just put Joey up on the table here I'll show you how it's done."

Joseph let out an indignant howl and tried to get up on his hands and knees rather than lie flat on the patterning table. It was starting out like one of our more difficult sessions back home. Dawn ignored this.

"A hurt kid needs to *feel* moving before he *can* move," she said. "It's like the way kids have to understand language before they can use it. So, Dad, if you'll stand at the end of the table and take his head between your two palms—."

I had already assumed this position, and Judy was standing by across the table from Dawn, holding Joseph's wrist and leg. We were eager to show that we were already veteran patterners.

"We did the homolateral patterning for about a month," I gushed. "But then we talked to Bruce Hagy on the phone and he said—"

"Wait a minute! Now, when you hold his head, I want your hands to be like this, with your thumbs above his ears and your fingertips resting along his jaw line. Be sure to lift when you turn it so his face will clear the table."

Judy said, "OK. And I'm supposed to bring the hand up when the head turns toward me."

"*Wait, I said!*" She stepped away from the table and crossed her arms, glaring at us. "Who's giving this demonstration, anyway?"

That time the message registered. Meekly, we let her lead us slowly and carefully through every detail of the routine. "This is not an exercise," she said patiently. "At least, not for Joey. It's input, and anything sensory can be done even when he's asleep. A kid *cannot* do patterning for himself. The higher a kid's level of understanding, the more likely he is to try and help you. Don't encourage that. All right, now let's change positions. I want to see each of you do this at each station around the table."

In spite of her gruffness with us, Dawn was extremely gentle in handling Joseph. To my surprise, he was actually falling asleep while we patterned him. "Remember not to hold too tightly," she said. "Adults tend to grip more and more firmly as they pattern, particularly if the kid is giving them trouble. That's often the reason he fights it."

Satisfied that we could pattern, she changed to the subject of masking. This time, Judy and I avoided mention of the fact that we'd already begun masking as well, and let her explain it. Joseph's pronounced tooth-grinding was a symptom of poor respiration, she said. Regular masking would address that. "I'm programming you for sixty-two maskings per day. Each will be sixty seconds long, and they will be seven minutes apart. You'll need to set a timer to count down the minutes. Do not mask him if he has a fever. If you discontinue masking for any reason, or if you have a problem with it, call me right away."

She concluded by discussing the balanced and varied diet that she wanted Joseph to receive, vitamin supplements to be given with each meal, and things to avoid (sugar, commercially processed foods, additives, and even excess fluids).

As before, all these requirements were recorded in detail on sheets that she gave us.

WHILE WAITING for our last consultation, we saw Lidwina crossing the common room. I flagged her down with a question that had just occurred to me. She'd said nothing about our inclined plane. Should we continue placing Joseph on the ramp at all?

"Nope!" She smiled. "He's already graduated from that."

"Oh." She and I stood there for a moment, looking down at Joseph. He was on his hands and knees again, moving slowly toward another child.

"I think Joseph is one of the kids who will make it all the way," Lidwina said.

Maybe she said this to all the parents. But I intended to prove her right.

10. CATCH THE SPIRIT

Before the trip, our reading led us to expect an assignment that included four to eight patterning sessions per day. But the program had evolved since publication of those books. Dawn had instructed us to do twelve.

Judy readily saw that this would mean a scheduling nightmare unless each volunteer agreed to stay for two (or more) sessions. Dawn had said to space sessions at least fifteen minutes apart. This interval became a time for developing relationships with our helpers and, we hoped, inspiring long-term commitments.

The program also required the rebreathing mask to be worn for one minute, at seven-minute intervals, all day long. So after five minutes on the table, we'd return Joseph to the floor and promptly slide a mask over his nose and mouth. With the mask secure, we'd look up and invite our bemused visitors to be seated. "Tell me again why you do that," they'd say doubtfully, cringing at the sight of a child with a plastic bag over his face.

Fully charged with enthusiasm, we explained everything happily. We paraphrased the lectures, recited Glenn Doman's stories. *Some* blind kids programmed by the Institutes had learned to *see*, we said. *Many* paralyzed kids had learned to walk. Maybe we didn't convince everyone that this would work, but our volunteers agreed with the objective and enjoyed our energy. If by chance we *did* accomplish something with this child, they would be witnessing a miracle, possibly even the first stirrings of a medical revolution.

"It *is* a revolution," we assured them. Doman had said we were in the process of exploding myths that the world had taken as fact. We quoted him now. "'Brain growth isn't predestined and unchangeable. It can be accelerated.' That's what we're doing here."

One priceless new helper was a law student named Sally Arguilez. She'd read Doman's books and, fascinated by his idea of raising a "renaissance child," was using his methods to teach her well seven-month-old daughter to read. She thought about kids constantly, and that was why she'd noticed my poster in the law school library.

"Your picture of a baby is what hooked me," she said. "That and your headline about teaching a baby to crawl! I had to come see what it was all about."

"My husband and I *argue less*," Sally joked, to help us remember her name. But there was little danger of forgetting her! She combined a jolly, ready laugh with an almost bossy, take-charge personality, and never beat around the bush. "How are you guys paying for all this?" she demanded.

Judy said, "We don't know, exactly. We're going through our savings. Eventually, I think we'll have to raid our retirement accounts."

"That's not right! You're already doing all the *work*. You shouldn't have to bankrupt yourselves into the bargain. And besides, this is going to take a while, right? Maybe you don't know how fast a family's savings can run out!"

"We're starting to learn," I said ruefully. In the last month we'd paid $480 to the Institutes and $200 to Dr. Frymann, none of which would be reimbursed. "When we get out of our HMO and enroll in a different insurance plan, I'm hoping some of these bills will be covered," I added. "It might be a battle, though."

"There's money out there for causes like yours. Look, I've been involved in fund-raising before. Let me contact some of the sources I know about. Have you been in the newspaper yet? Or on TV?"

Startled, Judy and I both cried, *"No!"* A year earlier we hadn't even told our families about Joseph's problem. Major-league publicity for it had never entered our minds.

"We need to fix that," Sally went on. "Leave it up to me, though. You're too busy. When do you need me next?"

By this point, Judy had acquired an oversized calendar, which she laminated with plastic and stuck on the refrigerator door. Some volunteers laid claim to a given block of time, and reappeared faithfully, week after week. We could expect Nancy at five o'clock every Monday, Wednesday, and Friday. Carolyn was a regular at seven on Wednesdays. Nell and Marge still came together in the mornings, while I was at work. But there were always gaps. Sally instructed Judy to write her name beside any uncommitted block of time that she could dovetail with her studies, her part-time job with the Sheriff's Department, and her family.

"We ought to have those little appointment cards to hand out, like they do in doctors' offices," I said half-seriously. But Joseph's inner circle of helpers never forgot a date, and stood ready to fill in when someone else did. Members of our crew appeared regularly at the door, singly or in pairs, throughout the day. I minimized our need for them by racing home to pattern every day on my lunch hour.

Shirley McKevitt, a petite, freckled senior at the college, always looked for blanks on our calendar. Each time, before leaving, she'd sign up for more slots.

"When I first started I didn't think I'd devote as much time as I did," she later admitted to an interviewer. "But when you see a little baby, who has potential to overcome his disabilities, and when you see the progress, it makes you want to keep on working."

Another student named Marzi Atwood liked to bring a friend to simplify things for Judy. And on rare occasions when she couldn't keep an appointment (when her car broke down and left her stranded, for example) she didn't cancel. She called various friends from a payphone until she found someone to replace her.

Sometimes volunteers showed up when I would have preferred a quiet meal. Sometimes I caught them frowning critically at the perpetual clutter and chaos of our house. Just a little privacy and free time would have been nice.

But when I stopped to think about it, I was awed and humbled by the readiness of all these people to help a stranger's child. One lady had come to our door directly from her mailbox, our appeal and all her other mail still in hand. Would *I* have stepped forward, if the tables were turned? No, more likely, I'd have let my good intentions become lost amid the ever-present concerns of the day. These people were truly special. And there were so many of them!

Within a few weeks, many of our volunteers began to feel like family. There were others who said very little. They came, they patterned, and they left. But as long as we could depend on them, they were welcome.

A few volunteers seemed to come because they were lonely and wanted to talk—about careers, philosophy, families, anything. Two of them discovered that, decades earlier, their grandmothers had lived in the same obscure Irish village and had undoubtedly known each other there. All this was fine, as long as the conversation did not distract anyone from the task at hand. People varied in their abilities to pattern correctly and keep up a steady rhythm. Occasionally Judy or I had to interrupt the chatter to remind someone, gently, that we were performing "closed brain surgery." This was vitally serious business, not a coffee klatch.

"Don't forget to keep the leg in contact with the table as you pull it back," we'd say. "Don't bring the arm up until you see the head turning toward you. No, look, if we get out of sync, the person holding his head *can't* speed up. Pause for a second and let us catch up with you instead." Sometimes, Judy tactfully pretended to be having trouble with it herself and asked them to help her concentrate. If necessary, all talk around the patterning table was banned.

MUSIC HELPED. Before every session, we put children's tapes on the stereo, and these kept Joseph entertained while providing a background rhythm for the adults.

> *Can you say the*
> *Se-ven days that*
> *Come in ev-ry week?*
> *Se-ven days,*
> *Se-ven days,*
> *Seven days in every week …*

For Judy and me, the singer's lilting voice, the simple tunes, and the light-hearted themes combined with our newly stoked optimism to push the last remnants of anxiety to the corners of our minds.

Still, we had to stay on our toes. If the tempo of a song picked up, some patterners responded by turning Joseph's head at a correspondingly faster rate. As if it were a dance, Marge tended actually to *stop* patterning any time a song ended! We kept reminding her to watch the digital timer that was counting down the minutes and to keep going until it beeped.

In addition to masking, the interval between patterning sessions served for crossing off a few more meters in the daily "creeping requirement." Our goal in Joseph's first week on program was a total of 20 meters of creeping per day. He achieved this with little difficulty. The following week the goal went to 30 meters, then 40, then 50, and in the fifth week it jumped to 100 meters per day. Now it was becoming a challenge.

The volunteers helped in this endeavor, too. One would crouch on the floor and entice him forward with a toy while slowly backing across the room. If necessary, someone else would crowd him from behind. A trip across the living room rug was good for two meters. Once around the patterning table was four meters. For variety, we dragged the sofa into the middle of the room and found that one lap around it was worth six meters. Judy kept a tally of the distances covered, and I summed it all up in the evening. Then I would herd him back and forth between his bedroom and ours in a last-ditch effort to accomplish his daily goal.

Practically speaking, Joseph was still immobile. That is, he seldom initiated creeping on his own. Given a chance, he still preferred to roll onto his back and stay there. If we left him in the antiroll device, he would merely rest his head on one arm and idly shake a toy with his free hand.

Sally said, "This business of always being on his tummy is interesting. I never thought about it before, but my daughter Jessica almost never rolls onto her back."

"There's no future in lying on her back," I said, again quoting the lectures. "It doesn't lead to creeping, or walking, or anything—except more lying."

"That must be right," she said thoughtfully. "It makes sense. Funny, though—no one ever said this before."

Then, satisfied that she knew what Joseph needed, she insisted that we take him to her house whenever helpers were in short supply. There we found large rooms and a long hallway. Pleased to find himself in new surroundings, he willingly covered longer distances. And when he tired, we plopped him onto a convenient table and patterned him along with Sally or her Mexican housekeeper.

The housekeeper pointed out that the Spanish word for creeping was *gatear*—literally, "to walk like a cat." Joseph grinned at this. We crept along beside him, meowing, and with that distraction he went on a bit more.

Gradually, we began to see changes. In six weeks, his capability for nonstop creeping increased from 2 meters in 30 seconds to 24 meters in three minutes. The Institutes had taught us to be obsessive about numbers like these. But little moments along the way are what linger in my memory. Once, standing in the kitchen, I heard a giggle. Turning, I saw Joseph peeking into the room from around the corner. He recognized this place, having been carried into the kitchen innumerable times, but this was the first time he'd arrived under his own steam. He looked giddy with excitement.

He began to find more reasons for creeping on his own. He'd go to the highchair to indicate that he was hungry. He'd even cross the room to Judy or me for a cuddle. Thirteen weeks after our trip to Philadelphia he was averaging 378 meters per day.

I wish I could say that he accomplished all these gains in good humor. The fact is that he often protested. We couldn't force him to creep. We had to enlist his cooperation, and so we constantly sought new rewards for his efforts. At the end of a particularly grueling stretch of creeping, I would scoop him into the air and cavort around the room with him in a rendition of the Mexican Hat Dance. This invariably brought giggles. He also liked his xylophone, and other musical instruments. But at the same time, little frowns indicated that he knew these treats were only bribes to make him work.

Late one afternoon when he was particularly grouchy and rebellious, the phone rang. Judy answered and spoke briefly. I heard her giving directions to our house, and assumed that we had a new volunteer. She hung up and shrieked. "That was somebody from Channel 8 News! They're on their way over right now to do a story on Joseph!"

Sally had warned that this might happen, so I just said, "Bring 'em on."

"The house is a *wreck*," Judy panted. "And listen to the way Joseph is yelling! But I didn't think I could ask them to make it some other night."

I'd barely started trying to clear the top layer of debris from our furniture when the doorbell sounded. Here already? They must have phoned from their truck! On the porch I found a tall, extremely clean-cut young gentleman who introduced himself as Stan Miller, anchorman for News Eight. On the steps behind him, bending under their load of lights and cameras, were a pair of technicians.

I backed up to let them into the house. Judy was upstairs, hurriedly changing Joseph's clothes and brushing his hair. Stan's assistants set to work deploying their equipment around the living room, and he flipped open a notebook. "Tell me what you folks are doing here," he said.

There'd been no time to prepare "a statement," so I began telling him whatever came into my head. I found myself talking fast, riding a surge of adrenalin. It was the same with Judy when she joined us. Stan tried at first to ask questions, but then he just let us talk. We even explained details to the technicians while they moved in to check the lighting and so on. They seemed taken aback by our energy, and perhaps also by the background noise level. Volunteers Joseph was learning to accept. But these new people who'd taken over his house with their brilliant lights and tangled cords were an outrage. He met it with a furious, sustained roar.

The front door opened again and Nancy appeared for her regular five o'clock patterning session. She froze in her tracks, amazed to find herself looking straight down the barrel of a TV camera.

"Sorry, Nancy," I said. "We didn't have time to warn you."

"Just look natural," advised the cameraman.

Nancy said, "Oh, sure. Easy." She hadn't budged.

I suggested that we proceed with the patterning, and the three of us took our accustomed positions around Joseph on the table. Joseph hadn't stopped his lusty howling, and a warning note sounded in the back of my mind. I turned to Stan. "He doesn't *always* carry on this way," I told him. "It would be easy for you to make it look like we're torturing this poor kid. I hope you won't, because that wouldn't be accurate." Stan nodded impassively, making no promises.

We patterned for the usual five minutes and then returned Joseph to the floor, all under the steady gaze of the camera. I explained the importance of the floor program, and Judy brandished Glenn Doman's book as our authority. She directed the cameraman's attention to the big wipe-off calendar where all our volunteers were scheduled. Another patterning session followed, after which Nancy gratefully fled;

and shortly thereafter Cheryl, our six o'clock patterner, arrived. The crew filmed every move we made, evidently deferring their decisions about what would actually be used. Finally they left. When things had returned to normal, Joseph and I concentrated on finishing his daily creeping goal, and Judy called all our volunteers and urged them to watch the eleven o'clock news.

Current events and current culture had faded from our consciousness, and the mere act of switching on the TV felt unnatural. I tried to imagine that we had a normal household again. But after coverage of developments in the Iran-Contra arms scandal, Cary Grant's funeral, and a blizzard in Colorado, Stan Miller began talking about us. "Coming up next we'll meet a San Diego family whose love for their child is doing what doctors say can't be done. We want you to meet a family whose never-give-up attitude has become very infectious." The scene changed to our patterning table. "Steve and Judy Gallup are determined," Stan said. "Determined to give their brain-injured baby a full life." He described Joseph's "unconventional" treatment and said, "A few months ago he could move very little. Today, he's crawling." Now the camera showed Joseph making his way somewhat unsteadily across the room. Fortunately, most of the audio was muted in favor of Stan's narration. Viewers all over San Diego could see that Joseph didn't look very cheerful, but hopefully they also saw the real story.

Judy's face appeared on the screen. She was saying, "It's such a difference to have a child who can move, after he just could not move at all. He can go and get things for himself now and that's just wonderful. That's what keeps us going." She nodded for emphasis. She looked down and nodded again, blinking back tears, when I said we intended to make our son well.

There was a short interview with Cheryl, who said she got "a sense of fulfillment" from helping him reach his potential, "although at this point we don't know what that is."

"Maybe Cheryl doesn't know what his potential is, but *I* do," Judy muttered to me.

The segment was ending, with Stan hinting that others might want to "catch the spirit" we were demonstrating: "A spirit that will someday help this child into the mainstream of life—not crawling, but standing strong and tall."

The phone rang. "Pretty good!" Sally crowed. "Did *you* like it? How come I didn't hear a call for donations?"

"We touched on that subject," I said, "but they didn't use it."

"Typical. They wanted a nice, uplifting bedtime story for their viewers. That's OK! This kind of thing never hurts. It'll provide credibility for other fund-raising efforts."

"And it might help some other family looking for answers for *their* kid," I suggested.

"You'll be hearing from a Catholic newspaper in the next week or so," she continued. "It's called the *Southern Cross*. I know the editor, and he wants to do a story on you since some of your helpers are Catholics. Also, I've written an article for a little community newsletter called the *Valley Voice*."

"Sally, you're a one-woman publicity department!"

"You *need* one." She went on to say bad things about a private school adjoining our condominium complex. The students there were supposedly encouraged to donate volunteer time to the community, and Judy had previously explained our need to a school representative. The initial reaction had sounded promising, but inexplicably, nothing had happened. On pursuing the matter, Sally learned that a pediatrician on the school's board of directors had warned them away. Patterning was a very bad thing to get involved in, he'd said, and the students should steer clear of us.

She concluded, "As long as people like that are going to throw obstacles in your way, you'll need people like me."

Every time we saw or spoke with Sally, she had more developments to report. When next she came to pattern, she said, "I just finished giving a talk at a Neighborhood Watch group. It's something I do as part of my job with the Sheriff's Department. I was telling the people how to burglar-proof their homes and so forth, and when I finished I asked if they had any questions. And then I said, 'OK, now I'd like to tell you all about a little boy I know.' I bet some of them call to volunteer."

"How can we ever thank you for all this?"

"Don't worry. I'm not doing it for *you*! I'm doing it for Joey!" She laughed and scooped him up—teasing us with a direct violation of our floor program—and gave him a smooch.

The top priority was improving Joseph's mobility, but that was by no means our only job. Any time we felt comfortable with our creeping goals, we had only to consult our daily checkoff sheet to see how much remained to be done in other areas, such as reading.

Judy learned to hate my habit of studying this sheet as soon as I came home from work. Invariably, something was amiss.

"Looks like we're behind on the patterning," I'd say grimly.

"Audrey cancelled again at the last minute. I couldn't find a replacement. What could I do? Marla was here, but I had to send her home."

I would scowl at the problem of fitting in two extra sessions in the limited time remaining in the day. Setbacks like this happened too often. "We've got to get rid of the people who let us down."

"I know that!" Judy protested. "Tell me something I *don't* know! Tell me how I'm supposed to find enough dependable people. Why give *me* a hard time?"

"We're low on word cards, too," I'd observe, sighing. "OK. We can still do it. I'll make up a bunch of new ones while you and Joseph are eating dinner, and then you can be showing them to him while I wolf down my food before Becky comes to pattern."

"No! We are going to eat together, as a family. Dinner is *one* time in our day when we're going to be a normal family."

Our worst disagreements probably came over the masking.

Joseph's immediate response when we put a mask over his nose and mouth was to begin breathing more deeply. This was natural and desirable, but after about forty-five seconds his breathing usually began to sound labored. One or both of us hovered beside him, watching the seconds tick away on our timer and sometimes arguing over whether to remove the mask early. There was a fine line between normal heavy breathing and panting, and Judy and I did not always perceive it at the same time. She accused me of letting Joseph almost suffocate. I replied that we'd been told to mask him for a full sixty seconds. Exasperated, she called the Institutes and described the problem to Dawn.

"I can't be there to decide," Dawn said irritably. "You'll have to use good judgment. If he's in distress, take the mask off early."

"Well, would you say that to my husband? He doesn't *have* good judgment."

"No, I'm not getting in the middle of that," Dawn replied. "The two of you will have to work it out."

We wondered about the other families we'd met in Philadelphia. How were they faring? One day near Christmas, Judy called a mother in upstate New York to compare notes. It helped.

Joan said, "We live on a secondary road way out in the country, and the snow is two feet deep. Our patterners can't even get here. We *were* relying on the grandparents, but now both sets of them have gone off to Florida."

So. We had problems, but apparently weren't alone.

Despite the turmoil, outsiders perceived in us a closely knit unit that was accomplishing miracles. The reporter from *Southern Cross* seemed impressed. I found her interviewing Judy one afternoon when I came home from work. She watched us pattern. She watched me flash word cards in front of Joseph's eyes. She asked questions as eagerly as we answered them. She even borrowed our copy of *Doran*, a British mother's account of life on program. The article, when it came out, compared Joseph to an athlete training for the Olympics. Various patterners were quoted testifying to the progress they'd seen him make already. It concluded:

Several obstacles keep Joseph from attaining his objectives at a faster pace.

'I need an extra set of hands,' Judy said, adding that she is 'physically drained' by 9 p.m.

She can use a total of 80 volunteers to supply Joseph with infusions of enthusiasm, which challenge him to record-breaking performances.

But she and Steve put these problems in perspective as they look back at their son's two-month winning streak. This team seems invincible.

This was the kind of publicity that brought results! There was even an editor's note that listed our phone number and invited readers to call us. Many did, and our pool of volunteers swelled.

We toasted in the New Year with Nan, Nancy, and Nancy's boyfriend Greg, who'd also joined the team. A few months earlier we had not known these people, and now they were among our very best friends. That in itself was cause for wonder. Together we finished the day's patterning, romped with Joseph on the floor until he was tired, and then tucked in the happy little fellow (still wearing his antiroll device, of course). Then we readied a bottle of champagne and settled round the table for an extremely rare bout of Trivial Pursuit, of all things. At some point in the evening I realized that Judy and I were enjoying ourselves more thoroughly than at any time in the last two years. Not only did we have a Cause, we were winning.

Never mind us. *Joseph* was winning!

11. MAKING THE WAY EASIER

The emotions sustaining my enthusiasm through those early months on program were a salad of joy and relief. From the very beginning, I'd believed that, if competent people only cared enough to address the problem, children like Joseph could yet claim their birthright.

We'd come home from Philadelphia confident of having found competent people. We accepted their ideas. At the very least, their ideas were plausible. I had no way of knowing whether they were right in saying that lack of oxygen is *always* the root cause of brain injury, or that creeping stimulates neural growth as opposed to being just a marker of it. The point is that they believed these things, and such beliefs formed the basis of a treatment program that seemed to work. We did not want to quibble.

Still, stuck in the back of my mind, there remained an exchange that took place during a question-and-answer forum at the end of the Institutes' lecture series. One of Glenn's points had to do with the structure of the brain being determined by its function. I'd given little thought to that, concentrating on less theoretical issues, but Judy wanted clarification.

"Doesn't the structure come first?" she'd asked. "If the structure isn't right, then won't the function be impaired?"

Of course, she was thinking about what Dr. Frymann, the osteopath, had told us. If Joseph was still in distress due to compression of his skull, then maybe that would block the effectiveness of the stimulation program we were beginning.

Glenn Doman's son Doug responded to that. "Oh, we had a doctor visiting here some time back who tried to say the very same thing. She—"

At that point, Gretchen leaned over and said to him in a stage whisper, "*They know her.*"

Doug's mouth snapped shut and he gave us a bland cat-ate-the-canary smile.

"Well?" Judy demanded. "Which comes first, structure or function?"

"People outside our walls may have a different interpretation of the problem," he said. "We aren't much interested in that, and we don't think you really are, either. If you liked what other people said, you wouldn't have come here."

Later in the week, we'd pursued the matter with the staff members assigning Joseph's program. We mentioned his upcoming appointments with Dr. Frymann.

"*Our* program is what Joseph needs," Lidwina had said gently. "Don't try to do something else on top of it. Believe me, you won't have time."

LIDWINA WAS CERTAINLY RIGHT that the program allowed no time for anything else. Accomplishing that alone looked like an impossible task, and so one of my first acts when we arrived home was to call Dr. Frymann's office and reluctantly cancel those appointments.

To my surprise, Dr. Frymann called me back.

"It's fine to do their program," she told me, speaking even more slowly and deliberately than usual. "And I know very well that it will keep you busy. However, your son is not going to make much progress, in *any* regard, if we do not address the structural problems resulting from his birth that I have explained to you."

Over the subsequent years of our acquaintance, I gathered that Dr. Frymann truly loved her little patients, while viewing benighted parents as the most trying aspect of her daily life. Her emotions were seldom easy to discern. But this time she really seemed to be pleading with me, to the extent she was capable of doing such a thing. Pleading on Joseph's behalf. So after mounting a half-hearted resistance, I conceded and let the appointments stand.

Somehow, we would have to fit the frequent trips to her office in with everything else on the schedule. And, if we hoped to stay on the program, nobody at the Institutes could ever know about this deviation from the plan.

DR. FRYMANN'S WAITING ROOM was always crowded, and the waits consumed precious chunks of the day. The only recourse was to take the antiroll device and the rebreathing mask and to do as much of the program as possible right there, in front of the startled people sitting around the room. Whenever possible, Judy commandeered the adjoining "chapel" (which was supposedly reserved for study and med-itation) and coaxed Joseph to log a few meters back and forth around the furniture.

Conversations ensued. She learned that a number of the children coming to Dr. Frymann were drowning victims, immobilized with twisted, rigid limbs. One boy had been found unconscious after chok-ing on food. Another had actually been strangled by a playmate. And some kids had simply been "born that way," as my boss put it.

As far as Judy could tell, they were *all* brain-injured. She couldn't resist the temptation to proselytize. Surely, Dr. Frymann was helping them, but what each of these children also needed was a full-time neu-rological program, just like ours. She described our routine and the rationale. Most of the parents heard her out with interest. However, although some had traveled great distances to see Dr. Frymann, they were not ready for the further sacrifice of starting a home program.

Meanwhile, Joseph improved—and not only in terms of his ability to creep. Although still irritable, he cried less than before, and slept more soundly. One evening, as he gratefully snuggled down into his bedclothes, I pulled a soft, blue blanket over the antiroll device that he wore all night and tucked it around his shoulders—and realized he was asleep already. I knelt, stroking his hair and listening to him breathe. Such a simple event, a two-year-old falling asleep! Moments like this were surely ordinary for other families. I wanted more of what they had.

I sat on the floor of his darkened room and leaned against the wall, just listening to his faint snore. Soon, Judy glided in and looked at him, too.

"There's my Sweet Pea," she murmured. She'd recently taken to calling him that.

WITH JANUARY came the due date for our first Interim Report of Joseph's progress. Paging through the questionnaire, I saw, "Overall, what is the worst thing about your child's physical program?" and "Describe the environment in which your child does his physical program. Include surface, clothes, dimensions…" The questions went on and on, for thirty-six pages. "Describe how you motivate your child." "Specify exactly how much program was lost" (which meant *To what extent did you fall short of your assignment?*).

This was going to take some thought. As far as I knew, we'd done a good job. We definitely hadn't missed any patternings. But Silvia had warned that the slightest lapse—in any area—would be viewed very seriously.

Judy and I felt most unsure of ourselves in describing progress with the intelligence program. Usually, Joseph seemed to look straight *through* his word cards, not at them.

Judy lined up his toy musical instruments on the floor. He loved music. How could this not work? First she showed him the xylophone. *BING.* "Xylophone!" *BING.* She showed him the word, in bold two-inch-high red letters: "Xylophone!"

One by one, she displayed the objects and then flashed the words across his field of vision: drum, maracas, cymbals, tambourine. Incredibly, he still didn't appear to notice.

Sometimes, he even turned away from the cards.

Judy called the Institutes about this and spoke to Rosalind, who said, "All brain-injured kids have visual problems to some extent. It could be that he has trouble focusing on the words. Experiment with holding your cards at different distances from his face. Also, don't assume that he's not looking when he turns his head to the side. A lot of our kids see *better* when they suppress the vision on one of their eyes. It's a way of reducing visual chaos when the eyes fail to work together properly. If that's the case, masking and creeping should begin to improve things for you pretty soon."

JOSEPH WAS STILL a client of the Regional Center, and subject to periodic home visits from their social worker. We understood by now that this organization would have no role in his recovery, but in hopes of demonstrating the value of what we were doing, Judy said they could document his progress. Accordingly, the social worker arrived one afternoon, with a nurse, to find a patterning session in progress. They sat patiently on the sofa and observed.

The nurse smiled patronizingly at Shirley and her little sister Cara as they left, then frowned at Judy. "These people you have coming in—I take it they're just volunteers from the community."

"Sure. They come from all walks of life. They aren't professional therapists, of course, but we instruct them on how to do it." Judy went on to assure her that all our patterners did their job well, and that despite their youth, Shirley and Cara were among the best. In any event, she said, we were seeing results. She explained Joseph's rating on the Institutes' Profile. "As you can see, he creeps on his hands and knees now. That's something we tried and tried to get him to do before we started patterning."

The social worker took notes, as always. The nurse wanted the record to show that she still had reservations. Our method of treatment was not endorsed by the medical community, and none of the people implementing it, including us, was a trained professional. Judy argued that she did have a degree in special education and that we were in the process of being certified as developmentalists by the Institutes. This did not carry much weight as far as the nurse was concerned. Standing on the front porch, she turned for a parting shot. "It's certainly true that he has made some progress, but don't you think he might have done so *anyway*, even without all this?"

This was precisely the response Doman had predicted we would hear. Masking her disappointment with a thin smile, Judy retorted, "You can think that if you want to."

Once an educator, always an educator. Having endured a year and a half with no clear direction for how to help our son, Judy now wanted to tell the world—other parents and professionals alike—that answers were possible. She wanted to make the way easier for others, and their lack of enthusiasm for the news troubled her.

"Look," I said when she repeated the conversation to me later. "I'm pretty sure the Institutes didn't ask us to go out and convert the world. So who cares what people say?"

"*I care* about all the other disabled kids, who're getting older while nobody is helping them."

"Yes, well, our *own* project, right here, isn't a done deal," I reminded her. "Be glad we don't depend on people like that nurse any more. The best way to bring them around is to succeed with Joseph."

"And then they'll say it would've happened anyway," she said bitterly.

"*And then* our son will be well! That's enough. That's *plenty!*"

OUR SUCCESS was, indeed, not a done deal. Joseph's performance suddenly began to slip. The daily creeping distances were falling off, and he was having more trouble than usual with the masking.

In fact, Judy suddenly realized, he was having trouble breathing at all. He'd become lethargic, and a quick check revealed that he had a fever.

The family doctor said he had a sinus infection. Again and again, his temperature soared to 102 degrees and a shade beyond. Judy popped him into bathtubs full of tepid water. We discontinued masking and started what Dawn called an "anti-stress diet," with greatly stepped-up dosages of vitamin supplements. Joseph's health remained shaky for several long weeks. He would start to recover and then get worse. Reluctantly—we used all medications reluctantly—we gave him the prescribed antibiotics and decongestant. Judy worried about his color, which she called "ashen." He seemed to have perpetual dark shadows under his eyes. Back we went to the doctor, who ordered x-rays and then diagnosed bronchitis and pneumonia.

Nan brought hot meals, and stern lectures. She insisted that we'd been pushing him too hard. "Give the kid a break! He's had enough!" Even Lidwina (back from a trip to Japan, where she'd been seeing more brain-injured children) seconded this advice. "If he's below par, just put him to bed and try again the next day. He'll pick up soon."

We had no choice. But it felt all wrong, especially as the days turned into weeks. Glenn Doman had *indoctrinated* us. Joseph could not afford to be ill! He was in a race with time and *had* to make every day count. Thinking positively, I referred to his condition as "creeping pneumonia."

Without immediate program challenges, I turned to wondering where he'd picked up the infection. From the beginning, we'd had a rule that any volunteer with a cold or sore throat was supposed to cancel. But sometimes people carry infections unknowingly. Our patterning table might be the nexus of a public health crisis. I had visions of volunteers standing around it wearing surgical masks and latex gloves. Would they still come if we required that?

Yet again we called the Institutes for guidance. "Everybody carries germs," Rosalind said. "When they touch something, they leave germs on it. It's unavoidable. Tell them to wash their hands before they handle Joseph."

"We do," Judy said. "And they say, 'Oh, I just took my hands out of soapy dishwater.'"

"Pooh!" Rosalind scoffed. "Send them to your sink and make them wash again anyway." She recommended stocking up on a surgical scrub solution used in hospitals. "Beyond that, you'll just have to build up Joseph's health so he can withstand the exposure."

His doctor prescribed other medications, but we were rapidly losing patience. Although we'd given up on the neurologists and pediatricians, we still relied on a family practitioner. He confessed that he knew nothing about brain injury. Because he had no bias, he'd offered no objections to our program. "If it works, go for it," was all he said. But now Joseph was languishing, and this doctor seemed willing to accept *that*, too. He cited different studies on the advisability of staying active during an illness. One indicated that bed rest contributed to recovery. Another showed that it made no difference.

Dr. Frymann offered to take on these aspects of Joseph's medical care as well, if we would agree to the idea of forgoing antibiotics. She never used them. Instead, she would give us homeopathic remedies.

I hesitated over this change in tactics, because I didn't understand how these more "natural" medicines worked. But on the other hand I had to admit that I didn't know all that much about prescription drugs, either. So we took the plunge.

For whatever reason, the health crisis subsided rather abruptly, within a week in fact. We resumed masking and found that he could tolerate it more easily than before.

As the program built back up to full speed, we observed that he was not as tuned-out, and was finding new ways of communicating with us. He opened a drawer and pulled out a blanket when he was sleepy. He looked at his word cards willingly. He even started making a few sounds that could pass for speech. I heard him say "up" and "down" when Judy showed him cards bearing those words.

I gazed at him, smiling in surprise. "You just said 'up,' didn't you, son?"

He lowered his long lashes modestly with a faint smile. God, what was he thinking? I'd have given anything to know. I sighed gratefully. Whatever problems this kid might carry forward, I thought, speech probably would not be among them. Soon he would be talking, and telling us exactly what he thought.

Encouraged, we began pushing the reading vigorously in an effort to catch up to our goal and added couplets: eat lunch, fig bar, peanut butter, drink juice. He did seem more receptive. Even better, we thought he was finally giving us better eye contact, however fleeting.

THEN CAME JACK, a reporter from the *San Diego Tribune*, who'd heard about us from Nan's sister. "This will be a great way to put your case before the public," she had assured us. "Tell this guy how much it's costing you to keep going. And don't be shy about it! Tell him what your income is. He'll know what to do for you."

I agreed to talk with the reporter by phone from my office, and again briefly at home one Sunday when he came with a photographer.

Jack began our first conversation with a show-me attitude. What kind of people ran these Institutes, anyway? Were they real physicians? Were their results documented? Why were we flying in the face of conventional medical wisdom?

It wasn't the line of questioning I'd expected. Now, like Judy, I found myself promoting and defending the program itself, rather than advancing the cause of a kid's uphill battle. By the time we said goodbye the reporter had softened, apparently willing to give this unusual project a fair hearing. But when I met him in person a few days later, his suspicions were in high gear once again. Unlike Stan Miller, and the *Southern Cross* reporter, this guy really wanted to argue. "I've been talking to a neurologist at Children's Hospital," he said. "And he told me this kind of treatment doesn't work at all."

I groaned. "I don't suppose the neurologist claimed to have any *other* course of treatment that works. Did he? People have to take responsibility for their own well-being. Obviously, we're the ones who live with the consequences. We can't turn Joseph over to doctors and therapists who don't expect anything from him."

"But what if the doctors and therapists are right? How do you know this isn't just a very difficult set of exercises that won't work?"

"If they're right, at least we'll know we tried. But they aren't right. Joseph has made more progress in six months of patterning than he did in the previous *eighteen months*."

"They say it's too expensive—," he began, whereupon Judy jumped into the conversation. "*We'll* decide if it's too expensive! *We'll* decide if it's too hard!"

"Well— how long will this go on?"

"I don't know," I admitted. "Right now we're hoping that he'll be OK in two years."

"What are you going to do if Joseph hasn't made any progress in two years?"

I actually laughed, because the answer that occurred to me was a flippant line from *The Importance of Being Earnest*, a play I'd seen many times in our former life. This skinny, buck-toothed reporter irritated me. I'd lost interest in his challenges, and so I went ahead and recited the line, no longer caring what he put in his newspaper. "That is a metaphysical speculation. It has very little reference to the actual facts of life as we know them."

"Maybe so," he said before I'd finished. "But what if he hasn't?"

I took a deep breath and repeated myself. "Joseph *is* making progress! I don't know for a fact that he'll be fully recovered in two years. It may take longer. But unless something better comes along—some approach to the problem that I don't currently know about—we will continue as we are until he's well. I fully expect to see him achieve that goal."

Jack closed his notebook. "Yes," he said slowly and pointedly. "I'm sure—*you* do."

The article he wrote steered a wide path around the intelligence program, although I'd explained very carefully how that tied in with the larger goal. The notion of teaching a two-year-old how to read was evidently too outrageous for a responsible journalist to touch. Jack had his hands full just balancing his contradictory input about patterning. He quoted the neurologist as saying that there was no proved benefit for our therapy:

> "About 5 to 10 percent of our patients eventually end up
> in patterning because their parents are seeking an alternative
> to what we recommend. Some improve, some stay the same."

Then to get a favorable point of view other than mine or Judy's, he quoted Jennifer, the mother who had given us her child's patterning board:

> "Joseph is a totally different kid. He's made a 180-degree turn."

The article returned to the doctor, who dismissed this testimony as "anecdotal" and issued the further warning that intensive home therapy programs could destroy marriages. Jack pursued that lead as well, concluding with a few words from the father of a drowning victim who'd died of pneumonia a year or two earlier while on the Institutes' program:

> "In our case, it brought our family closer together. Do
> you abandon your child to an institution or do you see if
> he might respond? What else would I have done with my
> time? Watched more TV? Gone to more movies? In evaluat-
> ing your life, you have to ask yourself what you've done for
> members of your family."

Ever cheery, Sally brought us extra copies of the article. "This is good stuff!" she declared. "It shows both sides, and lets people draw the obvious conclusion."

"Which is?"

"Ha!" Her eyes flashed. "I'll tell you what *my* conclusion was! I put down the newspaper and wrote a letter to that clown who said patterning doesn't work. I told him, 'Shame on you, Doctor! Instead of publicly criticizing something you don't understand, why don't you go to Philadelphia and see for yourself what's going on?'"

IN LATE FEBRUARY I called Lidwina to confirm our Revisit appointment.

"Great!" She said when she heard my voice. "I have Joseph's file open right now. I was just reading your latest update when the phone rang. His creeping sounds *good*."

"We have to prod him along all the time, though," I worried. "That goal of 800 meters in a day still seems so far off."

"I'm sure he'll make that before your Revisit date. But keep working to get his activity level up. You're going to need a large environment to get in long distances of nonstop creeping. You can do only so much indoors."

"That's for sure. You should see the size of our condo."

"Try getting him to creep outside. Some kids don't like putting their hands down in the grass, so you might want to take a carpet runner along and roll it out ahead of him."

She also wanted us to redouble our efforts on reading. "Joseph will need *many* more words," she said. "You should be showing him an absolute minimum of nine new words every day." She was silent while she reviewed our program and did some calculating. "Right now you are showing him twenty-five words per day, and he's seeing each word five times a day for five days."

"That's right."

"Observe his response carefully. I'd like you to decrease the frequency to twenty-one showings for each word, but only if he's getting it. Then you might try going down to three times per day for five days—a frequency of fifteen times. OK?"

"Frequency fifteen." I was taking all this down as fast as I could, hoping to understand it later.

"How about the masking?"

I told her we had been accomplishing the requisite sixty-two daily maskings before his illness. We'd built back up to about fifty, but it was hard to fit more into the day because he refused to wear the mask while creeping.

"To make the Revisit you have to be doing the whole program," she said firmly. "Try masking for shorter durations while he's active."

THE MOST OBVIOUS VENUE for outdoor creeping was a nearby easement beneath some power lines. Judy and I took turns carrying Joseph there for multiple short creeping sessions every day. At first, carpet runners did help ease the transition, but soon enough he was striking off on his own across the grass.

To keep him going, however, I had to get right down there on the ground with him, and creep as well. In this position, I felt a little like a mother horse whose foal is just taking to its legs. I nudged him along when necessary, and murmured encouragement in his ear. Also, I needed to stay alert. People used this area for walking their dogs. I had to ensure Joseph steered around the little hazards they left here and there.

IT WAS TIME to begin work on our Revisit Report, which even a cursory glance showed to be more formidable than the document we'd mailed in two months earlier. Still, as we pondered how to answer its many questions, we knew that time invested in this would contribute to fine-tuning the program and accelerating Joseph's progress.

We looked for evidence of headway in all of the developmental pathways. Under Mobility, we proudly recorded the fact that he had recently clambered up a flight of stairs without assistance. And of course there was his creeping. In November, he'd crept an average of 34 meters per day. This had increased steadily, despite the illness in January; and his average distance per day in March was 660 meters.

He finally achieved that goal of half a mile in one day on March 21, 1987—just nine days prior to our Revisit date. We placed two orange pylons 50 meters apart in the grass and simply chugged back and forth from one to the other, stopping to rest and praise him extravagantly every time we turned around. Each one-way trek took seven minutes.

Joseph, that staunch little hero, did everything we asked of him. But he refused to do two things at once. Wearing the mask while creeping, for even a few seconds, was out of the question.

Changes in the other developmental pathways were less obvious. Still, once we'd started, we couldn't leave the report alone until it included everything, large or small, that we liked or disliked about his status. We avoided mention of Dr. Frymann, of course, but found room to record an observation she'd made after an appointment one day: "He's coming alive."

He was almost twenty-five months old.

Preoccupation with Joseph saved me from much of the anguish I would otherwise have experienced regarding our finances. The balance in our bank account hovered in the neighborhood of $600, from which we were paying Dr. Frymann $55 about every ten days. Mortgage payments consumed one of my biweekly paychecks. And the Institutes' bill was growing by $411 each month.

For the moment, at least, I needn't have worried. Thanks to Sally's efforts as our publicist, articles about Joseph were appearing in various publications almost every week. She'd gotten him on TV again, along with scores of volunteers gathered to celebrate his second birthday. All this public attention provided supporting evidence that she used in lobbying every charitable and civic organization in town.

One evening when I came home from work, Judy met me with some good news. Sally had just called to say that the Deputy Sheriff's Association would contribute $400 toward the Institutes' bill. "That's great," I said slowly. "But there's something wrong here. She called me, too. I thought she said it was the Police Officer's Association. And the amount I heard was $200."

In fact, there were *two* gifts! Sally enjoyed messing with us.

The biggest breakthrough came when a service group called Nice Guys sent $1,400, with a note. "We hope the enclosed check will make things easier for you." It certainly would. Now we had enough to settle our entire debt at the Institutes. Excited, I called my parents in Virginia. "Nice Guys?" my father repeated, profoundly impressed. "Those really *are* nice guys!"

THE TV APPEARANCE also brought a phone call from a local mother who had been doing an Institutes program with her son for three years.

Judy was delighted, but surprised. "I thought we knew everybody in San Diego who'd been to the Institutes!"

"We keep a low profile," the woman said. She explained that their program had drawn unfavorable attention from neighbors, who'd even reported her as a possible child abuser. "When something like that happens, it makes you a very private person," she said. "But we didn't give up, and we're glad. When my son was five years old he was practically immobile. Now he's eight, and he runs three miles nonstop every morning!"

JOSEPH'S EXPECTED RECOVERY was a hot topic. The *Southern Cross* article won a journalism award and was reprinted in Catholic newspapers nationwide. The reporter began asking when she could return for a followup story.

"Wait till he's walking," Judy insisted. We'd had all the media atten-tion we could bear for a while, despite its benefits.

Help continued to come from unexpected directions. A long-lost friend in Ohio read about us and sent a check. Lew, our minister, went before his Kiwanis Club and brought back enough money to cover the airfare. Three ladies I knew at work organized a yard sale, and students at the college were selling candy—all to benefit Joseph.

To top it off, Judy's aunt in Philadelphia wrote to offer us the use of a car while we were in town. We could stay in their house again, and they would even provide transportation to and from the airport.

"Free lodging, free plane tickets, and a car—*and* money to cover our bill at the Institutes!" I said wonderingly. "How will we ever repay all these people?"

Judy sighed happily. "All we have to do is show them a little boy who's gotten well."

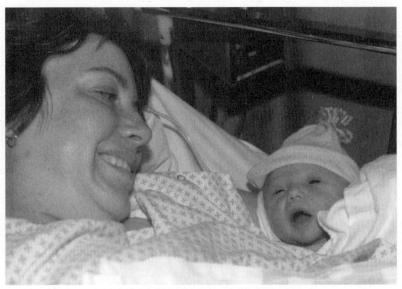

March 5, 1985 was a very happy day.

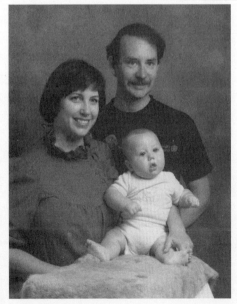

In early months following the hospital report, we simply hoped for the best.

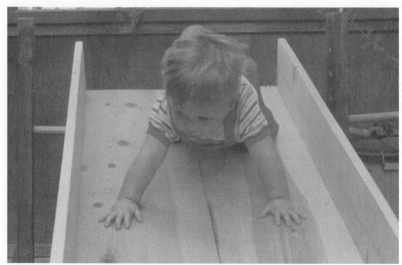

This inclined plane provided an environment
that encouraged mobility.

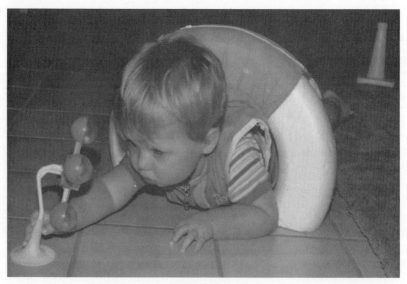

Judy cut a swim ring in half and attached it to a jacket to prevent
Joseph from rolling onto his back.

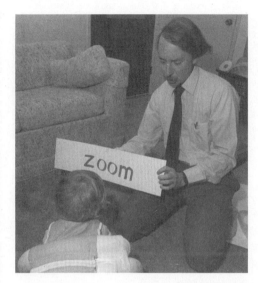

One of Joseph's thousands
of homemade word cards.
Photo by Sam Lucero.

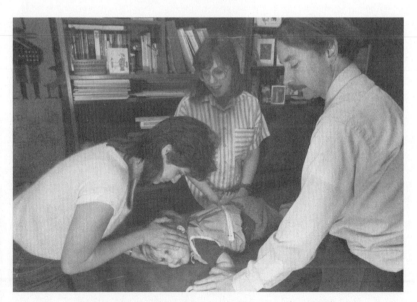

Patterning, with volunteer Sally Arguilez (left).
Photo by Sam Lucero.

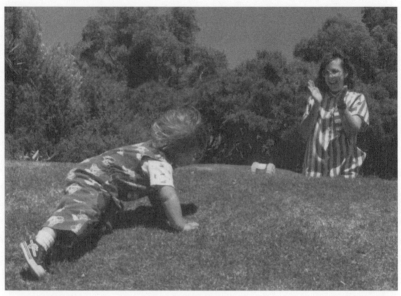

Joseph crept up to a mile on some days as part of his neurological development program.

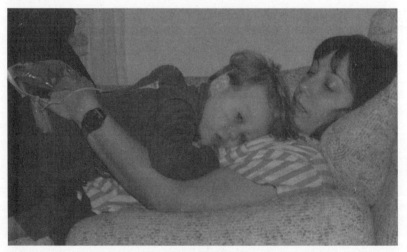

Fatigue

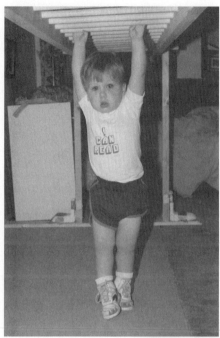

Joseph logged hundreds of daily trips beneath his overhead ladder in the process of learning how to walk.

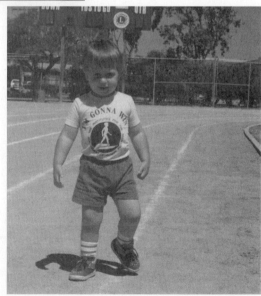

Joseph took his first steps at 39 months of age, and began distance walking shortly thereafter.

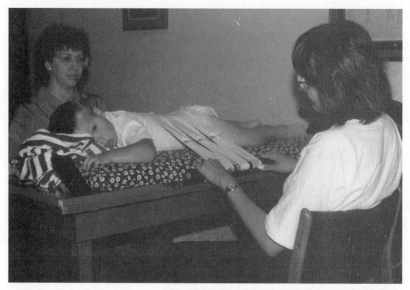

Manual respiratory patterning, with volunteer Isabel Sapien (right).

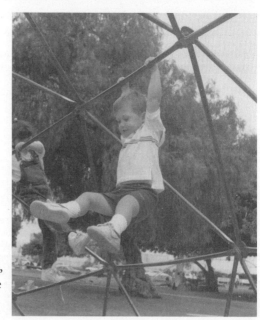

Playing in the park,
apparently just like
any other kid!

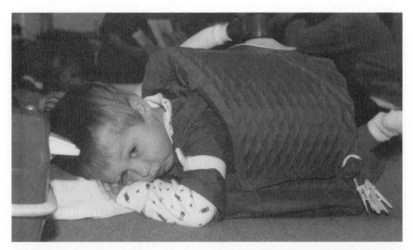

Trying for more gains, via the respiratory patterning machine.

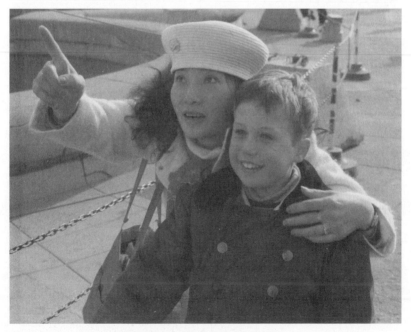

With Song Yi in Beijing, 1996.

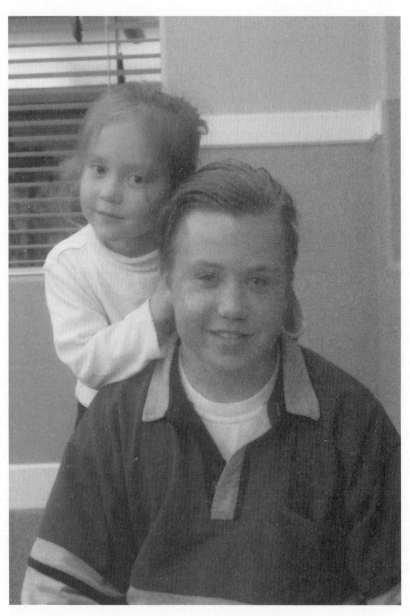

Susannah and her big brother, 2005.

12. REVISITS AND VICTORIES

Entering the Veras Building on the Institutes' campus Monday morning was like wading into the tumult of a convention floor. During the November visit, most families had held back shyly. What a change! This time we found everybody—at least, those who spoke the same language—eagerly and loudly comparing notes on how they'd survived the first few months on program. Meanwhile, timers continually beeped, prompting them to mask or remove masks from their kids as they spoke.

Joseph frowned, unable to process all the stimulation. Knowing he would very soon retreat from it into head shaking and whining, I hurriedly stowed our materials in a bench and took refuge with him in a familiar routine. Soon we were exploring that big room on hands and knees. Judy meanwhile had already spotted and hunkered down with her buddy Joan. Passing behind them a bit later I heard her confess, "Ice cream is *my* downfall. I reward myself with it at the end of the day. It's scary. I've gotten to where I need the stuff!"

A blast of chilly air drew my attention to the door. George and Elisabeta, the Germans we'd met last time, stood blinking at the room with befuddled expressions. I ran over and gave them a snapshot from that meeting. George accepted it absent-mindedly. I think he couldn't believe they'd crossed the ocean to this place once again. But the program must have been agreeing with their bright-eyed daughter, who looked far more charged-up than either parent. I recalled Lidwina telling us that the second trip to the Institutes was the point at which most families hit high gear with their programs. All of us would be seeing changes by now. All would have reason to believe that our kids were closing the gap that separated them from their well peers.

Not everyone we remembered from our first trip had returned, but in their stead were new faces. Soon, I fell into conversation with a South American couple, also here for their second visit. Both were physicians. The mother had given up her practice in order to manage their son's program, and now she spent her days patterning him and creeping around a track with him. They'd already met the goal of creeping an entire mile in one day. She explained that she motivated her son by placing a pet rabbit in front of him. The rabbit loped along just out of reach, the youngster scrambled after it, and the meters fell away behind them.

A little girl named Elsa had started walking during the last couple of months. Judy and I looked on enviously as she toddled around the room. "I can't find the words to say how badly I want to see Joseph doing that," I said, sighing.

Surprisingly, her parents showed no enthusiasm. Elsa's mother had retired grumpily to a corner to fill out their Revisit Report. I wondered why she'd waited so long to do it.

Also in this crowd were a few "senior families," people who had been through the basic course of six visits to the Institutes. They'd heard all the lectures at least once. Between visits they must have seen enough progress to justify settling into this program indefinitely as a way of life. We especially admired an active five-year-old named Kimmy, who darted energetically around the room and then, time and again, returned to crouch beside Joseph, as if to encourage him to do likewise. Her quiet parents radiated competence. Were they still patterning her, I asked? No, they'd discontinued the patterning after her Walking Victory. How long had they patterned? The father rolled his eyes and smiled. "Oh, we did it forever!"

Their big push now was developing Kimmy's ability to speak in sentences. To do that, they had to improve her breathing. She spent sixteen hours every day lying in a special respiratory patterning machine the Institutes had given them.

Every few minutes, a family was summoned to an interview with one of the busy staff members. Meanwhile, more familiar faces appeared. We recognized a young couple from Georgia as they emerged from an office and rejoined the group. They weren't smiling. The father shook his head ruefully. "Boy, oh boy, oh boy!" he muttered.

"What's up?" I asked.

"We told them we had done the program every day—except on Christmas Day. You know, you're not supposed to take any time off at all. But we thought, well, *Christmas.* Golly, for a minute there I thought they were going to kick us out!"

"You're lucky. That does happen," Kimmy's dad noted. "*I've* seen them send people away. And if they do, there's no appeal. Once they throw you out, brother, it's for keeps."

"That seems hard."

"Well, it is. But you've heard the argument. The Institutes can't afford to waste time on people who aren't committed to getting results."

"We are! But still," the other dad insisted. "*One day?*"

"One day off program leads to another. Look, you've heard what they say. If your house is burning down, you can take enough time from the program to call the fire department. Then you go next door and keep on patterning." He grinned. "See, if your priorities are straight you won't have issues like this."

On our previous visit, a mother had confided to me her misgivings about any regimen that would prevent her family from observing the Sabbath and keeping it holy. Remembering that, I scanned the room but didn't see her.

Then came our turn. A junior staff member named Nobuyasu Habara led us upstairs to an empty office, seated us, and began reading through our report very carefully. He asked several questions, and scrawled notations in the margins.

He didn't like our statement that we doubted whether Joseph enjoyed reading. "Let's see about that," he said. "Did you bring reading materials?"

We produced a fair-sized stack of word cards. I grabbed the topmost card and began jockeying for position in Joseph's field of view. As usual, I did not have his attention.

Mr. Habara said, "Let's try something different. Dad, you hold him in your lap. Now, Mom, take two cards and come around in front like this." He demonstrated how he wanted Judy to hold up first one word silently, then another, and then both words, side by side. She did so, showing first the word "duck" and then "chicken."

"Joseph!" she said loudly. "Which word says 'duck'?"

Without hesitation, Joseph looked at the card reading 'chicken.' Our hearts sank, but then he spoke! "Chi-," he murmured. Then he looked at the other card, grinned triumphantly, and said "duck!"

Mr. Habara and Judy both yelled as if somebody had scored a winning touchdown. As for me, my jaw dropped so far that the rest of my head had to follow it. *Never* had Joseph responded so positively to his intelligence program.

Judy went on to present Joseph with several more pairs of words. Each time, he singled out the word she named by looking at it, although he didn't say anything further.

Mr. Habara turned back to our report. "'Sometimes enjoys reading'?" he read aloud. He frowned, seemingly puzzled by our lack of perception. "This," he announced, "is a child who *loves* to read."

Well, it was news to me. I lifted Joseph from my lap. "Little guy, you've been holding out on us," I growled playfully.

"Now let's look at his creeping," said Mr. Habara.

I returned him to the floor, ran to the far corner, and beckoned. Joseph scowled at me and at the carpeted distance separating us, weighing the desirability of a hug against the trouble of making the trip.

"Come on, Joe!" I yelled. I pulled a ring of car keys from my pocket and jingled them vigorously. Now he came, and he did so at a good clip. Behind him, Mr. Habara watched his movements the way an art critic studies a canvas in a museum.

"OK. Can you also get him to crawl flat on his stomach?" he asked.

Judy and I looked at each other doubtfully. Crawling was an earlier developmental stage, but it did have a place on the Institutes' Profile. Each stage would need to be checked off before these people graduated him. "I don't know," I said. "We haven't worked on that. Come on Joseph, down on your tummy."

This didn't go so well. Either Joseph did not understand what was being asked of him, or he refused to perform tricks. He'd already crossed the room as I'd asked! Since the keys interested him, I tried placing them under a chair, but instead of squirming under it as I'd hoped, he crept around to the other side and stretched his arm until he could reach them.

"I wish you wouldn't use keys to motivate him," Judy complained. "That's such a baby thing."

"Hey, I'm trying to find something that works!"

Habara ignored this little flare-up. He now wanted to evaluate Joseph's tactile competence. He dropped a quarter and a small plastic toy into a cloth bag and held it out. "Reach into the bag, Joseph," he said. "Get the coin."

Joseph eyed him suspiciously. Long moments passed. *Please, just do it, son.* We hadn't worked on this skill either. But was it so difficult? After much prodding, he put his hand part-way into the bag, but he never withdrew anything.

"This is OK," said Mr. Habara. "I just wanted to establish a baseline of where he is right now. You'll be seeing more changes." He seemed very satisfied.

From there, we proceeded to a short session with Elaine, who carefully measured all Joseph's dimensions, as she had done five months earlier. She also took an arm and leg and patterned him with us for a few minutes, to ensure that we did it correctly. Apparently we passed the test, because she had no criticisms.

Dr. Wilkinson, the Institutes' medical director, gave Joseph a quick physical exam and worried about his heart murmur. Doctors back home had always dismissed it as "probably benign;" but she said it might explain his lack of energy. "Kids know instinctively when they should stop," she said. She wanted us to insist on getting a cardiac evaluation when we returned home.

Our final interview of the day was with Lidwina. She greeted Joseph warmly and told him he looked like her nephew. "That little fellow is named Joseph, too," she added brightly. "*And* he has blond hair. Just like yours." She held him in her lap a few minutes and studied him while he very studiously stroked her fingernails.

Reluctantly, she put him back on the floor and turned to us. She had two copies of a pink sheet of paper, one of which she pushed across the desk. It was headed DIRECTOR'S STATEMENT OF PROGRAM TO DATE. Someone had written numbers in a table at the bottom, but the top half of the sheet was not yet filled in. Lidwina asked Judy to act as the scribe and to write per her dictation, as she entered the same observations on her copy: "During Joseph's first five months of program, he has made good quantitative neurological growth and excellent qualitative neurological growth." She looked up at us and explained. "*Measurable* growth consists of both quantitative changes—movement from one stage to another on the Profile—and qualitative change, which is improvement within a stage—such as better crawling, or more words of speech. Joseph has moved up in two areas. He has achieved Victories in creeping—and reading!"

Then she referred us to the numbers. "We're really excited about his measurements," she said. She paused to let us digest the information. Values for Joseph's height, chest circumference, and head circumference were recorded, both those taken at his initial visit and today. The table showed that these were all well below the 50th percentile for kids his age. However, it also showed that they were increasing at much more than the average rate. "The growth of a child's chest is a measure of how much his breathing has improved," she said. "Joseph's chest has grown exactly one centimeter. In five months a well two-year-old's chest increases by only a half-centimeter; so he's growing at two hundred percent of the usual rate. That is just excellent, and it's directly attributable to the creeping he has been doing. Now, head growth is an indication of brain growth. As you can see, his head has grown at one hundred eighty percent of average. That, too, is excellent. He's still undersized, but at this rate he is bound to catch up!"

Judy and I grinned at each other excitedly.

"Now," she continued seriously. "What can you tell me about these head measurements?"

We stared at the figures again. I wondered guiltily if somehow they revealed the secret of the many cranial treatments Dr. Frymann had given him since our last visit.

However, Lidwina's question was innocent. Joseph's head circumference was 48.6 centimeters. His chest was 46.9 centimeters. Average figures for well two-year-olds were listed to the side.

"Well," I said hesitantly, "his head is bigger than his chest, but for a well kid it's the other way around."

"Mmm. Right. Joseph still has the proportions of a little baby. By nine months of age, a baby's head and chest *should* be the same size. At one year, and forever after, the chest should be bigger. So, we have to work on that chest even more. Until Joseph's chest is as big as that of an average kid his age, he won't be getting enough oxygen to function optimally."

I sighed. That made sense.

She looked at us thoughtfully, with a faint twinkle in her eyes, and asked a question that we would hear repeated on each of our subsequent revisits: "Are the results you're getting worth the effort that you're putting into the program?"

Judy and I spoke simultaneously. "You bet!"

Lidwina smiled. "Good. I think you'll like the lecture series this week." She handed us a list of the topics that would be covered, starting the next morning. The first was titled "How to Take Your Child to a Higher Mobility Level."

MOST OF THE FIRST DAY'S LECTURES were given by a dynamic, stocky young man who summarized everything the Institutes had learned over the years about mobility, and the techniques they'd devised to move kids from one milestone to the next. We paid particular attention to his discussion of the overhead ladder, also called the Bart DeLone program in honor of the first kid to graduate from it to independent walking. We knew this device was in Joseph's near future.

During one of the breaks, I found our German friends ranting about their translator. This week they'd been given a substitute who hadn't heard the lectures before. The information was new to her, and she was struggling to keep up with the pace at which it was being delivered. Her approach was to listen for several seconds and then summarize, instead of translating simultaneously. Elisabeta's voice rose in frustration. All day she'd been hearing a continuous stream of very rapid English and only short, halting bursts of the language she knew. The bells signaling the end of our break cut off her excited complaints. "*Ich muss nun englishe lernen!*" she cried, waggling both hands in the air as she hurried back to her seat.

On Wednesday we reassembled to hear Glenn Doman talk about his favorite subject, intelligence. Simply being human meant our kids could be *very* intelligent, he said. All they needed was the ability to read, the ability to do math, and a store of factual knowledge. Much of this we'd heard before, but repetition was intentional. Every parent had to be on board.

"The world can forgive paralysis," he told us. "But it won't forgive lack of intelligence. So for a brain-injured kid, the only protection against being thought stupid is to be so extraordinarily bright that the idea never enters anyone's head.

"Fortunately," he added, "that isn't difficult. In fact, I just wish it were as easy to make a paralyzed kid walk as it is to make a brain-injured kid bright.

"The human brain is the only container of which it can be said that the more you put into it, the more it will hold."

As before, he addressed some comments to his absent critics, as well as to anyone present who might still harbor their wrong-headed views. He especially wanted everybody in agreement that high intelligence was a *good* thing.

Because the pursuit of intelligence in a child was easy and fun, it encouraged progress toward other goals as well. "High motivation is a product of success. Low motivation is a product of failure. We're going to teach you how to make your kid a winner, largely through an intelligence program, and *that* will make him highly motivated to achieve anything!"

To my right, Judy was scribbling notes—not what Glenn was saying but rather new ideas for improving our program that occurred to her as he spoke.

"Remember this," Doman admonished us. "In the first six years of a kid's life you can teach him *absolutely anything* that can be presented factually. And he learns it without any difficulty at all. The time before he is six is precious. Use it!"

On the pad in front of me I scrawled a note of my own:

I am so glad we came to this place!

This program didn't ruin lives. It was the best thing we had ever done.

Joseph still had a long way to go. I knew that normal two-year-olds routinely say cute things as they expand their vocabularies. Joseph had emitted very little speech thus far, so whatever intelligence he had was still bottled up inside. But in the context of all his other deficits, this was not too scary—especially since he was now finally becoming mobile. He would get there.

Thursday and Friday were devoted to learning our new programs. As before, the families assembled in the Clinic and the staff began rotating us from one office to the next for individual conferences.

"I've really enjoyed your little guy these last two days," Lidwina began. "I feel like I know him much better now. He's a real character. Especially when it comes to food! Every time someone brought in a bowl of fruit or something, Joseph was the first to see it coming." She described how he scrambled over the bodies of other nonwalkers in order to be the first to eat.

Judy laughed. "He does take his eating seriously. We don't want to use food as a reward, but nothing gets his attention faster."

The object of our discussion was romping energetically on the floor and making a good deal of noise. I thought he smiled at what Lidwina had said about him. She gazed fondly at him for a long moment before handing us the sheets of paper on which we would write the new physical program.

"The purpose of Joseph's physical program," she said, dictating while she herself wrote, "is to continue to mature the midbrain and to prepare him neurologically and physically for walking. Mum and Dad, you must: *(A)* provide Joseph with the opportunity to creep, and creep, *and creep*; *(B)* start him creeping in a 'clambering' environment to give him the vestibular input to go from the quadruped to the biped position; and *(C)* continue patterning him to improve his coordination. But you can reduce the patterning to ten times daily."

"Why is that?" I asked.

She smiled knowingly. "Oh, we think you'll have your hands full accomplishing the rest of what we're going to give you." She handed more papers to us, with detailed instructions for keeping records of the distances he would be covering. "Work up to creeping a mile in a day. Sixteen hundred meters. That's your Revisit goal. I want you to do this a minimum of five times before you come back."

Then she gave us plans for constructing our own overhead ladder—a structure suspended parallel to the floor at just the right height so he could reach up and grasp the rungs. "The purpose of the overhead ladder is to put Joseph in the perfect environment for walking." She explained that she wanted us to begin by having him simply stand under it, holding one rung, for two minutes nonstop. Later, we could prompt him to start moving his feet and reaching from one rung to the next. At that point, we would also begin keeping track of the distance covered in this mode. "The more walking he accumulates using the ladder, the sooner he will walk out from under it."

I studied the diagram. Kimmy's father had given me some pointers on how to build this device, and that part didn't look hard. But it was supposed to be four meters long—a little over twelve feet. *Where were we going to put this thing?*

Our next session was with Dawn, who expressed concern with Joseph's health, diet, and especially his "auditory competence." She didn't like the fact that he seldom looked up when called. "Something is not right in that pathway," she complained. "And it's keeping him from being as bright as he ought to be. I want you to expose him to a wide variety of sounds and to watch closely for his response. We need a very clear evaluation of his ability to locate the source of a given sound, and his ability to hear low volume. Does he understand something when you say it only once? Pay close attention to that, and keep records of what you observe."

Then she showed us a new type of mask, which we were to use in place of the ones we already had. It was a long, tubular plastic bag—the same mask Silvia had demonstrated in Mexico several months earlier. We were to hold it over his mouth and nose for periods of up to two minutes. The maskings were to be done exactly five minutes apart, in groups of four to ten maskings each. This would increase the depth of his breathing for longer periods of time.

Back in the waiting area, Elisabeta told me in alarm that their daughter's new program looked almost impossible. I foolishly assured her that she would achieve her goals easily. My impression so far was that our own program would be fun. The reality would not sink in until after we had been under way for a week or two.

Teruki, who had prescribed the original plan to teach Joseph to read, now met with us to devise a full-fledged intelligence program. "Congratulations on the Reading Victory," he said pleasantly. "Joseph has a functional ability to read. His next goal is to read homemade books for information and pleasure." He showed us examples of what he meant. He examined our reading materials and suggested trying a slightly smaller print size. After performing some calculations on a pad, he said we were to add 560 new words to Joseph's reading vocabulary. Using these, we should then make 330 phrases and sentences for him, and 32 books.

That was just a beginning, of course. The time had also come for building the encyclopedic knowledge and math skills that Glenn had recommended in his lecture. This would mean teaching groups of related facts, in the form of large pictures pasted onto cards. "Our goal here is to grow the cortex of Joseph's brain and increase his store of knowledge," Teruki said. He wanted us to teach at least 510 such "bits of intelligence" by our next visit. "As you cover different subject areas, you'll find that they supplement each other. For example, you might show him maps of all the countries between the U.S. and, say, Brazil. Then you could make him a very enjoyable book entitled 'Joseph Creeps to Brazil.'"

"Creeping to Brazil?" I scoffed. "That sounds pretty far-fetched."

"Not if you add up all the creeping distances he's supposed to be doing. Lidwina tells me he's going to be one busy little boy."

We turned the page in our instructions and saw the math assignment. Judy said, "Good! Joseph likes math." We believed this to be true because, in our eagerness before the first trip we'd already exposed him to these other parts of the intelligence program.

"Yes, well, when you started we asked you to wait on the math and bits because reading is more important," Terry said. "But now that Joseph has demonstrated the ability to read, he's ready to branch out. I'm not surprised to hear that he likes math, because little children have a very easy time with it. Since you've already exposed him to the concept of quantities, you can just review them quickly now and move on to numerals and then equations." He gave us a list of sample equations that demonstrated the four basic functions—*and* fractions, decimals, squares and square roots, and simple algebra! We looked up in amazement. "He should be at about that level when we see you again," Terry said, smiling.

BACK HOME, in the course of obtaining the requested cardiac evaluation, Judy and Joseph ended up in the office of another pediatrician. On the morning before they went in, I warned her, "You're going to be told to quit this."

"How could anybody tell us that now?" Judy demanded, wide-eyed. "We are *cooking!*"

"When you hear it," I continued, "just ask what we're supposed to do instead. Should be interesting."

Excited by the recent victories and all we'd been told, Judy walked into the doctor's office with a lot to say.

This doctor scoffed at Judy's claim that Joseph could read, and refused to let her demonstrate the mask or antiroll device. "We don't approve of that program," she said. "And the best advice I can give you is to discontinue it."

Forewarned, Judy was able to respond. "What do you recommend instead?"

"I think he would be happiest in a day-care setting, with other children."

"Day care? *Day care?* If I left him in day care he would just lie on his back all day and roll his head from side to side. Are you saying that's what he should do?"

"If that's what he *wants* to do, yes. You see, a child needs 'downtime,' in which to just do what he wants."

"But, Doctor, the problem is that he doesn't have the *option* of doing other things! We're trying to give him more options. That's the whole purpose of the patterning and the creeping and everything else we do."

"It hasn't been proved that patterning and creeping have any effect whatsoever on development."

"But surely you've observed—haven't you?—that when older kids have problems learning, for example, that these are often kids who never crawled." The doctor stared at her expressionlessly. "Well anyway, *at the Institutes*, they've observed this. I understand that they have seen about fifteen thousand brain-injured children over the last thirty or forty years; so they must have *some* basis for their position. Doctor, have you seen fifteen thousand brain-injured children?"

"Of course not."

Judy tried to soften her counterattack. "The Institutes are a resource that we feel we have to use. You are another resource. We want to listen to what everyone says, so we can make the most informed decisions. But I think it's obvious that if Joseph is ever going to catch up, I have to make every day count for him."

The doctor continued looking at her silently.

"One reason I wanted to talk with you today," Judy continued, faltering a little under that impassive stare, "was that I need to explore ways of getting funding for the program. We've been filling the gap with donations, but there must be some government or social agency that can help."

This was not to be. The doctor told her that state funding was not available for any treatment being administered outside of California, and furthermore, it would most certainly not be forthcoming in our case. "The American Academy of Pediatrics has issued a position statement on this subject," she said. "Patterning has no medical justification, and therefore nobody is going to support it."

"I see."

"Did you have any other questions?"

They were glaring at each other by now. "No," Judy said coldly. "We just need the referral for the cardiac test, if you don't mind."

13. THE BENEFITS WERE OBVIOUS

Meanwhile, I had been assembling the overhead ladder downstairs in our garage. With the space limitations in our house, I suggested keeping it there. However, Judy protested that she would need continual access to it throughout the day. Finally, we moved our living room furniture to the garage instead.

The first day it was in place, Joseph stood under the ladder ten times. On the second day he actually reached from one rung to the next. He seemed to enjoy it. For once, something was easy. I grew optimistic. "This is great! I know he'll be walking in just a few months!"

Visitors coming through the doorway always bugged their eyes and took a step backward the first time they saw that incongruous scaffolding where the sofa had been. But they believed my prediction. Exciting things were about to happen.

After a week, Joseph was making twelve daily trips along the entire length of the ladder. We helped by showing him which arm and leg to move next. Sometimes he went from one end to the other in less than two minutes.

On the other hand, this progress seemed to occur at the expense of the creeping. The hospital test indicated that, despite the heart murmur, Joseph had "functionally normal cardiac status," which was good news, of course. But how, then, could we account for the fact that his daily totals were dipping to figures below 300 meters? We just could not motivate him to do more.

In fact, he grew increasingly exasperated with us for asking more of him. Matters came to a head one Saturday morning in May, when I urged him to start yet another series of laps around the room. Joseph abruptly threw himself face-down on the floor, screamed hysterically, and refused to go another inch. We waited until he was calm and then Judy tried, with the same result.

These efforts were at a standstill, and that's how they were going to remain until Lidwina could be reached by phone.

The first person we spoke to, however, was Silvia, who happened to call from Mexico just then.

"How is your program going?"

"Horrible!" Judy said bitterly.

"*Horrible?* Has Joseph made progress?"

"Well, yes …"

"Then it can't be 'horrible.'" They talked for several minutes. After ranting about Joseph's stubbornness, Judy described the recent confrontation with the doctor, since that still troubled her. Finally, Silvia said, "Whatever you do, don't get so discouraged that you give up. And *don't* let anyone tell you to quit! Remember that when you're working hardest is when you see the best results."

Later that same morning, our next-door neighbor Mike came to pattern and stayed on a few minutes after we had finished. Joseph stretched and climbed up from the patterning table into his arms.

"Wasn't it good of Mike to help us!" I said. "Can you give him a pat?"

To everyone's surprise, Joseph did just that. He patted Mike affectionately on the shoulder.

I was delighted with this unusual responsiveness, but Mike seemed uneasy about something. Whatever it was, he was having trouble finding the right words.

Nell arrived early for the noon patterning session, and we introduced them. It was time for Mike to go, but now he finally spoke up and asked if we'd seen the news on TV.

"Oh, I know what you're going to say," said Nell grimly. "That was a tragedy, what happened with that family in Pennsylvania."

Judy and I looked at them blankly. We seldom caught more than the bare highlights of current events.

Nell explained that an Institutes family had been unable to keep up with their program. The child had been sick. He wasn't achieving his goals. In a desperate and irrational state, the mother had shot and killed him.

Mike finally made his point. "I just want you to know that any time you guys need a break, or you feel like you're losing perspective, I'll be happy to keep Joseph over at my place for a while. I mean that."

"The same goes for me," cried Nell. "Free babysitting!"

"Gosh, folks," I said doubtfully. "Thanks for saying that, but—we aren't all that stressed out. Are we, Judy?"

"We don't need time off," she muttered. "We just need to get this boy well."

"Well, the offer stands," Mike told us. "Don't wait till you're desperate." And thus unburdened, he left.

Naturally, this revelation was uppermost in our minds now, but Judy wouldn't let Nell talk about it further as we patterned. "Joseph doesn't need to hear this," she insisted. Then, bending over and speaking to him, she said, "That boy's mommy made a big mistake. She was wrong. But *we love you, Joseph*! You're getting better every day, and so are we!"

Several other patterners had also seen the item on the news, and suddenly they all wanted to ease our load by looking after Joseph. A secretary in my office brought in a short article about it from the local newspaper. It began:

BROOMALL, Pa. (AP) – A mother who enlisted 70 volunteers to help teach her severely retarded 2 1/2-year-old son to crawl had considered suicide before she shot him to death, her lawyer said. "She was unable to cope and unable to handle the whole situation." ...

The article continued with an account of how the mother "telephoned her husband several minutes after the shooting. He drove home, found the boy's body and called police, authorities said. Paramedics found the boy on the floor where he usually napped, a pacifier 6 inches from his mouth. The parents were on the front lawn, crying."

Although we wouldn't talk about it in Joseph's presence, we did want to understand how the thing could have happened. The family lived in a suburb of Philadelphia, so Judy called her cousin Michael to see what he could tell us. He responded by mailing several lengthy articles from the *Philadelphia Inquirer* that appeared over the next several weeks. Reading these, we saw that in many ways this child's program had been like Joseph's.

> Every 20 minutes, she put the severely brain-damaged child on a table and, for five minutes, turned his head from side to side while the volunteers pumped his legs.
>
> She held a plastic mask over his face to increase oxygen circulation in his brain. She flashed cue cards at him. She crawled beside him on her hands and knees.
>
> And when she was done, she did it all over again. Every 20 minutes. Every day.

He had been born 9 1/2 weeks premature. At five months, his brain injury became evident because he wasn't reaching normal developmental milestones. And so the family "set out on a yearlong odyssey that included physical therapists, doctors and a nursery school for disabled children." Nothing had worked, and "the last hope for their son, who could not sit up or roll over at an age when other children can run, was the Institutes for the Achievement of Human Potential."

Reporters interviewed patterners and neighbors, who described the rigid schedule the family had followed. The mother "had no time for anything else," one said. "Somebody must have shopped for her because we could see the groceries left in the hall. Everybody wondered how they could keep up the pace." Another said that the mother "was just exhausted. I wish she would have taken the time to run a comb through her hair … When did she clean? When did she wash? The house was in shambles."

In spite of the strain, the family had been ardent believers in their son's program. "Something about it clicked for them intellectually," one patterner said. "They said it just seemed right." As usual, the authorities were less enthusiastic. One article concluded:

> Physicians and psychologists are frequently critical of the Institutes' program, condemning it as scientifically unproven. At worst, they say, it can raise parents' expectations beyond what is possible for their child to accomplish.

A physician was quoted as saying, "When I heard about Eric's death, my own personal reaction was that I wondered that something like this hadn't happened earlier."

"Now that is a callous, cowardly reaction," I raged, throwing down the paper. "What has this guy done to help brain-injured kids recover? He's just protecting the status quo."

"If these experts got behind the families on program, they could make a difference," Judy said bitterly. "With organizations like the Regional Center, that supposedly exist to help, we should have been able to call somebody when we came back from our first trip to the Institutes, to get support. That's what Doran's mother did in England. She may have been a single parent, but she had dedicated helpers assigned by a social agency. But we have to waste our energy always trying to prove we're legitimate. If it weren't for ordinary people who think for themselves, and know a worthy cause when they see it, we never would have gotten started. I think the experts *want* to see us fail!"

THE STORY SEEMED TO TROUBLE JUDY more than it did me. She even spoke of writing to the unhappy woman, although I couldn't imagine what there could be to say. The wholesale offers to baby-sit did not tempt us, but we did invest one evening's time in going to a class on stress reduction. It was sponsored by the support group for parents of disabled children, and Judy saw several familiar faces from the previous year.

"Are you guys patterning now?" one asked her.

"You bet! We've been to Philadelphia twice. Joseph's doing great!"

"We pattern sometimes, too."

"Good! How often?"

"I don't know. About ten times a week. I'd like to do more, but my husband and I both have jobs. So …" She shrugged apologetically.

We found the evening enlightening, but not because of the presentation. The speaker talked about stages of grief and various coping techniques, such as music and mutual support among family members. "There's a tacky bumper sticker you may have noticed around town," he said. "It reads, 'It used to be wine, women, and song but now it's beer, the old lady, and TV.'" He smiled sadly. "I'll bet everyone in this room could come up with variations. Such as, 'Now it's physical therapy, IEPs, and late-night runs to do the grocery shopping.'" He paused. "Our lives are totally different now because of our children. It's good for us to recognize and acknowledge the sacrifices we've made—and especially the sacrifices our spouses have made. Whether it's bowling or playing bridge with friends or some hobby, these things can be an important part of a person's life and self-image. People tend not to really notice when somebody gives up an activity that used to be important. But sometimes it can make a big difference if you just put an arm around your spouse and say, 'Honey, I've noticed that you never do—*whatever*—anymore.' Moments like that can be beautiful."

A young mother just behind us asked him to suggest anything that could keep her going. "I know my son is never going to improve," she said in a dull, matter-of-fact tone. "And after a while it just gets hard to keep on going through the motions, day after day." The speaker gave her a lingering, sympathetic smile. Then he said, "It's quite possible to have a successful, happy life in spite of problems and disappointments. And so, even though you say your child will never improve, it's important to remember that you're still very important to him. How does he feel about you and about himself? No matter what problems he may have, he'll have something very important going for him if he likes being with you and doing things with you. Together, you can still look forward to meeting the challenges of life as they come up."

The lady Judy had spoken with a few minutes earlier volunteered that she relieved tension by unloading her pent-up frustrations on her child. "He's nonverbal. He probably can't understand. So it doesn't matter what I say to him," she said.

The room was uncomfortably quiet for a moment after she spoke. I turned in my seat, uselessly trying to reconcile her good looks and apparently upbeat attitude with this confession.

The speaker's wife took the floor next to demonstrate some yoga exercises that might ease tensions more constructively. She recommended finding a quiet corner of the house, and even blindfolding oneself while practicing daily "restorative asanas," which, she said, could promote a healthy immune system. She emphasized the importance of beginning such a routine *before* one became too debilitated by tension, and warned that prolonged, unrelieved stress could open the way to dire physical and emotional maladies.

When the formal part of the evening was over, everyone clustered around the refreshment table. One mother was selling subscriptions to *Exceptional Parent* magazine. Paging through sample copies, I saw ads for wheelchairs and similar devices for accommodating to disability.

Judy's old pal Peggy, from the parents' group, materialized beside her. "Hi! I didn't know you were here!" she enthused.

Judy said, "We don't get out often, but we made an exception for tonight." Then she asked about Peggy's six-year-old son, whom we had last seen at a support group meeting in his wheelchair.

"He's doing really good. He had that surgery on his legs, you know, where they cut some of the muscles? Now his legs aren't all twisted up, and he can stand with a walker. So—he's learning to walk!"

"Great," Judy said feebly. Inside, we were both cringing at the idea of putting a child through such a procedure. I was hearing Glenn Doman's emphatic voice. *Brain injury is in the* brain! *Not in the hands, not in the legs, in the brain!* Almost apologetically she added, "Joseph's walking under an overhead ladder."

"Really?"

"O yes. He's up to thirteen trips a day now." Inevitably, her enthusiasm overtook her, and she began reciting more details about our program than any casual acquaintance would care to hear. Then she produced a snapshot of Joseph standing up tall and straight, with his hands gripping a rung of the ladder.

"Isn't that wonderful. It was good seeing you." And Peggy turned away as abruptly as she'd appeared. She was standing with her back to us, apparently deep in conversation with someone else, before Judy had time to put away the photo.

"Golly," she said as we walked out to the car. "Do you think I offended her, bragging about Joseph?"

"She may have felt that you stole her thunder."

"I only mentioned the overhead ladder because she said they're using a walker. It's so much better to use the ladder because reaching up expands the chest for better breathing, and it enables the child to stand up straight. We went through a lot to learn that. I thought she'd be interested in knowing about it."

"She chose a different route." Without covering any new ground, we debated again whether we had any moral obligation to share the facts, as we understood them, with such people.

"Well, at any rate," I said, "we discovered something tonight. You don't have to be on program with the Institutes to be stressed!"

"As if we didn't know. These other parents are just as worn down as we are. And *they* don't have the hope of one day seeing their kids recover!"

FINALLY I GOT IN TOUCH WITH LIDWINA and described Joseph's refusal to creep. "He's probably bored," she said. "But you have to win."

"Bored. I guess that's it. But he was crying so hard we worried that there still might be some physical problem."

"Is he creeping at all?"

"He *can* come like a shot to the kitchen when I offer him a banana."

Lidwina laughed. "Try putting him on a steep grassy slope outside," she said. "He should find it easier to creep downhill. It's OK if you carry him up to the top of the hill. Let him just creep down it. That should get your distances back up."

I knew just the place for this—Presidio Park, on the hill above historic Old Town San Diego. We took him there, and I placed him at the top of a long, very steep grassy slope. I felt sure he welcomed the change in venue. I got down on my hands and knees beside him, noticing the added weight on my arms.

As with the inclined plane we'd used a year earlier, the way ahead was so steep that forward motion was easier than staying put. From this elevation we could see a long way across Old Town and the freeway, and all the way out to the ocean. Just ahead lay a broad, grassy expanse, dotted with eucalyptus and olive trees and the occasional sunbather. I'd paced off a distance of fifty meters and, as before, Judy marked both ends of the course with orange pylons. She was waiting by the marker at the lower end.

"Well, Joseph, my boy," I said brightly. "Let's go."

We were making progress again!

Judy hugged our little boy when we reached her, and gave him a little snack. Then it was her turn to take him down the hill. She carried him back to the starting point, and I waited for them to return, beckoning energetically whenever I thought Joseph was looking my way.

After an hour of this, we'd accomplished only 300 meters.

Even so, we went home feeling greatly encouraged. We were going to achieve that mile after all.

From that point on, at least one of us took Joseph to the park every day. We became intimately familiar with our hillside there. Judy found a sturdy waterproof coverall for Joseph to wear when the grass was wet. On hot days, we modified our course to take advantage of the shade trees. On weekends and the Fourth of July, when the park was crowded, we adopted a circuitous route that avoided all the picnic blankets while still maintaining a downhill direction. Joseph invariably wanted to invite himself onto blankets we passed, especially when food was in evidence. He howled in protest when we steered him away, but saved his most pitiful complaints for the benefit of any grandmotherly types who might sympathize. We certainly drew our share of puzzled looks from these people. Judy and I just kept our heads down and drove him on past all distractions.

The knees of our jeans wore through quickly, as did the patches Judy sewed over them. Joseph's pants showed rapid wear, also. Judy contacted a seamstress, who made him two indestructible canvas creeping outfits with padded knees.

After a month, Joseph was covering 100 meters nonstop in as little as eight minutes, and we were up to a thousand meters per day. I was becoming obsessed with the challenge of making that mile, but the days just weren't long enough. Some evenings after work I'd take him back to the park for his second or even third time of the day. We'd make our way down the hill together and I'd carry him back to the top. And we'd creep down again, until the daylight was fading and the ground was becoming cold.

Still, the next morning he would start at zero, facing a goal of sixteen more downhill trips.

The daily patterning requirement still consumed an appreciable amount of time, since we had to meet our volunteers back at the house. Unfortunately, patterning often had to conform to their schedules rather than ours. More than once, Judy found them waiting on the doorstep when she and Joseph rushed home from the park.

Afterwards, quite often she'd load him into the car and race back to the park for another hour or two of creeping, only to have him fall asleep in the five minutes it took to drive there. Sometimes she was convinced he did this on purpose.

Repeatedly carrying Joseph up the hill became a real chore—especially for Judy. In fact, carrying him *anywhere* was becoming a problem she couldn't ignore, since his weight was aggravating an old back injury.

Lidwina suggested that we designate one day a week as our "marathon creeping day" and make all-out distance efforts then. We chose Saturdays, when I was home, and this arrangement took some of the strain off her.

"Now I've *really* got an incentive to get this boy walking," Judy groaned one day, pressing palms against her aching lower back.

Nell, who had come to help with patterning, said, "Use a stroller! The Institutes will never know. Think of yourself!"

"But if I use a stroller, he'll learn that mobility is something other people do *for* him, and not something he does for himself. Also, by carrying him around, I have a vested interest in seeing that he walks. Because I *know* I can't carry him forever!"

"If you carry him or use a stroller, either way, he's not doing it for himself," Nell rejoined reasonably.

"Maybe," I suggested, "the theory is that they don't want us to get comfortable with this situation. Like Judy says, we've got to stay motivated to change it."

Nell gave me a withering look. Most of what she said these days betrayed a distrust of those people at the Institutes who were behind all the pressure being manifested in our lives. By this point, I think she was more concerned with Judy's well-being than Joseph's. If I sided with the Institutes, then I was suspect as well.

Likewise, Mike had told us he "didn't like" the Institutes. We never complained about them, but several of our friends had concluded that the organization was altogether too rigid. Nancy had seen Glenn Doman interviewed on TV and thought him smugly self-righteous.

The general feeling was that he'd set up a potentially damaging situation for families that were already highly stressed. We chose to ignore that point of view, of course. The benefits of sticking with the program were still obvious.

JOSEPH'S SPEED under the ladder improved steadily. By the middle of June he could make a trip in as little as 48 seconds. We were well on our way toward the Revisit goal of ninety percent independence. On the 22nd he went three consecutive rungs with no assistance at all. Lidwina said we could hasten progress even further if we lowered the far end of the ladder by an inch or so. This accomplished our purpose, and within two weeks he was walking the distance while we stood back and cheered. I still felt confident that he was nearly ready to step away from it and just stroll across the room, but Lidwina reminded me not to push for that before he crept the mile.

THAT BREAKTHROUGH occurred on a Saturday in early July. Joseph and I logged 800 meters of creeping in the morning and then came home for lunch. He fell asleep during a patterning session. Judy then departed to run some errands, leaving me to look back and forth nervously between my napping son and the clock.

Dorothy was scheduled to join us for patterning at three o'clock, but if we hoped to make our goal we would have to be back on the slopes by then.

Perhaps Dorothy and another patterner could be persuaded to come now, while he slept!

Dorothy's phone was busy, and remained so. I called Nancy and Greg, and they were happy to fill in. Joseph awoke at the end of the second patterning session. Now we could return to the park, but Dorothy's line was still busy! I called a neighbor, who agreed to knock on her door and cancel her appointment for me.

Then Joseph and I were off. He completed his first mile that afternoon.

I gave it a tremendous buildup as we approached the pylon for the final time. "This is it!" I sang. "Just twenty meters more! Just ten meters! Joseph *is* going to do it! A whole mile in one day! *Sixteen hundred meters!*" I hoisted him high in the air and danced in a giddy circle. He giggled. So did I. Horns blared bombastically in my head, as in the movie *Rocky* when Sylvester Stallone sprints to the top of the stairs.

And we still had fifteen minutes in which to return home for the next scheduled patterning session.

It was the major accomplishment of the year.

Of course, daily creeping did not end with this achievement. Lidwina confirmed our Revisit date at the Institutes when I told her the good news, but she reminded us to do a minimum of four more one-mile days in the interim. Surprisingly, these were no longer difficult. We even managed to work in short dips in a swimming pool as rewards for Joseph between creeping and patterning sessions.

Such rewards really helped motivate him, and clearly, that was important. A helpless parcel no more, Joseph had become an active participant in his program. His cooperation was vital.

"How on earth do you get him to *do* it?" my parents asked. Surely, from an outsider's perspective, it seemed strange. We crept right through groups of people tossing Frisbees. We crept past startled sweethearts, necking on their blankets. We even found our way, inadvertently, into people's vacation snapshots and home videos. Who knows what they said about us? On the other hand, who cares?

Thanks to the daily contact with our volunteers, we didn't feel as estranged from the rest of the world as we might have otherwise. Also, occasionally we exchanged short letters with the families we'd met in Philadelphia. These were generally helpful, but one day we received an unexpected message from Elsa's father. He wrote, "We have, as you might imagine, been having difficulty taking care of everything. We were scheduled for our Revisit in August but have decided to discontinue the program. The strain was too much on us." They were now busy renovating their house and making plans for another child—upbeat pursuits to be sure, but the tone of his letter was glum.

On the other hand, our former neighbors in Virginia, who had the child with Down syndrome, were now well under way with an Institutes program of their own. "Thank you so much for telling us about it!" they wrote. "This is so exciting, and we've nothing to lose."

Anticipation mounted for the upcoming third trip to Philly. We too were excited, and events continued to justify that. One night Judy sang the Pat-a-Cake nursery rhyme, modifying the words slightly.

"… and put it in the oven for Joseph and Mommy," she concluded.

"And Daddy!" Joseph insisted.

"And Daddy! You're right!" She cried, hugging him and laughing. "Joseph and Mommy, *and* Daddy!"

There was a new feeling in the air that we were all on the same side.

14. NORMAL?

We arrived in Philadelphia during what must have been an unusually brutal heat wave. Certainly, it was brutal by San Diego standards. Judy's aunt and uncle had fled to the seashore, but they'd said we could share the house with their grown son Rob. We saw little of him, as he had closed off one wing of the house (the air conditioned part) and ventured out only on quick sorties to the refrigerator for beer. Fortunately, as always, we spent most of our time at the Institutes, where things were much cooler. We actually looked forward to that frigid lecture hall.

Our first meeting there was with a young "black jacket" named Matt Newell. We had read about Matt in the Institutes' magazine, but this was the first we'd seen of him. We spent an hour getting acquainted, as he studied our documentation and evaluated Joseph. The moment of truth came when he tried to test for reading and understanding using our intelligence materials. Joseph correctly identified a painting called *The Baptism of Christ* over another choice, but he squirmed and looked away the rest of the time.

"This is pretty typical," I told him sadly.

Matt wasn't perturbed. "I'll talk it over with the rest of the staff during the week and we'll give it some thought. But he's obviously made real progress, especially with his primary goals. There are still some weak areas in the auditory pathway. But you've done good work!"

As before, Elaine checked Joseph's measurements. She announced that he had less body fat and that he showed generally increased dimensions. Then she handed us off to Lidwina for the summary.

We found Lidwina looking relaxed and pleased with our results. The most dramatic physical change was a chest increase 371 percent of normal. "This is what we like to see," Lidwina told us. "He's getting a big 'tank' now for better respiration, and believe me he's going to need it to support his increased activity level.

"Now, Mum and Dad," she continued. "We need to try and establish what it is that is keeping Joseph from walking. Is it strength? Is it vision? Is it balance? Is it coordination?"

She waited patiently for us to sort through these choices. Judy and I eliminated some alternatives, such as insufficient strength, right away. Finally I made a stab at the answer. "I would have to say that the main problem is balance."

"I think so, too. Later on this week we'll be showing you some activities that will address the balance areas of his brain."

THE MOST NOTABLE LECTURES this time were devoted to the key subject of respiration.

"If you were deprived of food," Glenn said, "Eventually you would experience a range of injuries resulting from malnutrition. The same would apply if you had no fluids. Now, hypoxia, which means insufficient oxygen, results in the brain injury, and the brain dysfunction, of virtually every kid who comes to the Institutes. What's worse, because of *continuing* respiratory problems due to their brain injuries, brain-injured kids remain victims of chronic hypoxia. All of them! Their problem is that they can't breathe and do anything else at the same time."

To illustrate the point, he recommended sprinting until we were gasping for breath and then trying to complete a simple task like singing "Happy Birthday." He even demonstrated what the result might be.

This, he said, was the one problem holding our kids back from greater progress.

"In the case of a midbrain-injured child, this condition actually gets worse as he grows bigger, and his need for oxygen increases. One result is that he will be smaller than other kids his age. Another result is that his function will not improve. In fact, he may lose abilities. A brain-injured child who looks normal and speaks normally today may by adulthood be rigid, strapped into a wheelchair, and unintelligible to anyone other than close family members who have been with him over the years as his condition gradually worsened.

"If I could take all the midbrain-injured children and put my hand on their heads and say, 'Kid, breathe properly,' I expect that we would graduate them from the Institutes within six months. I can't do that. But we're accomplishing it the hard way."

He moved on to a survey of methods developed at the Institutes that improved breathing—various forms of masking and respiratory patterning, which he called "passive" measures, and the "active" measures: crawling, creeping, walking, running, gymnastics, and brachiating.

Later that afternoon, Matt and other staff members arranged what they called a Practicum. We returned from a break to find an enormous overhead ladder suspended about seven feet above the floor at the front of the auditorium.

Our mission, Matt explained, would include brachiating the entire length of the ladder and then walking a balance beam.

As far as the dads in the room were concerned, this looked like fun. But Judy approached the ladder with dread. "I don't think I can do this," she muttered.

"Come on! Everybody else is managing."

"So? It'll be that much worse if I can't."

I'll always remember seeing Judy swinging hand over hand all the way down the ladder, and I'll always remember her startled smile afterwards.

"You looked so graceful!" one of the mothers assured her.

We returned to our seats. "I decided it wouldn't be fair for me to ask Joseph to perform if I weren't willing to try new things myself," she whispered to me.

"And see! You did fine! This is probably the way it feels for a kid when he faces a new challenge." I thought about it and added, "Bet that's the main reason they had us do it."

We were already anxious to get back home and resume work. All we needed was specific guidance on what to do next.

On Thursday, Lidwina led us outside to see how Joseph managed in a "clambering environment." We placed him on a steep, grassy hillside and watched him inch his way up it. The purpose was to transfer more of his weight to his legs.

Then she wanted to see him perform beneath their overhead ladder. We set it to 94 centimeters, the same height he was accustomed to at home, and I helped him grasp the first rung. Several staff members gathered to applaud his efforts, which obviously spurred him on.

Finally, she demonstrated several forms of "vestibular stimulation" that she wanted us to begin giving him. "Spinning around and somersaulting and being upside-down are all ways of growing the balance areas of the brain," she said. "What you're doing is putting the child in as many different positions as possible with respect to gravity. Normal kids do this to *themselves* all the time. In fact, they *love* to do it. They jump on beds and roll down hills and do cartwheels and ride on swings. Often, brain-injured kids aren't able to do this for themselves. And in fact, they're handled like little china teacups. What they need, however, is double or triple the ordinary dose. So in addition to more clambering and ladder walking, I want Joseph to start getting *lots* of vestibular stimulation. Be sure to vary the intensity and duration of each procedure so you'll continue to challenge him. The brain gets accustomed to something very quickly, and then it's no longer a challenge. Later we'll move to actual gymnastics, which is a high-level balance development activity."

Between meetings with the staff people, we circulated among the other families, as before. The children in our group were all continu-ing to show encouraging progress, especially a tiny boy with Down syndrome from Belgium. His mother told Judy that the program con-sumed two-thirds of their income, but we could easily see why they stayed with it. Again we thought of our former neighbors in Virginia and their son, now on program. We mentioned them to Lidwina dur-ing our debriefing.

"Physically and intellectually, those kids do quite well on program," Lidwina said. "Their main problems are physiological. Those problems can often be corrected, and when that happens you start to see a kid who really shines. We now have some who are entering the realm of total wellness!"

Then Judy broached the unavoidable subject of the mother who had shot her own child.

Lidwina shook her head sadly. "Eric had been making splendid prog-ress. In five months he began crawling for the first time, *and* crawled a total of twelve miles. So the problem wasn't that the program wasn't working for him. And we can't say that it was too difficult, either. Thousands of parents have done the program with their kids, and this is the first time anyone reacted that way. Of course, we try very hard to screen families before they begin, as you know."

"I felt a lot of empathy for the mother when I first heard about it," Judy said. "I know it's easy to lose your perspective and become dis-couraged."

"And that's another reason we want you to stay in touch," Lidwina said.

BACK HOME, we perceived a pattern that recurred with each of our trips East. There'd been a time when all our volunteers felt good about coming to help this little boy. Some of them didn't feel that way now. *This was taking too long.* They continued showing up, usually, until our week away broke the momentum. Afterwards, they couldn't seem to get started again. Judy recognized the signs of discontent and made it easy for them to go. They'd given many hours of their time, and we said goodbye with no hard feelings.

And of course people's circumstances changed. Shirley had graduated from college and found a job back East. Marge said her family had drafted her to look after the grandchildren. (Actually, we learned later, a family member had been diagnosed with AIDS and Marge was afraid of adding to Joseph's problems by possibly exposing him to that.) Whatever the reason, we found ourselves contemplating a lot of blanks in the patterning schedule.

Recalling the formula that had worked so well before, I made a new flier with the heading, 'HELP A CHILD LEARN TO WALK!' and posted it at the college.

"The people who start now will see the real miracles," I predicted. "But they won't understand how far we've come."

Fortunately, our patterning requirement was now down to a mere six sessions per day. And we still had some diehards in Nancy and Greg, Nell, Sally, Dorothy, Marzi, and Carolyn. Four ladies with whom I worked, Ruth, Elaine, Betty, and Isabel, were also in for the long haul. They filled in the gaps in our schedule, and we persevered, regardless of what happened. Even a power outage just meant that we patterned by the cozy glow of candlelight.

To get started with the balance development activities, we needed several pieces of equipment, including a swivel chair. Judy took care of locating these items on our first weekend home. Joseph and I returned from a morning of clambering up hills at the park to find her attaching a seat belt to a bar stool that she'd found in a thrift shop.

"It only cost one dollar!" she crowed.

I gave the seat a spin. "Well, it's perfect." The object was to secure Joseph in the chair and to rotate him at different speeds, frequently alternating the direction. This was called "upright vertical pirouetting." It was to be followed immediately by upside-down vertical pirouetting, and to accomplish that Joseph had to hang from straps looped around his feet while we spun him from an overhead swivel hook.

Joseph let us put him through these gyrations without complaint. I believe he enjoyed them. But we found that making the transition from the chair to the hook was a little awkward, and Judy vowed to improve the setup.

At some point during Joseph's program, I recognized an important difference in the way Judy and I approached things. It was my nature to grit my teeth and forge ahead through all difficulties. I was the one who accomplished the major goals with him, such as the long-distance creeping. But as the program became progressively more involved, I had less mental energy for analysis.

Judy, on the other hand, constantly looked for ways to improve our operations. In the short term, this made her less productive, and I berated her for wasting time on schemes that often led nowhere. But occasionally she redeemed herself in a big way.

She wrestled with the problem of how to suspend Joseph from the hook until one day she had it. Joseph needed a table on wheels! Then she could move him from the swivel chair to the table, roll it into place beneath the hook, attach the straps, and push the table away—all without endangering Joseph or straining herself.

Andy and Donna, a husband-and-wife team who patterned with her on Wednesdays, donated an old metal cart. This, it turned out, could double as a patterning table. The heavy wooden desk we had been using was thereby rendered unnecessary, and it followed the rest of our furniture to the garage.

PHYSICAL EXCELLENCE was still Joseph's top priority. To achieve it, he had a new schedule of creeping distances, to be achieved in an uphill-and-downhill environment, and an ever-increasing number of walks under the overhead ladder.

The months passed, and autumn was turning into another of San Diego's mild winters. Now that we spent so much time outdoors, Judy and I congratulated ourselves on living in a place where the climate was predictably good. We took Joseph clambering every day. One area in the park offered an expanse of steep, grassy mounds, which actually covered the ruins of an old fort. Here, Joseph began experiencing the sensation of going up on his hands and feet—"elephant walking," as Lidwina called it. Judy or I would get him started up a hill in this manner and then run ahead to hide behind the crest. On good days he would laugh and scramble after us. We noted that he was showing increasing independence; we guided less and followed more, letting him pick his own course.

By Interim Report time, Joseph had surpassed his goal of 130 daily trips under the overhead ladder. He was doing twelve trips nonstop in as little as four and a half minutes, while Judy or I walked alongside providing encouragement. I was disappointed that he had not progressed to standing alone, but there was always the challenge of meeting the next day's goal to keep us occupied. Lidwina said to begin weekly marathon days under the ladder, beginning with 160 trips and adding thirty trips to the previous total each week.

PHYSIOLOGICAL EXCELLENCE continued to run a close second place on our list of objectives, and we were now attacking that with yet another kind of breathing mask. Elaine had given us a variation that had an opening covered by a cloth screen. A child wearing this could breathe in all the fresh air he wanted, but he had to make a strong inhalation to pull it through the fabric. This exertion trained him to breathe more deeply. Also, because it was possible to wear this for a longer time than other masks, the benefit was greater. Our program called for twenty such maskings per day, each one five to ten minutes long. After the first month, Joseph was able to tolerate it for the full ten minutes.

And finally there remained the goal of intellectual excellence. We continued making Bits and showing them whenever Joseph seemed receptive. I felt that the reading had to become more interesting, and we kept looking for ways to spice it up. "Joseph!" We'd cry. "Here are five words that describe your walking. It's *wonderful, outstanding, incredible, marvelous,* and *terrific!*" Judy flashed word cards bearing each of these adjectives with the speed of a faro dealer—and Joseph regarded them with poker-faced inscrutability.

We had been directed to move into written sentences, preferably sentences that conveyed factual information. Every night after Joseph had gone to bed, Judy and I would sort through the growing collection of Bits that we had already showed to him. Then we'd select pairs of related pictures and write a statement about each. "The pug has a curly tail." "The chow has a black tongue." We showed each set to him twice a day for no more than five days and then replaced them all with new material. "The bulldog is friendly but looks grouchy." "Schnauzers like to run and play." It was a great way to introduce new words. "The rhinoceros is a solitary animal." On the other hand, "Sea lions live together in large groups called colonies."

We learned a few things, ourselves, too. For example, endeavoring to distill something from an encyclopedia entry about William Penn, I spotted the origin of that promise on the Pennsylvania license plates. As a Quaker, he had been in the Society of *Friends*! It was fun to learn—or to be reminded of facts I had once known. It was important, however, to avoid the trap of doing research for our own enjoyment. Joseph needed a variety of discrete, easily digestible facts for the next day, and somewhere along the way *we* needed to get some sleep!

Our biggest hurdle was finding information likely to appeal to him. The chance to see new intelligence materials still did not constitute a reward—something Joseph would exert himself to earn. Eventually it would, everyone at the Institutes still insisted, and we wanted to believe them. In the back of my mind, however, I worried. We were muscling him through the physical activities well enough, but I didn't know how to get more performance on the intellectual side.

"He says new words from time to time, but doesn't continue to use them," we complained to Lidwina. One morning Judy had straightened the bed and then commented, "There! That looks neat!" Joseph agreed. "Looks neat," he said. Judy rushed to the phone and called me with the news that he'd spoken. But that was a one-time performance. Days would go by with no speech at all. Then, on a Monday morning, after coping with two overcharged parents all weekend, he would glance at the door and say, "Where Da?" "Daddy's at work today, Joseph." Judy replied. "He goes to work on Mondays." Joseph would nod, as if that was the answer he had expected, and Judy would call me again. And then again more wordless days or weeks ensued.

"Inconsistency is common with all children at this stage of mobility," Lidwina told us. "My advice to boost language onward is simply to get in maximum creeping." And it was back to the park once more.

Judy kept looking for encouraging signs of progress every day. Sometimes she even manufactured them. There was one evening, for example, when I found little handprints all over the mirror doors of our bedroom closet. It was a mess that might have sent some mothers running for the Windex. But Judy had propped Joseph up against the mirrors and created the smudges intentionally, just to make things look more normal.

We did still aspire to being a normal family.

There was no space available in our house for erecting a Christmas tree, but Judy improvised by hanging lights and ornaments from the framework of Joseph's ladder. One Saturday morning I was encouraging him back and forth under this newly decorated structure when Carolyn appeared at our door.

"I've been addressing our Christmas cards, and I got to your name," she said. "I thought it would be better if I just came over and gave this to you personally rather than putting it in the mail." Inside the card was a huge check, made out to the Institutes.

I looked at her, totally speechless. She and Ric had previously donated a smaller amount toward our bill, but the generosity of this gift, coming from a single family's budget, eclipsed anything we had ever anticipated. I knew that I shouldn't accept it. It was too much. From time to time, Judy's parents and mine had given us money, too, but Carolyn wasn't even related. We couldn't accept it. But we did. Our bill at the Institutes was continuing to mount, public interest in our campaign had tapered off, and several charitable organizations had recently declined to help. Sally's early prediction regarding our savings had been accurate, and I felt that there was no choice.

Carolyn smiled at my embarrassment. "Ric and I support what you guys are doing. We *want* to help. Well, anyway, I've got a lot to do today, so I'd better run. Merry Christmas!"

I probably didn't even speak as she left.

ANOTHER PART OF THE ASSIGNED INTELLIGENCE PROGRAM was called the "Family Law." Joseph was to learn that it was no longer acceptable to yell or cry. If he became too loud, he had to go away from everybody for a few minutes. I'm not at all sure he viewed that outcome as a penalty. At any rate, he still yelled and cried at times. Again we called on Lidwina for help. "It is very hard on Judy and me to listen to screaming while marching him back and forth under the ladder, for example," I said. "Our own judgment and effectiveness suffer."

She suggested eliminating certain foods from Joseph's diet. Three weeks passed, with no dramatic changes in his irritability. Then we tried adding a calcium-magnesium dietary supplement, which if anything, made matters worse.

We would be at the limits of our patience, and then, inexplicably, Joseph would have a good day. One marathon day in late January he performed 530 trips under the ladder. The total time spent walking in this manner was 162 minutes, and Joseph was cheerful and perfectly cooperative throughout.

The next evening was different. He began by whining, and the volume of his complaints built up steadily until I could not ignore them.

I stopped and hugged him. "Joseph, I know this gets tiresome for you." He laid his head on my shoulder and let me rub his little back.

"You're a real trooper to keep it up so faithfully. I promise that you won't have to do this ladder walking much longer. Only until you learn to walk by yourself! Then we can take the ladder down! And, boy, walking will be a *lot* of fun."

Joseph was quiet, listening. I decided to explain things further.

"You see, Joseph, you have what is called a 'brain injury.' That's why it's hard for you to do the things other kids do. But this program is going to fix that for you. The ladder walking, and the patterning, and the creeping, and the masking, and—"

As I listed his many chores Joseph began to cry again. It was a forlorn, desolate whimpering, and it broke my heart to hear him. "Hold on, son! Remember that these are *good* things to do! They help you, even though they aren't always fun. Your Mommy and Daddy sure do admire the way you keep on working to accomplish your goals. We love you so very much, and we'll be so happy when you're well. You just don't know how happy we'll all be."

We took a short break, and then he was ready to go on again.

SEVERAL VOLUNTEERS WHO PLAYED MUSICAL INSTRU-MENTS were now coming by to give demonstrations. Judy had devised this variation on the intelligence program, based on her observation that Joseph responded well to music. We hoped it might serve as auditory stimulation as well. Accordingly, in intervals between patterning sessions, these volunteers treated us to occasional live performances on banjo, flute, oboe, and slide trombone. Joseph's reaction to the latter was especially rewarding. He'd been in a very foul mood, and continued fussing, at nothing in particular, while the musician assembled the instrument. But with that first *bwamp-bwah-bwaa*, his protests stopped, and in moments he was laughing and bouncing with excitement. Never had I seen him change gears so fast.

But this innovation drew no approval, or even comment, from Philadelphia. "Use your time to best advantage," Lidwina ordered. She'd just seen a videotape we'd mailed in that showed a session of dogged plodding back and forth under the ladder. "Show him Bits while he's walking! Hold word cards in front of him as he goes. Make it fun for him!" She sounded vexed with us for failing to grasp this critical point. Then I too became a little vexed (privately). Lidwina surely knew what appealed to the typical kid on program, but so far Joseph was not altogether typical.

Still, if it could be possible to enjoy the ladder, we were well advised to try, because this part of the program continued to take up more and more of our day. On February 25, Joseph spent over three hours in the process of logging 630 trips. Sometimes he barely touched the rungs as he passed beneath them. But he still seemed to lack interest in trying to walk alone. We were on a plateau; we *knew* he would walk. But how soon? What else would it take? We had been told at the Institutes that all kids walked away from the ladder before they reached 1,000 trips in a day. That was not entirely comforting. Even at the present rate of increase, we were a long way from 1,000 trips.

Distant friends and family members did not help morale by calling with the question we hated most. "How's the *baby*? Is he walking yet?" Judy patiently explained, several times, that at age three Joseph was no longer a baby and that, furthermore, when he did take his first steps, we would probably hire a skywriter to announce the fact.

In thinking back on those days, I remind myself to avoid what Judy derisively referred to as "pop psychology." Even more than questions about "the baby," she hated to hear people hypothesize that we might be motivated by guilt, or indeed by anything other than the simple drive to help our son.

"They don't understand Joseph's problem, but somehow they're experts on us," she huffed indignantly when such views were expressed in her hearing.

I don't know what prompted her to insist at this point that I was not handling the situation. One might hazard a guess that she was projecting her own feelings onto me, but it's also possible that I deserved it when she told me one night that I needed to get out of the house and change my thinking. She'd read about a support group for fathers of disabled kids, and wanted me to join.

"You should see yourself!" She said. "You're so tense that it's upsetting Joseph and me. So go! These guys might give you some ideas for how to cope." Perhaps noting a suspicious expression, she added, "Don't worry. I promise to keep doing the program while you're gone."

I WAS THE LAST TO ARRIVE at the meeting. The front office was dark, but a note taped to the glass directed me down a twisting corridor. A murmur of voices grew louder, and I found a cozy room that contained several men seated on a collection of worn-out furniture. One of them was talking; so I exchanged a few quick nods and took the nearest available chair. The speaker was describing a confrontation with his son's doctor. Evidently, he had taken the child to a new doctor and had gotten a more encouraging evaluation. Now he was trying to convince the first doctor to revise the prognosis.

When he finished speaking, there were greetings and introductions. They explained to me that it was their practice to take turns describing whatever challenge happened to be uppermost in their minds. Charlie, the group leader, would then attempt to identify a central theme in the concerns expressed and encourage further discussion on that.

Tonight everyone seemed to be thinking about wives. One father thought his was near the breaking point. "She already spends four days every week taking our son to speech therapy, physical therapy, and all the other special things he has to go to. Sometimes he has two appointments in one day. And now they want him to go to occupational therapy on Thursday, the only day she has free. She's generally a wreck when I come home in the evenings. I have to watch my step. It's easy to set her off." Smiling for the first time, he said they liked to relax in front of the TV until late at night. This was their way of putting the day's tensions behind them.

Another man said he had solved all problems with his wife very neatly. "I hardly ever talk to her," he said. "That works! She keeps the house in order and makes sure both our kids get packed off to their respective schools in the morning." He paused to explain to me that he had *two* handicapped children, one with "CP," as he put it, and one who was "mildly retarded." "Different vans come to collect them," he said, "because my little girl goes to a school downtown and my boy goes to Schweitzer. And it seems that there's always a different driver. So she has to take both kids out when she sees the first van come, and she asks the driver where he's going. Then she puts the appropriate kid on board and waits with the other kid until the second van arrives. As for me, I get satisfaction from my job. I spend as much time there as I can." He laughed. "My wife generally calls in the evening and asks if I was planning to come home. I'm always surprised to see how late it is."

"What do your kids do in these schools?" I asked.

"Beats me! My daughter was going to this place where they give her physical therapy, but then they decided she needed some academic stuff. Now I think she goes half a day to one place and then they bus her someplace else and she spends the rest of the day there. Unless she returns to the first school to catch her ride home again."

I wondered silently if these children were getting any benefit from all this logistical maneuvering. I felt uneasy. Did I have any business suggesting a way out for them? I thought I owed it to the children to try, but the fathers around me didn't seem to be searching for new ideas. One said, "If I had the choice of seeing my kid develop, say, eighty percent of the capacity to be like other people, and doing so would mean that he didn't develop the capacity for *love*—well, I'd rather see him at only forty percent, or even twenty percent, as long as he can experience love." He didn't say why there had to be a tradeoff.

When it was my turn to speak, I chose my words carefully. "My wife and I don't see eye-to-eye on everything," I said. "She thinks I'm too critical, and sometimes I think she needs to push harder for what we both want. But we're on the same team." I briefly described the Institutes program. None of those present knew anything about it. "We work together," I said. "We have to work together, even when we're having a fight, because the program requires both of us, and additional helpers too."

"How long will it go on?" asked Charlie.

"The Institutes' ultimate goal for any kid who goes there is a full recovery. I expect to keep working at it until he's well. Normal." I shrugged. "No one has promised that we'll make it all the way, but even so the highest objective seems to be the best one."

"Oh come on!" one father scoffed irritably. "*Normal*? What's so great about being *normal*? Do you mean to say you want your kid to be just like *you*? No offense, you understand—but I've had it up to the gills with that word, 'normal.'" He laughed bitterly.

"Actually," I offered, "I hope he'll be *better* than me. I'm no benchmark."

That wish dropped like a pebble into a deep pool. When no one responded, the focus shifted to the next father, who lamented that it was almost tax time. As usual for this time of year, he and his wife were in dire straits. Some years earlier, they'd won a lawsuit against the hospital where their daughter was born. They'd been awarded an enormous sum of money, but the stipulation was that they couldn't touch the principal or interest until she was grown. They were, however, responsible for paying annual taxes on the earnings.

Everyone proposed ways in which he might address this problem. Uninformed theories and complaints about tax law dominated the discussion until Charlie checked his watch and called a halt to the meeting.

We stood. The father who didn't like the word "normal" grinned as he zipped his jacket. "Next time, I hope to report to you that my boy has finally gotten his motorized wheelchair. We've been trying to get that thing for *months*. You wouldn't believe the amount of paperwork that has to go through for the funding."

"Is it that expensive?" I asked.

"Is it expensive! Man, it's thousands of dollars."

This seemed hard to believe.

"It shouldn't be this way, but it is," said Charlie. "We really need a Henry Ford in the wheelchair industry."

"I take it your son can't walk at all," I guessed.

"Oh, he could sort of bear weight on his feet and teeter around, but it was incredibly hard on him. Hard on me, too. I tell you, I couldn't stand to see it."

We had reached the sidewalk outside and people were saying goodnight and dispersing.

"My son Joseph doesn't walk yet," I said, "but we expect him to learn." I mentioned the overhead ladder.

"Listen, you don't know. You haven't seen the CAT-scan of my kid's brain. Hah! If I got pictures like that from the photo lab, I'd want a refund. It was nothing but black!"

"Joseph's CAT-scan was upsetting, too." I said. "But the brain has a lot of spare parts."

"It was a hard decision for us to make," he said, sorting through his car keys. "Jason could stagger across the room in a half-assed sort of way, but he'd be so mentally exhausted by the time he got where he was going that he wouldn't be able to *do* anything. We figured, what was the point? With a motorized wheelchair he'll be able to zip around as much as he wants."

I GAVE THE FATHERS' GROUP a fair try. Jason did get his wheelchair, I learned. At the next meeting his dad spoke proudly of the gouges it was putting in their furniture. But after that I told Judy that the group wasn't for me.

She meanwhile sought perspective through increasing attention to prayer. Her sister Pat called frequently from Virginia, urging her to *claim* wellness for Joseph. "God is greater than evil. He wants us to follow his Word and be healed. So have faith in God to break the yoke of disease and lack. Don't be moved by what you see. Walk by faith."

This advice was easier to prescribe than to implement with any visible effect. And as weeks passed with no change in our circumstances, Pat began taking a more aggressive tone. "Treatment has its place, but you're taking this program too much to heart. I think you must be turning your back on the real source of Joseph's healing. 'God's words are life to those that find them and medicine to all their flesh.' That's from Proverbs."

"But we feel the program *is* the right thing to do," Judy argued. "We were led to it, I feel sure."

"In that case, why isn't it working faster? Listen. God can make Joseph well today! He says so in the Bible. 'Whatsoever ye shall ask in my name that will I do.' So there must be something wrong about the way you're asking."

Judy thought about it. We needed so much help, and indeed we had received so much help from others. Still, we always needed more. Maybe we were supposed to give something in return. Could we expect to continue receiving if we didn't? Could *we* help anyone?

A name occurred to her, and she found an old address book. We'd once met a very elderly widow who lived in a retirement community. The poor lady had outlived every single relative she'd ever had. Surely she was lonely. Possibly Judy could do something for her.

On checking, she found that Jeanette's situation had deteriorated. She was now convalescing in a foul-smelling nursing home, having broken some bones. She'd managed to lose her possessions to an unscrupulous "friend" and, for all practical purposes, was destitute.

Judy set her mind to finding a remedy. Jeanette was a Swiss citizen, and an inquiry to the consulate in Los Angeles revealed that she qualified for a government pension. This unexpected income enabled her to move to more comfortable quarters.

Judy visited Jeanette when I was available to work with Joseph, and helped her get out of bed and on her feet again. Perhaps victories achieved on her behalf compensated, in Judy's mind, for slow progress at home. They remained close for the remaining months of the old lady's life.

WHEN I BACKED AWAY from the issue of walking, I could see that Joseph was changing in other areas. He had developed a more intellectual sense of humor, and he laughed readily at anything he perceived as a joke—such as the idea of "looking at music" (sheet music) as opposed to listening to it. He established eye contact with people more readily. Outdoors, he grinned back at strangers when they waved. Sometimes he even said "Bye-bye" to them. They smiled indulgently and strolled past with no idea that they'd been treated to a rare performance. People who knew Joseph but saw him infrequently assured us that they now saw a knowing, sparkly glint in his eyes. He looked "smarter." When they visited, he actually seemed proud of his program and wanted to show off his ladder-walking skills.

To bring out language, we kept presenting him with choices. Did he want to wear the red shirt or the blue one? Did he want juice or water? He didn't seem to care. Then Judy asked if he wanted to wear his breathing mask or walk under the ladder. His reply—"No"—was not what she'd expected, but it did represent a choice. That one, regrettably, we could not honor.

In addition to the ladder walks, I was now propping Joseph up in a corner several times a day and stepping away from him. I would crouch and hold out my arms. "Come on, son. It's just a step, and I'll give you a *big* hug when you get here! Believe me, you can do it!" He fell forward into my arms a couple of times, but the exercise made him very nervous. Evidently, nothing was going to happen fast. Perhaps some new ideas would emerge when we returned to the Institutes. And so we made plans for our fourth visit, still without a Walking Victory.

Adding to the uncertainty, a letter arrived from Judy's Aunt Julie in Philadelphia. "Things here at that time are going to be rather unsettled," she wrote. "In fact they are a bit confused right now as people are coming and going for the next couple of months, and I can't plan on having you folks."

This was unsettling news. The Institutes had provided a list of private homes in the area that offered accommodations for families, but at this late date they had no vacancies. And motels were out of the question. We were already relying on a second donation from the Kiwanis Club for our airfare.

Judy called her aunt in hopes of resolving the problem. Possibly the next-door neighbor, whom we'd met on previous trips, would agree to take us in.

"Don't do that!" Aunt Julie protested. "OK. We'll make adjustments, and you can stay here."

"Well—but we don't want to create a problem."

"Really, it's no problem. We're looking forward to seeing you again."

Misgivings abounded but we took her at her word, seeing no other choice.

15. THE LIFE PLAN

It was that week, in places where they have real seasons, when yellow stripes of forsythia blazed their brightest across wet green lawns, and the new dogwood blossoms were just turning white. Early Monday morning I drove our rental car between the stone pillars at the Institutes' gate, feeling like an old hand at this business. I parked behind the Veras Building and we hurried through a light rain with our sample word cards and Bits, and our Revisit Report.

By now, we'd fallen back into a different group of families. There'd be a lot of new faces in the waiting area, but Judy wasted no time in making friends with the first couple she saw. Mark and Terry were from Spokane. They sat on a blanket beside a bright-eyed little girl in an antiroll device. "This is the week when they tell us about the Honeymoon," Terry said.

"Already?" We remembered reading that for Institutes families a "Honeymoon" was an extended break from the program, a time for resting and reassessing. The concept seemed alien.

"Hey! How are ya? Remember us?"

It turned out that we were surrounded by families whom we hadn't seen since our first trip, seventeen months earlier: Laura and Paul from Ontario; Joan and Michael from New York; and some fellow Californians named—?

"Sarah and Bob! And Nikky!"

"Of course! Say, it's good to see you guys again." This family wielded cameras, and a photo album documenting the progress of everyone they'd met at the Institutes. We even saw snapshots of ourselves taken during that first, intoxicating week. Judy and I looked younger and fresher in the pictures, I thought (as did our clothes—we were still wearing the same outfits). However, the most apparent change was in Joseph. The puffy-looking baby with a vacant stare in the photos bore little resemblance to the energetic kid with us now.

Their daughter Nikky had recently begun creeping, but she generally preferred a five-point stance, with the top of her head resting on the floor between her hands. Sarah explained that this represented a balance problem. "Our advocate told us we'll get a balance development program this time," she said.

"Who's your advocate?"

"Matt."

"Ours is Lidwina."

"She's fantastic, isn't she?"

"She keeps us going."

The day's evaluations brought no great surprises. Joseph had moved up a level in manual competence, which translated into a slightly increased neurological age. On the other hand, his auditory responses continued to be unsatisfactory. Dawn blasted an air horn that made Judy and me jump out of our skins, but Joseph remained totally unimpressed. This absence of a vital response to threatening sounds meant he didn't have sufficient auditory awareness to save himself from danger.

"When anyone hears a sudden noise like that, he should be jumping across the room without stopping to think about it. At the very least, a baby who's immobile should cry for its mother."

"Maybe he heard you warn us that it was coming," Judy suggested.

"No. Listen, this doesn't go through the higher brain levels. He *should* have responded!"

The failing represented a "hole" in his auditory pathway. Although

WHAT ABOUT THE BOY?   213

his Profile reflected the fact that he understood at least twenty-five words of speech, at the level of an average eighteen-month-old, lower-level problems like this would inhibit functioning all the way up the chart.

GLENN'S LECTURES this week included a talk entitled "The Life Plan."

"Our objective has always been to make each of your kids well," he said, pacing thoughtfully at the front of the room. "The only reasonable goal is to make your kid completely well, in every respect. Maybe we'll succeed and maybe we won't, but that shouldn't change the goal.

"At the Institutes, we've had goals for ourselves, too. Some of these were achieved on or even ahead of schedule. Some weren't. And we achieved *some* things we hadn't even expected. The fact that goals aren't always achieved doesn't mean we shouldn't have plans.

"Of course, you can always give up!" He pointed to the exit at the back of the room. "The way out is always open. Quitting doesn't take any effort. It's doors going the *other* way that close. So let's not worry about that option. Let's go for broke.

"What's the goal for your kid? At the Institutes we have arbitrarily picked college graduation as the thing to shoot for. Maybe you've got something else in mind, but just for the sake of argument, let's assume everybody wants to graduate from college."

I recognized what he was doing, because this was the same kind of thinking I used in my job when scheduling a new project. The idea was to start with the target date and work backward through the necessary milestones that led up to it. I did some hasty arithmetic. If all went well, Joseph would graduate from college in the year 2007. To do so, he would have to enter college in September 2003. To do that, it would be necessary for him to graduate from high school in June of that year. He would have to enter high school before that; in the normal course of events that would be in 1999. Of course, this goal presupposed finishing grammar school and being neurologically well — at the top of the Institutes' Profile.

"It's better to plan to go to college and fail than to plan to go to an institution and succeed," Glenn concluded. The lecture was over and he started to leave the room, but Judy jumped to her feet.

"Glenn, before you go, I just want to say that you give everybody in this room so much hope, and a feeling of direction that we wouldn't have otherwise." She was speaking nervously, with a charge of emotion that had evidently been building all day. "It's—well, it's a privilege to know you, and it's always a joy to hear you talk. And I just think we should all try to show what you mean to us."

The room exploded into enthusiastic, prolonged applause, with everyone standing.

"OK. OK. Thanks. Thank you very much, but stop that," Glenn said, embarrassed. He returned to the front of the room for a moment. "As you may know, I just got back from Europe a few days ago," he said. "Several members of our staff are still over there, setting up a satellite branch of the Institutes. You'll be hearing more about that soon. Last week I had a press conference in Stuttgart, in West Germany. A gentleman from the French press asked me, very respectfully, 'Mr. Doman,' he said, 'Can you tell us why it is that the French Academy of Pediatrics has issued a statement saying that the Institutes' form of therapy does not work?'"

A few parents guffawed expectantly.

"And I answered him, just as respectfully, by saying, 'I have never been to the French Academy of Pediatrics. I don't know any of its members. Frankly, I don't know what they do. Therefore, it would be improper of me to offer an opinion of them or their work, and I would expect the same courtesy in return.'"

We all laughed now, but Glenn wasn't finished. "The reporter persisted. 'But Mr. Doman,' he said, 'The statement of the French Academy of Pediatrics is based on a similar statement that was made by the *American* Academy of Pediatrics.' And I said, 'The same thing goes.

I've never been to the American Academy of Pediatrics, and they have never been to the Institutes, in spite of the fact that they've had a standing invitation for several years.' Then to top it off, a journalist from the local paper wanted to know why I hadn't been to Germany before. 'Oh, but I have,' I told him. 'I *shot* my way through these streets in 1944 so that everybody would have the freedom to say what he thinks.'"

More laughter and applause ensued. It was a rare celebration of togetherness and common cause. Bob and Sarah, the self-appointed photojournalists, took advantage of the opportunity to organize everyone for a snapshot of Glenn standing with our group (a copy of which they later mailed to us), and then we disbanded to collect our kids from the Veras Building.

This was always a happy moment for me, coming directly from an inspiring lecture to reclaim my boy. I couldn't love him more, but these trips to the Institutes helped me see him in the right perspective. Joseph was already a hero. He had already done many very difficult things, things very few other kids ever did. He was a winner.

Judy and I took turns hugging him tightly, spinning around as we did so. Around us, other families were carrying on in similar fashion. The big room echoed with a glad clamor, which tapered off as everyone dispersed.

Soon it would be time to roll up our sleeves and get busy again, on whatever assignment we would now be given. In the dining room we found places at a table with the Canadians and the New Yorkers. They were talking about the difficult transition period of learning a new program.

Paul said, "I've found that the best way to start is to get away to someplace quiet. I fix myself a nice stiff margarita, and then I look at all those papers that spell out what we're supposed to do. I read the number of Bits we've gotta teach and the patterning and the masking and all the meters of this and hours of that. And I say, 'Aw, now *this can't be!*'"

Everyone nodded and rolled their eyes. He was telling our story.

"Then I down the margarita and look again," Paul continued. "Finally I say, 'Yep.' And then we do it."

JOSEPH WAS VERY, VERY CLOSE to independent walking, and in fact Lidwina confessed that she'd half-expected him to take his first steps during this week at the Institutes. "But I'm sure he'll walk before the middle of June," she said.

The main obstacle was still his balance, and she outlined an even more involved balance development program than the one we had been doing all winter. One day every week was to be designated "balance development marathon day," and on this we would devote twice as much attention to the vestibular activities as on the other six days. This meant six complete sessions of vertical pirouetting instead of three, 100 somersaults in each direction instead of fifty, 200 meters of rolling instead of 100, and so on.

"After each activity, get Joseph back into the vertical position," she said. "*Constantly* challenge him to use his balance."

Next she told us to set up a "cruising environment," to enable him to travel around the house while steadying himself with a series of nipple-high packing boxes. She showed us photos of another family's cruising environment. We saw a very nice home, cluttered with rows of cardboard boxes placed several inches apart. It looked like they were packing for a move.

"Continue to widen the distance between the boxes," Lidwina said. "Eventually he will have to take independent steps between them. You'll find that it helps to put interesting objects on top of boxes across the room from him so he'll be motivated. Give him things he can do constructively—shoeboxes to open, for example. Inside, let him find things like a little box of raisins, or a cap to put on.

"In addition to that, there is still the overhead ladder," she continued. "Joseph's present ability on the ladder is terrific. He handles it like a breeze. So write this down: Five days a week, I want him to do five hundred trips under the ladder. One day a week will be a ladder marathon day. Increase the number of trips by thirty each week. Then, on balance development marathon day, he can just do four hundred trips."

"That adds up to a lot of walking," I murmured.

"We will provide Joseph with the opportunity to walk the overhead ladder, and walk the overhead ladder, and *walk* the overhead ladder—until he walks away from it."

Finally, until he started walking, we were to continue organizing his midbrain for better understanding through more creeping.

Lidwina smiled. "When he does walk independently, your Honeymoon begins. That will be the 'no-program program'—zoo trips, walks on the beach, kids' parties—anything that will stimulate him, socially or physically or intellectually."

"Wonderful!"

"While you're on the Honeymoon, look for ways to create a normal life. It's a time for resting up and taking stock of the situation. Observe all the changes that have taken place. By the end of the Honeymoon you must have the same enthusiasm for resuming the program that you had on Day One."

AS ON PREVIOUS VISITS, we spent this day and the next moving between the waiting area and offices of various staff members. Phyllis gave Joseph a new intelligence program. Elaine switched him back to the reflex mask he had used originally. "He's done quite well with all the masks," she said. "What we do after this will depend on the progress he makes with language."

We knew speech would be the next major hurdle after walking. Judging from the rate of progress thus far, I expected this to be another long, hard campaign. But it was too early to worry about that. Lidwina had explained that language development naturally took a back seat to mobility; we couldn't expect much talking from Joseph until after he had firmly established himself as a walker.

LONG DAYS AT THE INSTITUTES meant that we never saw much of our hosts, Judy's aunt and uncle. That was especially true on this trip. They had the house to themselves all day and most of the evening, but alas, Joseph still made our presence known late at night. Jet lag and unfamiliar surroundings combined to make him excitable when the rest of us wanted to sleep. I still worried about being a nuisance. Even so, we were startled to receive a letter from them immediately after arriving back in San Diego.

Aunt Julie wrote that it would no longer be convenient for us to stay at their house. By breaking the news well in advance of our next appointment, she said she was allowing us ample time to find other accommodations.

It was embarrassing to realize that we had overstayed our welcome. We tried on a few other emotions, too. But all we could do was put the matter behind us. Judy wrote to her aunt once more, thanking her for having helped us four times, and then began the search for affordable lodgings. Mark and Terry recommended a widow who rented rooms to Institutes families. A phone call revealed that she had a vacancy for the week in question, and we gratefully reserved it.

WITHIN A FEW DAYS, we had learned the new routine and were back in high gear. Joseph generally awoke at seven o'clock, about the same time I left for work. Judy began masking him immediately, and recording everything on the daily status sheet. After breakfast, Joseph began his walks under the overhead ladder. Judy yelled encouragement and presented Bits and word cards as he patiently made his way back and forth, back and forth. Between ladder walks, she placed him in the cruising environment we had set up, and worked in more maskings there. In midmorning they began concentrating on balance-development activities. I still returned home during my lunch hour on most days so that we could join forces with a volunteer for two patterning sessions. Afternoons were spent creeping and clambering in the park, after which he napped. I was home again by five o'clock for more patterning, balance development, masking, intelligence materials, and an intense effort to finish the requisite number of ladder walks before Joseph called it a day at nine or ten o'clock.

When he had not walked independently after a few weeks of this, we tried Plan B, which meant sawing out alternate rungs from the ladder. This *forced* him to trust his own balance as he ventured along it the last few times.

One of our favorite patterners during this period was an aspiring physical therapist named Carla. She joined us for the midday session and asked intelligent questions throughout.

"When you get to physical-therapy school, you'll probably hear some negative talk about patterning," I said. "I hope you won't accept everything they tell you without question."

"Don't worry!" As we spoke, Joseph was standing between two tall cardboard boxes, steadying himself against one with his left hand and stretching his right arm toward the next box, which was just out of reach. Carla grinned. "It's obvious that you're onto something."

The program worked by giving him an ideal situation. When I slowed down enough to think about it, I reflected that all people could improve their circumstances to favor maximum health and achievement. I could easily imagine ways to improve my own life. I needed to be more physically active, for example. I needed more sleep and much less anxiety. I always told myself, as I suppose others do, that there'd be time to address all that at some point in the future. In Joseph's case, however, it was not optional. He *had* to have the best arrangement possible, and he had to have it now.

Our ability to provide that seemed absolutely feeble at times. How much help would we really need to do his program perfectly? For starters, things would be better if we had a cook, so there'd be no need to take time out for preparing meals; if we had a corps of research assistants, to provide a steady flow of refreshing new material for the intelligence program; if we had a carpenter, a seamstress, and someone to recruit and schedule fresh patterners. At the office, I looked around at the various specialists in my department, all working in their different ways toward the common goal of completing projects. *That* was what we needed: a full-time dedicated work force! What wonders might we achieve then? Succeeding on program meant being a problem-solver, but the solution to this one still eluded me. Judy and I forged ahead, doing our best with the resources at hand.

Breaks came from unexpected directions.

Several employees at the County Planning Office took a very gratifying interest in the cause. One of them, Rose Garduño, had been a regular patterner ever since reading one of Sally's articles about Joseph. Now her coworkers stepped in as well. Throughout the week, they took turns driving over on their lunch hour to support our noontime patterning session.

Judy visited a new church, where she made friends with Frank and Evelyn Kleber—two more enthusiastic volunteers.

These were some of the people on *our* staff when Joseph achieved his breakthrough.

16. WHAT TO DO ABOUT THE RHINO

"Lidwina, I'm calling to let you know Joseph has started walking."

"*Super!*"

Then Judy backpedaled, feeling she'd made too bold a claim. "I mean, he can take a few steps independently if you place him in a standing position. He still can't get up by himself if he's in the middle of the room—."

"Hold on, there," Lidwina laughed. "Let's back up a minute. You say Joseph is walking?"

"Well—yes!"

"That's fantastic! Now, when you say 'a few steps,' how far is that?"

"We were just out on the sidewalk, and he went sixteen feet in about ten seconds."

"Already? Well, that overhead ladder just works miracles. Have you celebrated yet?"

"No."

"Stop right now and take the rest of the day off! This calls for champagne! Oh, and thanks very much for calling. News like this always makes my day."

We had permission to start our Honeymoon at any time, but Judy and I decided to carry on a bit longer with the patterning, at least, and the vestibular techniques. We'd promised Joseph that walking would mean the end of his involvement with the overhead ladder, and he held us to our word, refusing to go near the thing. In place of that part of the program, we added an escalating schedule of very short walks that Lidwina had outlined on the phone. A couple weeks of this would establish him more firmly in this new mode of transport, and enable all of us to enjoy our break more thoroughly. We set July 1, 1988, as the target for resuming normal life.

Eagerly, we spread the tidings to everyone who had taken an interest in Joseph over the last eighteen months, the donors of money as well as the volunteers. We knew some had lost interest in the project, but we wanted them, especially, to know that their efforts had borne fruit.

"Whoever would have thought we'd see *this*!" marveled a neighbor named Diane. She and her husband Phil had patterned Joseph in the earliest days of the program. His victory was theirs, too, but I wondered what she did think we'd expected.

It was a heady, upbeat time, and patterners arriving for the last few sessions were inclined to celebrate with us. The gang from the County Planning Office took photos of Joseph beaming delightedly in his new two-point stance and presented Judy with a framed enlargement.

Joseph didn't need to be told that he'd crossed an important threshold. Yes, at 39 months it was very late. But from a mobility standpoint, this still meant full citizenship at last!

Despite profound satisfaction, we still had a demanding schedule. As always, every day brought reasons, both large and trivial, for departing from the program. The car would suddenly have a dead battery. Judy would have a doctor's appointment. I would be called upon to stay late at my office. And so on. But these were minor hiccups. We persevered.

BUT THEN word came that my 81-year-old father was in the hospital with an inflamed pancreas. At first, it was not considered serious. A few days later, however, pneumonia had set in. He was losing touch with reality, and suddenly the prognosis was less optimistic. The family members I spoke with seemed to be in shock. After all, despite his age, Dad's health had always been good. He was still the strong one, the anchor, for all of us.

Maybe the time to lose him had arrived, but I wanted to determine that for myself. So Judy called in extra patterners, and I grabbed an overnight flight to Virginia.

Dad had never understood Joseph's program, although he approved of the objective and rather liked uphill battles in general. He'd recently mailed us a newspaper clipping that described a father's desperate (and successful) attempt to save a child from a charging rhinoceros, of all things, by leaping into the animal's path and waving it away. He saw a parallel between that apparently senseless act and what we were doing. Self-sacrifice for your loved ones was only natural, even if it defied logic. All my life he had taught me by example never to shrink from necessary confrontations. I'd been a slow learner in that, but having a brain-injured child had finally brought the lesson home. So if I was going to lose my dad now, I intended to lose him fighting.

I arrived in Charlottesville just in time to join my two sisters for a conference with his doctor, an austere old Southern gentleman who clearly meant to disabuse us of any hope that this patient might ever be his old self again. Dr. Taylor described Dad's condition as "acute," and said there were various possible explanations for what had brought it about. None of the tests he'd ordered confirmed anything, however. The most disturbing development in recent days was this abrupt onset of confusion. He called it "metabolic encephalopathy," and said it often occurred in older people when things start to go awry. They had done a CT-scan and had noted a loss of brain tissue. But this was typical for someone Dad's age and did not account for his condition. The doctor's feeling was that, once the immediate medical crisis had been addressed, Dad should go directly into a nursing home.

I thought of Jeanette, Judy's elderly Swiss friend back in San Diego, and her vulnerability and helplessness. I could not imagine my father in like circumstances. "That's not going to happen," I said bluntly.

The doctor aimed an indignant expression at me. "Are *you* going to be around to look after him?"

"If necessary, I will see that arrangements are in place for a companion. But please understand me. He's going back *home*, and he's going at the earliest possible moment."

We weren't hitting it off. The doctor looked offended. I regretted that, but I no longer harbored illusions that anyone speaking as he did offered what we needed. Already, this looked like a replay of our early experience with Joseph's providers.

I THEN HAD A CHANCE to assess Dad's condition for myself. I found him propped up in bed, speaking to Mom in a hoarse monotone. Little or nothing of what he said made sense. After delivering a string of disconnected phrases, he'd say, "In other words—" and then trail off into total incoherence. I strained to identify a theme in his discourse. Did he *think* he was telling us something? Maybe the problem wasn't in his understanding so much as in his ability to express himself. Who could say? Maybe there was some parallel between his situation and Joseph's. Both were now locked up in bodies that prevented interaction with the world.

After some time, the others departed. I remained standing beside the bed, admiring my father's familiar shaggy white eyebrows and his tousled cloud of extremely fine hair. He was staring intently into space, thinking – *what*? If only I knew! I felt as if a brick were hanging inside my chest. Now *two* people I cared about were unreachable!

What had happened to him? Just two weeks earlier, Mom had said, he'd been up to his usual rigorous activities, climbing into a tree on his extension ladder and sawing limbs with a chain saw, for example. He'd called to congratulate us on Joseph's first steps and had sounded perfectly all right then. "I've always believed you were on the right path," he'd said. "I just have a strong feeling that good things are in store for all of you." Now he gave no indication even of knowing where he was.

Another doctor breezed into the room for a quick examination. Dad took no notice of the man's prodding, so he addressed himself to me. "This old fellow is really skinny!" he said, impressed. "I can feel his descending aorta when I put my hand on his abdomen!" Then, abruptly, before I could think to respond, he was out the door again.

In recent years I had developed an attitude toward medical people in which I presumed a sort of equality with them. The original idea had been to offer myself as an ally in whatever course of treatment would benefit Joseph—to encourage their candor and perhaps inspire them to give his case more thought than they might otherwise. When treatments were not forthcoming, and I found other ways to help him, there seemed still less reason to show them the kind of deference the rest of my family displayed. Perhaps this had prompted the doctor's unguarded remark to me.

I caught up with him at the elevator. I cared nothing for hospital protocol, which dictates that all questions should be fielded by the patient's primary physician. I wanted opinions!

"Doctor, what is going on with my dad?"

"Well, the problem that put him here in the first place has pretty much cleared up."

"I mean mentally."

He looked uncomfortable. "That's not my area. I'm a gastroenterologist. But a lot of these old-timers have a pretty loose grip on reality, even in the best of circumstances. When you change their surroundings, change their routines—." He shrugged. The elevator arrived and he stepped on board.

"Then if he were home again, in *familiar* surroundings, he might recover?"

"That's possible. I really couldn't say. It's been nice talking with you." The doors hissed shut.

I couldn't say either, nor could I call this *my* specialty. But as the next few days unfolded, I set out to see what could be done.

Judy, ever the health nut, had packed my suitcase with teas and herbs that she assured me would support Dad's recovery, plus special whole-grain oatmeal that she'd mixed with ground nuts, and plenty of high-dosage vitamins. Hospital food might or might not be adequate. We rather suspected it wasn't, and the first meal I saw there, including canned fruit cocktail and instant pudding, confirmed this.

At her suggestion, I'd stopped at a grocery store on the way in from the airport to load up on fresh produce. When someone brought in Dad's dinner tray, I deftly substituted a plastic container of finely chopped carrots, tomatoes, and sprouts, dusted with vitamin C and zinc to promote healing, B-complex vitamins for energy (B_{12} deficiencies had been blamed for confusion in older patients, I'd read), and a trendy new amino acid preparation that supposedly heightened mental alertness. I knew I was grasping at straws. But if I grabbed enough, they might make a raft.

He admired the fresh food, out of long habit, perhaps. But the idea of actually eating it held no attraction. Getting him to swallow anything took forever. I gathered that he was sufficiently aware to see that he was in a jam of some description and that he was at a loss for how to fix it. He apparently thought that doing nothing—not eating, for example—was probably as good as any other approach. Every time I got something good into him, I mentally danced in celebration.

As he took the last bite of one meal, I jovially exclaimed, "Finito!" Still chewing, Dad muttered, "Finio, finias, finiat." He pondered that, sighed, and continued, "Finiamus, finiatis, finiant, finbam ..." His voice trailed off.

"What was that, Dad? Latin?" He didn't reply, and indeed seemed to have forgotten my presence.

Like everyone in his generation Dad had studied Latin as a child, but I'd never heard him use it. Presumably, some long-dormant neural synapses were coming back into play. Was that good? What were the prospects for his more recent mental activity?

If Dad remembered his Latin, maybe other aspects of his early life were accessible to him. When I had his attention again, I began prompting him with references to various old stories he'd repeated too many times over the years. He looked interested. Beyond that, there was no immediate reaction. After a day or two of this, however, he was recalling the time the goat had butted him in the stomach when he was a little boy. He remembered tampering with his uncle's alarm clock, and the furor that ensued when it went off in the middle of the night. Slowly, and with effort, he pieced together these old narratives, and even added details I'd never heard.

On Sunday, Mom brought the funny papers to him. I told her that was a great idea. Anything familiar from the outside world *had* to be good. She showed him his favorite comic strip, "Hägar the Horrible," and he actually chuckled at it. For the briefest moment I glimpsed the Dad I knew.

On Monday morning, I situated myself at Dad's bedside before he woke. I'd brought a new homeopathic remedy that Judy had express-mailed from California and an audiotape with subliminal healing messages. I was just hitting the Play button on the tape player when Dr. Taylor stopped in on rounds.

"The X-rays indicate that we've just about licked the pneumonia," he announced. "How's his mental state?"

"Improving!"

He scowled at me doubtfully. "We're going to try and get him to spend some time upright, now. I'll have the physical therapy people check in with him later today."

Dad was awake. He blinked up at me as the doctor left.

"Did you hear that exchange?" I enthused.

"Why, yes—."

Apparently, he had not. There was more disjointed speech, as he sought to organize his thinking, and finally he said, "I'm afraid I've been pretty ignorant here lately."

"Not *ignorant*, Dad. But they say you *have* been feverish." I slipped the remedy into his mouth as I spoke. It was supposed to be taken first thing in the morning. He accepted both the clarification and the pill placidly, while he wrestled with some idea that he couldn't express. Eventually he found the words. These *people* had been coming in and out of his room, he said. They seemed like nice enough folks. But the trouble was—they seemed to know him. And he didn't know them.

"Well, Dad, would you like for me to tell you who *I* am?"

"That wouldn't be amiss."

So I launched into a detailed account, not just of my history, but of the entire family. I cited all the dates and place names defining his career that came to mind. He looked thoughtful. "Yes," he decided. "That sounds right."

But he continued to worry. "I haven't been very smart," he said dejectedly. I couldn't tell whether he was referring to the life I had just summarized or the fact that he now found himself in a predicament. Still struggling with his words, he talked about how you go as far as you can with what you know, and then you have to guess about the rest.

"Dad, that's true for *everybody*!"

Matters continued in this vein for several days. The family members saw him in shifts, because when too many of us were present he seemed to tune out. I tried to be there during meals. He showed new interest and vigor when the physical therapist stood him up behind a walker. Dad had always been physically active, and I felt sure this development would help point him back toward his life.

Still, other things simply were not clicking. When prompted, he could quote snippets of Shakespeare and Milton, passages someone had made him memorize decades earlier. But aside from these old mental tracks, something was missing. Some kind of connective mechanism for putting everything into context just wasn't operating. During dinner one night he started raving about *gasoline*, of all things. He thought there were several drums of the stuff in the room, and that he was responsible for getting out a shipment to somebody. When an orderly came in, Dad thought he was the deliveryman. I couldn't get him to shake the idea.

"Dad, you've *never* been involved in gasoline!"

"I haven't?" He looked incredulous.

"No! You were a chemist at the Bureau of Standards, in Washington. And then you ran the lab at Reynolds Metals, and you were a consultant—." Desperately, I ran all the facts past him again, trying to connect. He just smiled wryly and shook his head at the list of jobs I said he'd held. Clearly, the whole litany sounded to him like a lot of foolishness. Then he noticed the food I was cutting up under his nose.

"What's that?" he said distastefully.

"Chicken."

He shook his head sadly. "You mean a chicken gave up its life, for *this?*"

I tried to laugh. "Not willingly, I'm sure."

Dad gestured for me to take the plate away, and no amount of coaxing would change his mind.

My bright ideas were coming to an end. To use Dad's way of framing the problem, I'd taken what little I knew as far as it would carry me, which wasn't far at all. It wasn't enough. Like Joseph, Dad was beset with an invisible, poorly understood adversary—one that could not be waved away as easily as some stampeding beast. Every night, I prostrated myself before the highest power—call it God or whatever you like; I couldn't pretend to understand that, either. I begged for the privilege of having my father back just once more, for an encore, if you will.

"I know everybody has to go sometime," I pleaded in the dark. "But I'm not ready to lose him yet. And not this way! Don't let him go out this way. Please, give him back to us just a bit longer. One more good visit with him, anyway. One more chance to—to interact with that strength and perspective and good humor. I still need him. Please!"

This was the man who had drilled me on the multiplication tables, who'd designed and built a two-story clubhouse for me in the backyard (complete with a fireman's pole), who'd taught me how to swim, use tools, think critically, and play the violin. He had taken pains to ensure I would not forget that my parents were my best friends and that there would never be a problem I could not bring to them.

Although stronger now, he still talked sheer nonsense most of the time. At least, it *sounded* like nonsense. I wondered if it might not actually be very profound. At one point, trying to cross the line from ordinary reality and meet him on his own terms, I actually climbed into the bed with him. (His roommate, a good-natured old farmer, was surely getting an earful of our crazy talk.) But almost stubbornly, Dad resisted my attempts to pull him back. I kept describing the man he'd always been, using adjectives he'd taught me to value—*self-sufficient, vigorous, alert*—in hopes of striking a chord.

I thought he was preoccupied with the futility of his life work, or even of any work. "Just scrap it," he grouched when I urged more vitamins on him. Then he added, "You can scrap ninety percent of all human endeavor."

"What about the other ten percent?" I suggested, maneuvering the spoon to give him one more bite.

"Scrap that, too."

Another evening, the topic of human striving struck him as being simply quaint. I had wheeled him out to a lounge, and through the open screened window we heard the surging drone of traffic in the humid summer twilight. He seemed to think the noise was coming from the rectangular shelter at a bus stop, which he took to be a car. His face creased in a benevolent smile. "The people over there aren't giving up," he said with admiration. "But they can't make that old thing run." Motors roared again with every change of the traffic lights, and he chuckled at what he took to be persistence in trying to get the jalopy moving.

His attention wandered. Periodically, he interrupted the rambling flow of his thoughts to hand me nonexistent objects for safekeeping. It still wasn't altogether clear that he knew who I was, because he referred to me in the third person. "I asked Steve to recommend a good electric razor," he mused, idly stroking the stubble on his cheek. "Thought he'd be up to speed on that. But he said he never used the things." It was true. We'd had that conversation a few months earlier. But whom did he think he was talking with now?

Even so, a coherent theme, perhaps even a philosophy, seemed to be emerging. All the worrying and striving that people engage in is just so much foolishness. The poor saps! He seemed genuinely to pity them. The fact was, he said, "You can throw out a lot of horseshit and the world will take it for gold." Or conversely, "If you tell 'em you're a stupid bastard, they'll believe you."

In a way, he was perfectly coherent. Suddenly I realized that he was very seriously offering some advice about "Little Joe," the pet name for his only grandchild. "Don't sell him short," he urged me. All my forth-right talk about brain injury over the years must have troubled him, although he'd never mentioned it before. "I'm not saying Li'l Joe will have any kind of lasting problem, mind you," he said, fixing me with a level gaze. "But in any event, people are going to start finding fault with him soon enough. That always happens. No point giving them ammunition."

This was more like the dad who'd taught me so much. I realized he must have been the source of the notion to keep Joseph's problem a secret during the first year. Encouraged, I continued making my pitch at every opportunity, essentially calling on him to *please recover*. I said his recovery was important—to *me*. He heard that, but said my efforts were misplaced; I should be thinking about my own happiness.

"But we're in this together! How could I go off and lounge on the beach while my own family needs help?"

He considered this, perhaps recalling the story about the rhino. "One's highest duty *is* to his family," he finally said. I took this as an opening. Perhaps, I think now, if Dad saw no point in continuing, it wasn't fair of me. I didn't see it that way at the time.

So I tapped into a much more recent memory. Four years earlier, he'd had a cardiac arrest while undergoing minor surgery on his knee. For ninety seconds his heart had been stopped, and the attending physi-cians had just about concluded that he was dead. He'd known that, because he heard them talking as they worked to revive him. He'd even glimpsed some tired-looking old guy on a table and realized with a jolt that he was looking down at himself.

"We've lost him," one of them said flatly. And then: "Well, he's gone."

For a moment, he'd been willing to accept that pronouncement. It was like falling asleep, he told me later. It felt so easy—and so attractive—just to drift off into nothingness. But then he changed his mind. *No!* He wasn't ready for that! Then, having made up his mind about that, he focused everything he had on breathing again, on getting his eyes open. And he succeeded.

"You remember that episode, don't you?" I said gently.

"Oh yes," he said softly. "I came—back from the brink."

I let the memory settle and then said, gently, "Dad, listen. I'm asking you to do that again. Come back."

He focused on me with a wondering expression. "I hadn't realized I was such a worry to everyone."

Suddenly, he *was* back. It was that easy. The realization dawned on me in a golden moment, triggering joy so intense I had to resist an urge to just get up and *leave*—to go find a quiet place where I could try to absorb the miracle that had just occurred and savor my delight. I stayed, however, and Dad continued demonstrating a sustained awareness of who he was, where he was, who I was, and what we all needed. He spoke of "the necessary cessation of life," a prospect that held no terror for him. But, he graciously promised, "I'll try to pull things together for a little while longer."

I understand that sentiment today in a way I did not then. Now, I begin to see that a man can love the people in his life and yet no longer have what is needed to cope with that life day after day. But then I looked right past it, past the possibility that I might be selfishly compelling my father to reshoulder a burden that had grown too great.

The next day he went home. Waking up to life once again was an ongoing process, enhanced by the simplest acts, such as pushing his arms through the sleeves of his shirt for the first time in two weeks.

"*What the hell has been going on?*" he demanded. "I must have been really sick!" He vowed to demand an explanation from Dr. Taylor. He was still very weak, but the tide had turned. For now, at any rate, he would be all right.

I don't know why he recovered. To be fair, without medical intervention the pneumonia alone might have been fatal. But something else was working on his behalf. Emotionally exhausted, I wondered if there were any lesson here that could be adapted to Joseph's case. Prayer? I'd also prayed for Joseph, of course. Directly asking the patient to get well? That, too, I did with Joseph. Daily.

IN SAN DIEGO, there were other fences to mend. In my absence, the little guy had gone "on strike" and refused to walk, to Judy's great chagrin. The Honeymoon was upon us, however. We let him revert to creeping, and soon enough he was ready to walk again. I'll always remember the gratification we shared when he began roving the house, enjoying freedom both from the daily routine of program, and from the floor. There was so much for him to see, and so much catching up to do! Well kids began satisfying their curiosity in this way at half his age. He especially liked stretching to reach objects on bookshelves.

A volunteer urged Judy to join a playgroup with her and her son. The children were younger, but Joseph fit in with them reasonably well. They yelled, and talked, and jumped—and *ran!*—and stacked up impatiently behind him on the sliding board ladder while he methodically made his way to the top. Their clamor made him withdraw into himself. Sometimes he responded with an unpleasant siren-like noise of his own, which drew unkind stares from passersby. And he showed a peculiar fascination with *sand*, digging his hands into it while the others were dashing away to ride the swings. His problems weren't all solved. But the time had come to let him try engaging with the world on his terms.

A family in our original group at the Institutes sent their congratulations. "We were in Philadelphia when you called Lidwina about Joseph walking. Everyone was so excited!" Their letter went on to say they had a new baby. At six months she was already up and creeping. "It's amazing to see babies doing this stuff without anyone showing them how," the mother wrote.

Amazing, yes, and also humbling, I thought. By now we understood something about how to affect child development. We could do it with a lot of hard work. But I remembered the ease with which my little sister Angie had zipped through all the milestones, without receiving any unusual help, and I knew we'd barely glimpsed the processes at work.

JUDY'S SISTER PAT arrived for a visit. During the day, while I caught up on matters at my job, they toured the local attractions. A system evolved in which they took turns walking a few paces ahead of Joseph and then waiting while he tottered in pursuit. He steadied himself for a moment against a convenient leg and then tried again. In this way they leapfrogged their way through Southern California's popular attractions. He stopped by the dolphin petting pool at Sea World, where he managed to get soaking wet. He stroked the coarse fur of a miniature gazelle at the Wild Animal Park. He'd always loved to swim, but he scarcely knew what to make of the beach, with its frothy, roaring waves and their way of sucking firm ground from under one's feet at the water's edge.

Meanwhile, the distances he could walk rapidly increased.

It was a perfect time for a Honeymoon, and a perfect time for a house guest (our first in two years). Judy and I hadn't fully realized how very quiet we both were until her talkative big sister joined us. Over time we'd fallen into a way of communicating almost telepathically and speaking in a kind of shorthand that our younger volunteers found amusing. *The archetypal old married couple!* Although efficient, this didn't provide the best environment for a child learning to speak.

But with Pat on hand, everything was tirelessly discussed, described, analyzed—usually in a way that included Joseph in the conversation.

WE HAD NO FIRM DATE for resuming program activities. That was weeks away still, but the playgroup outings confirmed that the battle wasn't over. Brain injury gave no honeymoons. This—not the program—was the real cause of our stress and anxiety.

But the program was *tough*. And its demands kept escalating. I wondered what challenges were likely to be assigned next. I wondered if we'd be equal to them. Could we improve our efficiency? The Institutes always gave parents free rein in deciding exactly how to accomplish the goals they set for us. Scheduling our time, assigning responsibilities, and finding and organizing materials was strictly up to us. And that was as it should be, except for the fact that our resources felt so woefully inadequate.

Again, I compared our capacity with that of a huge organization like my employer's. Several times per year, the company delivered rockets for launching satellites into orbit, and inevitably some launches did not go well. But when anomalies occurred, extremely detailed investigations into the cause immediately followed. My job included preparing the final drafts of the reports: root-cause analysis, recommendations for corrective action. Clearly, that was the best response to any setback, and I wondered how to adapt it at home.

Unfortunately, Judy and I were the only people likely to improve our operations, or even to discuss them in any detail. Others readily agreed that our project was *hard* ("arduous" had been Pat's word for it). Incredibly, we still encountered some who thought it was *wrong*. At any rate, there could be only limited value in brainstorming between just two beleaguered parents, even with the benefit of several weeks' rest. *And as for mishaps!* The biggest, of course, was the one that had hurt Joseph. Since we didn't know the cause of his brain injury, we had no assurance that it wouldn't recur.

And that was a concern, because Judy had begun talking about having another child.

The idea terrified me. It put me into an absolute funk.

We knew so many kids with developmental problems. In fact, I'd come to think of families without disability as some privileged and elite minority. But what made the difference? I still fumed at the memory of Dr. Mulligan saying that Joseph's condition had "just happened." How could anyone in his position live with such an unscientific conclusion? There *had* to have been a cause! I knew, as well as I knew anything, that it was a normal and constructive impulse to seek that cause.

We stirred through the possibilities again. As a two-year-old, Judy had lived on an Army base not far from Hiroshima, only seven years after the bombing. Her latest hypothesis was that radiation might have damaged her, genetically. If so, any further kids she bore might also be disabled. She took the question to her doctor.

"I need to talk to you about having another baby," she began.

He smirked, or at least a smirk is what she saw. "Better take that up with your husband, not me!"

"No! You don't understand. If there's something wrong with me—some reason why I had one disabled child—I need to know about it now. Because we can't take on another."

The doctor shrugged. "I wouldn't know how to *begin* to plumb that mystery," he said. "It's true that if you were to get pregnant, it would be regarded as high-risk—so high-risk, in fact, that I wouldn't want to keep you as a patient. But nobody can quantify that risk. We certainly can't eliminate it."

"I understand that there's always risk," she said. "I just want to minimize it."

"Wait till you get pregnant," he said. "We'll talk about what to do after that."

"Look, we're not into abortion!" She protested, but he just shrugged. She had gone to the doctor for a pre-pregnancy exam and guidance.

His refusal to provide either amounted to the final straw. A long time would pass before Judy saw another MD for herself.

"HAS IT BEEN A GOOD HONEYMOON?" Lidwina asked on the phone a few days later. The date we'd set for picking up the program was fast approaching. *Were we ready?*

I claimed that we were. "The problem with being on Honeymoon has been that we don't have that structure built into our day," I told her. "Now that we've taken away the things Joseph normally *has* to do, he tends to fill in the gap with stupid stuff like banging the closet door repeatedly, or just pulling on a loose thread in the carpet. He won't sit still in my lap to read books, and we can only do so much romping on the floor! I'm afraid I don't know how to interact with my kid."

Judy amplified that. "Joseph doesn't know how to direct himself. We have to work every bit as hard to occupy his time in a meaningful way, so—we might as well be on program!"

Lidwina reminded us that the vocalizing and random behavior were attributable to the brain injury and were not entirely under his control. (The creeping was supposed to have eliminated this self-stimulation, I recalled, but didn't say.) At any rate, we'd just have to live with it a while longer. And we *were* too frazzled to resume the program, she decided. "Wait until after you've come back for the Revisit. Until then, just try to spend some quality time together. His pathway to wellness will be increasingly intellectual from here on, but first you need to build up good times together to carry you. Remember, he *is* just a little fellow. Keep your priorities straight, and give him your love and respect."

I observed that we'd "declared war on the brain injury, but not on the kid."

"Well put." Lidwina added that she was leaving to consult with senior families in Italy and would therefore miss us when we returned. "I'm anxious to see the little guy walking, but he'll be getting around even better the next time you come."

So there were a few extra weeks of Honeymoon. We let Joseph pick his level of activity. We even left him with Sally while we took an overnight cruise to Catalina Island, our first night away from him since he first came home from the hospital.

Judy felt moved to join Frank and Evelyn's Unity church, drawn by its message of *practical* Christianity. All of us were entitled to "have life, and have it more abundantly." All of us had a great deal of control over how well we succeeded in that. Positive thinking became a watchword around our house as we tried to turn our focus from the impediments to the destination.

Then, at the end of that summer, Lynn returned to San Diego, bringing our parents with her for another visit. She'd stayed with them in Charlottesville the last several weeks, ensuring that Dad continued eating properly and remained mentally engaged in his surroundings.

Old age had caught up with him at last. Sometimes I had the impression that he pretended to be in step with events around him when in fact he wasn't, quite. But that didn't seem to bother him. Perhaps, like the pseudo-experts he'd always scorned, he now enjoyed faking it.

And then, sometimes he was still completely tuned in. I remember relaxing with him on a bench at a shopping mall while Judy, Mom, and Lynn were browsing in a store.

"Let me buy you something," he said, gesturing at a window displaying fall fashions. "How about a sweater."

Touched, I protested. "Dad, I don't need anything."

"Well, I know that. But let me get you something anyway."

"Oh, Dad." I wanted to touch him, but we were never close like that. I thought he probably felt sorry for me. He too could see how far Joseph still had to go. Maybe I should have let him give me one last gift. But I couldn't accept anything more. That prayer had been answered.

17. FOUR-POINT-EIGHT MONTHS IN SIX

Mrs. Sweeney offered rooms in an aging stucco house just a block from the Institutes' gate. She told us this location made her especially attractive to foreign families who wanted to avoid the problem of renting a car.

"For me, doing this has been a way of traveling around the world without leaving home," she smiled. "And believe me, I've seen it *all* in the years I've been taking families. I'll always remember one family, for instance, that came from Japan. The mother was just a tiny thing. Their son was almost as big as she was. I looked out my window in the morning to see them hurrying down the sidewalk to their appointment. That lady was carrying their child on her back. *And* she was lugging all their other stuff—the word cards and devices and extra clothes. There she went, loaded down like a pack horse. And the *father!* Well, *he* was walking about ten paces ahead of her, with his hands free! I guess there's something about their culture, where men don't do certain things.

"But I told him that night he'd better start lending her a hand. I don't think it had ever occurred to him to do that, but from then on, he did start sharing some of the load. At least while they were staying at *my* house!"

Although not associated with the Institutes in any formal way, Mrs. Sweeney seemed to know everything that went on there, including behind-the-scenes scuttlebutt concerning the staff. She told us someone we knew had just resigned because the long hours and low pay had led to disagreements with his wife. "They spend every waking hour on the job, you know," she said. "The only way it can succeed for those who're married is for both spouses to work there. And, of course, that's what most of them do."

Likewise, she knew very well what life was like for the families. We spent some time discussing the unique relationship that existed between parents and staff.

"I had an Hispanic family come back recently for their Revisit. I just love those people. They've become like my own family. And they were so excited because their daughter was getting ready to have her First Communion. This was an older, well daughter, not their brain-injured one. You may know that, for Catholics, a girl's First Communion is a major event. So they were going to ask their advocate for permission to take that day off from the program."

"Hmm," I said doubtfully.

"'Hmm' is right! I told them, 'Look, if you really want to take that day off, do it! But don't expect the Institutes to approve.' I said it would be better to say nothing, unless they wouldn't mind having the idea shot down. If I've learned anything in the years I've been doing this, it's that families have to be intelligent about what they say. You've got to do the program, of course. But you've got to keep the family together, too. And it doesn't do a brain-injured kid any good to have his parents kicked off program."

Her words came as no great revelation to Judy and me. Actually, our recent dealings with the staff suggested that they might be disposed to grant such a request—more so than in our early days, at least. Presumably, we'd passed a probationary period, and had attained the status of partners with them. Even so, we had no wish to bring in unnecessary problems.

MONDAYS AT THE INSTITUTES always meant evaluation. This time, Joseph faced an international panel of staff members—Marlene Marckwordt, a Guatemalan, and Dr. Ernesto Vasquez, who came from Mexico, as well as an observer visiting from a related clinic in Australia. The Walking Victory was a foregone conclusion, but they were delighted to grant it to him. The most exciting part, however, came when we deployed our intelligence materials. Since the last visit, we had begun teaching Joseph to read in Spanish, and this naturally pleased his current audience. "Let's start with some single words in Spanish," Dr. Vasquez suggested. We presented Joseph with word cards reading *abrazo* and *beso*, asked him to identify them— and roared approval as he unhesitatingly made the right choices.

Another pair of cards came out. I held them up, and Joseph crossed the room to touch the word I had named. He laughed happily at our excitement. Maybe he was surprised, himself, that it was so easy.

After several more Spanish and English words, Dr. Vasquez wanted to try the same thing with complete sentences. "Joseph! Which card says, *'You are a wonderful boy'*?" No problem. By the time we got to the Bits, however, I sensed that all this was beginning to get a little old. Once, Joseph touched the right card with his *foot*. Another time he looked at the right card but deliberately touched the wrong one, and laughed at the joke. Or he touched both cards. But that was OK. He'd satisfied everyone present.

At the end of the day, Matt took us into his office for the verdict. These summaries also acknowledged qualitative improvements that did not amount to Victories, but the bottom line could be discouraging. In terms of actual numbers, he told us, Joseph had moved up *two* Profile levels in the mobility pathway, from Creeping to Walking without needing his arms for balance. This translated into a neurological gain of 4.8 months.

The trouble was that six months had passed, meaning he was now further behind than ever.

Matt could see my disappointment. "Joseph's progress is like a flagstone walkway," he said. "Each time you come back, he's a little further along. Sure, he's not well yet, but we didn't expect him to be well. What he *has* accomplished is very significant! You should have been sitting here the night Lidwina got your call! I remember she ran past all the offices shouting, *'Joseph Gallup is walking! Joseph Gallup is walking!'* All of us stopped what we were doing and went out for ice cream to celebrate." He grinned. "Now, that's the attitude *you* need to cultivate. Joseph deserves to be told how great he is."

"OK! *JOSEPH!* It's time to come learn about the hugging program!"

It was Thursday morning, and Dr. Vasquez was yelling and banging his hands together like a soccer coach.

The hugging program?

Earlier in the week Judy and I had been asked to monitor Joseph's breathing and to complete a short questionnaire. Was his breathing easy to see? What percentage of the time did he breathe with his mouth open? What was his breathing rate at rest? We could easily see that it was irregular. There'd be a couple of deep breaths and then some so shallow that we argued over whether he had inhaled at all. Sometimes he held his breath for several seconds and then gasped. I'd never given it much thought, but apparently he always breathed that way.

Also, he wasn't always able to coordinate his breathing with his eating, which meant choking incidents were not rare. There'd been one this week, in fact. Dr. Wilkinson had been summoned in case he needed CPR, although as it turned out that wasn't required.

The implication of all this gradually became obvious, and Dr. Vasquez now proposed to introduce us to respiratory patterning. He said, "The reason for lack of improved function in almost all brain-injured children is their less-than-satisfactory respiration. Brain injury is caused by lack of oxygen. And Joseph's current status in the path toward wellness is still limited by his ability to deliver enough oxygen to the brain. He does get *some* oxygen, of course, but the amount varies. That's why he's not always alert. If we can improve the availability of oxygen, we can improve his functioning across the board."

This sounded simple enough, as did the means proposed for addressing the problem. To Joseph's great indignation, he found himself once again on a patterning table! He clearly thought he'd outgrown that procedure. Actually, he had. There was to be no more *cross*-patterning, but the new program required even more patience.

We'd heard about respiratory patterning from other parents, and had gathered that it was not a favorite pastime. A child receiving this treatment lies on a table between two adults, with a specially fitted garment wrapped around his torso. Straps lead out in opposite directions to loop around a pair of dowel rods, which the adults grasp like handlebars and pull rhythmically. The effect is to squeeze the child's chest and force him to exhale. The effect is very much like old-fashioned artificial respiration, and in fact, that is what it had evolved from. The main difference was that it consumed several hours every day.

Dr. Vasquez emphasized the importance of synchronizing our pulls and maintaining a perfect rhythm, which was established by an electronic metronome. "The pull must be sufficient to affect your child's breathing but not enough to hurt him," he said. "Pull smoothly; don't ever jerk it. Be aware of the child at all times. With the other kind of patterning, there's room for variation. But in patterning someone's breathing, there can be no monkeying around. Pulling in and out would be no big deal if the object in the middle were not a human being. But since it is, you have a huge responsibility to do it right."

Respiration had suddenly become the key to everything else. To demonstrate, Dr. Vasquez took us into an adjacent room where a machine measured the levels of oxygen and carbon dioxide in Joseph's bloodstream. When we first hooked him up, the digital readout showed an oxygen level of 77 mm Hg. Dr. Vasquez told us that the usual reading—for a well child—was about 85. So this represented a measurable physiological shortfall. During the test we tried masking Joseph, and observed that this quickly drove his oxygen level down to 51. But once the mask had been removed, the reading soared into the 80s, dramatically demonstrating the potential for improving things.

Masking may have been a strain for Joseph in the early days of program, but he handled it now without a thought. So, however dull and time-consuming this next stage might be for Judy and me, we were *ready*. We had everyone's assurance that visual convergence, language, coordination, and use of the hands would all improve with better respiration.

Several sessions of respiratory patterning followed throughout this day and the next, until Dr. Vasquez thought we had the hang of it. Joseph's prescription would be a minimum of three hours daily—more if possible. The more we did, the more input Joseph would receive on how it felt to breathe properly.

The optimum *rate* at which he would be taught to breathe had yet to be established. Judy and I would have to watch him closely, adjust our rate of patterning up or down as we saw fit, and report all changes in his performance to the Institutes every month.

And of course, we left with an array of other assignments, as well, including a graduating set of goals for distance walking, new vestibular techniques to improve his balance, a new auditory stimulation program involving blasts of an air horn, and a stepped-up intelligence program aimed at independent reading and problem solving.

RIDING HOME on the airplane, I drafted a letter to our remaining volunteers. "There is no more cross-patterning!" I wrote gleefully. "We may be asked to do more of that at some point in the future, but his mobility and coordination are so much improved that we can discontinue it while tackling other things." I didn't know how much help we'd need with the new program—or how willing they'd be to stay involved. But I wanted to reassure them once again that they'd accomplished something.

Judy and Joseph dozed in the seats beside me, lulled by the muted thunder of jet engines. Below passed a stately procession of farms and golden-brown fields, readied for winter and yet another cycle.

And here we go again.

18. THE HUGGING PROGRAM

The walking parts of our new program made us intimately familiar with all the contours of our neighborhood. We sought out and scaled the steepest driveways and grassy hillsides as well as exploring rough terrain and level paved areas. Three times a day we sallied forth for a thirty-minute walk in these varied environments. At any given moment during the next few months, passers-by could expect to encounter a few people walking their dogs, a jogger or two—and Joseph.

We bought a rollertape, the kind used by surveyors, and pushed this along to keep track of distances covered. At first, Joseph barely exceeded a thousand feet in twenty minutes of steady walking on level sidewalks, but that figure went up quickly.

During all the months of patterning and creeping and ladder walking, I'd yearned for a time when we could do this kind of program. Upright, independent walking! Something normal! And indeed, strangers we met along the way saw nothing out of the ordinary at all. Here was just a little boy out for a stroll with his mommy or daddy—except for that peculiar stick on wheels that the adults were pushing. Now, *that* part was odd—.

Then there was our strange insistence on keeping this little guy moving. Joseph tended to dawdle, finding distractions in every shrub or flower. Sly smiles hinted that he might be teasing us, or testing our resolve. Well, we still had plenty. We maneuvered him past every potential stopping point, constantly asking for more speed.

"Come on, Joseph!"

We probably used that phrase more than any other.

"Come *on!*"

The words seemed to hang in the air, like subtitles in a foreign-language movie.

Come on to wellness. And faster, please!

Thanksgiving arrived, as did another film crew from Channel Eight. Someone thought it was time to reflect on how far we had come and to draw conclusions. Stan Miller asked leading questions. How did I feel about all those doctors who had let us down? I shrugged at this and mumbled something unusable. The experts we'd once relied on were not relevant. They must have known, far better than Judy or I at the time, how serious Joseph's problems were. But they hadn't tried to help him. They'd stalled us with advice to wait and see, when intervention was urgently needed. I could have hated them, but I preferred to forget them.

Anyway, regarding his future, we hadn't proved them completely wrong just yet.

Stan thought otherwise. For the piece that was aired, he used some old footage from an earlier broadcast while he reviewed Joseph's story in a voiceover. Then he cut to a sequence of Joseph venturing out the front door of our house and strolling easily along the sidewalk accompanied by our cat, Bandit. Judy was allowed an opportunity to publicly thank all the people who had helped make it happen, and this led to a touching musical interlude, showing patterning and then walking—all in slow motion—with a song about bringing joy into the world. The piece concluded with me saying, "When Joseph walks, it's something I'll never take for granted."

A fitting note for Thanksgiving eve.

We *didn't* take it for granted, but perhaps the time had come to adjust our relationship with the world around us. The very next day a roving photographer for the newspaper snapped Joseph's picture as we logged some mileage through a deserted shopping mall. It didn't even occur to me to mention brain injury when he asked for our names. Earlier, I would have seen an opportunity to advertise our program. But sooner or later Joseph would be joining the ranks of normal people, and I must have already decided to begin the transition.

The transition would involve many changes, especially an end of our heavy dependence on others. I relished that prospect, but didn't accomplish it gracefully. As I look back over our story, there are points along the way where it now appears something went wrong. This, I think, was one.

We'd felt compelled to take a course of action broadly condemned by established authorities, and now it seemed obvious that we'd been right to rebel. In other respects, however, we were rather conventional. Circumstances had made us dissenters, albeit in the cause of achieving normal life for our son and ourselves. In such a case, how does one reintegrate oneself into the mainstream that had been so disappointing? How does one begin reconsidering the possibility of learning anything from it? We wouldn't have known where to look for new ideas, but we were so deep in a groove, we didn't even consider whether we needed them. We were burning bridges.

The volunteers who'd joined us along the way, however briefly, would always deserve anything of us they asked. But from this point on, the idle curiosity of outsiders began to meet with a chilly response. Far too many had taken up our precious time with questions that served no purpose. Increasingly, we resisted being treated as a sideshow. Joseph did not benefit when some smiling neighbor, who'd never bothered to introduce himself, slowed his car to match our pace, rolled down his window, and called out, "How's he doing?"

How are you doing? is the most normal of everyday greetings, and I might have taken the question that way. But I'd grown defensive. I bristled. What did those people expect? Did they want to hear about his respiration? Did they want to hear how far behind we had already fallen in preparing reading words and Bits? No. They wanted more hearty assurances that miracles were continuing to unfold. Find your own miracles, Buddy.

With the lessons Judy was bringing home from her new church, not to mention motivational courses provided by my employer, I might have known to use such opportunities and give those assurances. Theoretically at least, an important component of success is putting on a show of optimistism, even when you don't happen to feel that way. Already I lacked the energy.

"No more publicity!" I vowed. "We've been on public display long enough."

WELL, EVEN GIVEN THE REDUCED INTERACTION with others, Joseph's victories ought to have kept us in a more upbeat frame of mind. I wonder if our dour attitude came from the hours and hours of respiratory patterning.

We had been instructed to avoid distractions such as visitors or TV so that we could provide a steady rhythm of inhalation and exhalation. That was good advice, because in the early days it took real concentration for Judy and me to synchronize the timing of our pulls, even with the aid of a metronome.

Our day began at six o'clock. One of us would lift Joseph carefully from his bed and carry him downstairs to the patterning table. There was no need to turn on lights; if he stayed asleep, so much the better. We silently laced the straps around him, took our seats, and set sleepily to work. After forty-five minutes, daylight was beginning to seep in under the curtains and Joseph was beginning to stir. We stopped at seven, leaving me half an hour in which to shower, dress, and hurry off to my job.

We patterned for another hour when I came home in the evening and again at bedtime. Once Judy and I felt comfortable with the technique, we relaxed a little and began conversing about other things. She said she enjoyed having my undivided attention for such long intervals.

At length, we ran out of things to say and then began playing tapes. Joseph showed interest in a collection of passages from Shakespeare's plays, looking at the tape player with an expression that said, *Here is something new!* For variety, we tried recordings of Robert Frost's poetry and miscellaneous recorded books. The library had several of the Jeeves stories on tape, and Judy and I enjoyed these bits of nonsense. If Joseph didn't follow the humor, it nevertheless did him good to hear us laugh.

Judy claimed to see an immediate improvement in his level of alertness. She said he stayed happier and more energetic all day long, and was more fun to be with, and that he cooperated as never before. And at night he climbed into his bed with a happy smile on his face and snuggled down into the covers—like any kid ought to do! So although the practice of repiratory patterning was more than tedious, the apparent result was worth it. *Why hadn't we started this sooner?*

His lack of speech, however, did not change. There had never been much, of course, but now there was less. We tried to be patient, remembering the time when we'd been desperate to see him walk. If three hours of patterning per day were good, then four or even more hours would be better. Lidwina suggested a weekly marathon day of five hours.

But now miscellaneous little problems such as aching elbows and stiff necks began to plague us. We were patterning later into the night, until one of us was on the brink of nodding off, and it became harder to get up and do the early morning session.

Nancy and a few others were willing to help, God bless them, but found it a challenge. Some people simply could not understand the necessity of pulling hard enough on the stick and sustaining the pull for the right duration. Conversation was definitely out, unless they had mastered the technique, and it was a rare volunteer who could endure this for more than twenty minutes.

For some, it was a physical impossibility. In truth, we hated asking anyone to make the sacrifice.

A few offered to help in other ways, such as making intelligence materials. Marzi began coming by frequently with stacks of Bits that she assembled at her apartment: types of snakes, famous sailing ships. Everything she did became a welcome supplement to our own efforts. Her fiancé, a young engineer named John, watched us pattern one evening when she made a delivery and said, "There's got to be a way to do that mechanically."

Well, of course, the Institutes did have motor-driven respirators, although there'd been no discussion of letting us have one. Judy had also tried unsuccessfully to draw up plans for a homemade device—perhaps something with pulleys and levers—that would enable one of us to accomplish the task alone. Being freed from the chore of finding helpers was a wonderful motivator.

According to Mrs. Sweeney, a German family had already invented what we needed, but that was a big secret. Fear of a rebuke from the Institutes prevented them from telling their advocate or sharing the design with anyone.

As the bills from our last trip began coming in, I recognized that something else was lacking too. We needed more money—a lot more of it—if we hoped to see Philadelphia again.

Therefore, in spite of the desire for privacy, Judy took our case before her new church.

Very few of the people there knew our situation. Judy had enjoyed just blending into the congregation. Even more, she enjoyed the church's message that success, peace, and health were realistic objectives for everyone. She heard lessons to the effect that one can take any divine idea, such as health and perfect functioning, and acknowledge it as true even in the absence of objective evidence. One only had to believe in it, affirm it, be open to it, and give thanks for it. And the idea would be manifested in life.

This did not necessarily relieve one from also taking whatever concrete steps seemed appropriate. So, one Sunday morning, while Joseph and I were concentrating on the usual walks and other program activities, Judy stood up in the church and described our plight.

"There are lots of different ways you can help us," she said. "Take your pick!" She talked about the intelligence program and the respiratory patterning, about the multitude of little projects that could make our life easier, such as arranging our thousands of retired Bits in such a way that we could access them for review. And then, of course, there was the inescapable question of money.

She didn't expect an immediate response, but as soon as she sat down the minister's wife, Meredith, was making a suggestion.

"I will take the responsibility of coordinating pledges," she said. "Judy says the airfare and lodging cost them about twelve hundred dollars each time they go back to the Institutes. If a hundred people here in the congregation can each contribute twelve dollars, that will solve the problem! You can make your checks payable to the church."

We learned, later, that Judy's appeal touched off a certain amount of behind-the-scenes debate, since some church members were opposed to acknowledging that brain injury even existed. Presumably, since it was not a manifestation of a "divine idea," it was not real and should be ignored. However, there were enough people who felt otherwise. In no time at all the money had been amassed, and the church had made out checks to the travel agency and to Mrs. Sweeney.

Our former patterner Evelyn was among those who heard this appeal. She came back to help with the intelligence materials but then became discouraged, she said, because our standards were so high.

"They're probably *too* high," I agreed. "The Institutes tells us to stress *quantity*, not quality—to just get in as much information as we possibly can. But we've always tried to make perfect Bits so we'll have the best chance of grabbing Joseph's attention. That's why we go for pictures that are as big and as bold and as bright as we can possibly get."

Our expectations were too much for Evelyn. But in consolation she gave us a collection of old magazines to mine for usable pictures, and topped that off by ordering some ready-made Bits for us from the In-stitutes bookstore.

Late into the night, after the day's patterning was finished and Joseph put to bed, Judy and I would sit at the kitchen table, paging through books and calendars and magazines in search of materials. We still taught facts about the world in sets of related Bits; so it was necessary to plan ahead. I might come across an excellent picture of a spider monkey, but unless and until we had accumulated several other pri-mates, it would have to bide its time on the shelf. Here was a great, full-page view of the Leaning Tower of Pisa! I realized famous build-ings—or even just famous towers—would make a worthwhile category and alerted Judy to keep her eyes open for more examples. Surely, even in those pre-Internet day, such things had to be archived somewhere, with clear images of Big Ben and the Eiffel Tower and the Seattle Space Needle and all the rest on file and ready for use. Magazines, alas, were not laid out with the interests of the Bit maker in mind. We'd find great pictures—but they were only two inches high, partly obscured by type, or cluttered by extraneous, distracting stuff in the foreground. When we did come across something usable, translating it into a Bit took careful work. Say it made up a two-page spread in the *National Geographic*. To get both halves out of the magazine intact, I had to peel back the cover, pry open the heavy-duty staples, knife out the two sheets along the centerline, smear rubber cement on the backs, and carefully—oh, very carefully (because the tissue-thin paper tore easily if you lifted it up again once it was stuck down)—mate them edge-to-edge on the cardboard.

But wait! Better scan the text of the article first, because it might contain information that we could relay to Joseph when showing him the picture (how tall, how old, how far away—).

When I was really up to speed, I might get five such Bits assembled in an hour.

Five Bits! We could run those past Joseph in about ten seconds the next morning. Hopefully, he would look at them! On good days, a fleeting glimmer of interest did show in his face.

We had the choice of worrying about all the times he did not respond, or rejoicing that at last he was starting to discriminate—to show a preference for certain topics. Lidwina assured us that it was not at all uncommon for a kid who walked as much as he did to lose interest in Bits, due to mental energy being diverted. Our task was simply to carry on and not get discouraged.

But we still hadn't found a picture of the Washington Monument! Or the CN Tower in Toronto! As long as we were on the subject, it would be wrong to overlook those landmarks. You'd think finding such pictures would be easy. Could I write to some news agency for them? Or was there a book—something affordable, not one of those fifty-dollar coffee-table editions—that I could slice up for the pictures?

It was a mild craziness, to go about my day preoccupied with the question of where to find more pictures. I knew that. But I had a project. Whenever my energies started to flag, I recalled how badly we'd wanted a course of action that would help our son.

Then, frustrated with that, I'd get on a kick of assembling Bits that were entirely homemade (or office-made, when the workload there permitted). Joseph should learn the logos of the different auto manufacturers, I decided. Everybody can recognize the emblems for Chevy, Mercedes Benz, and the rest. Being able to do so makes one just that much more aware of the surroundings. Several new makes of cars had appeared on the streets while we'd been engrossed in the program (Saturn, Acura, Infiniti), and I had to learn their logos myself. Anyway, it turned out to be an enjoyable exercise, creating plausible copies of the designs and (as always) typing the name in bold one-inch letters to glue on the back.

Four categories of five Bits each, taught for four days and then replaced by new stuff. Plus facts about those pictures, and homemade books, math, problem solving—every day. Did they really think we could keep up that pace? We taught whatever materials we had, but producing the prescribed quantity on schedule was another matter.

WHAT ABOUT THE BOY?   255

THE REQUIREMENT for auditory stimulation involved ten daily sessions with a sudden, loud noise, such as a blast from the air horn. We
gave him thirty blasts in each session—or as many as possible until the
freon caused the horn to freeze up. At this rate we were going through
canisters of compressed gas faster than the marine supply store could
keep them in stock. Joseph typically gave a violent start at the first blast
(as did the cat, if we forgot to let it outdoors first, and anyone else who
happened to be in the vicinity). After about ten blasts, he seemed to
be looking for a way to escape. That wasn't good enough, however.
We were supposed to see an instantaneous, gut-level fear reaction. I
began to wonder if the whole question of his hearing might be totally
misguided.

JOSEPH'S WALKING continued to improve, but he remained un-
steady on some surfaces. To improve his balance, we had to see that
he accomplished ten daily sessions of forward somersaults, building
to twenty somersaults each; another ten sessions of twenty backward
somersaults, and five sessions of log-rolling, one hundred meters in
each direction. For this, Judy and Joseph found their way back to the
neighborhood YMCA. Glen, the gymnastics coach there, welcomed
them enthusiastically, said they could use his facilities every day, and
then surprised us with his own article extolling Joseph's progress for
the "Y" newsletter.

WEEKS PASSED. At some point during the winter, we realized that
we'd all become sick. There was a half-hour conversation with Lidwina,
who decided we needed to take a week off from the program. "Don't
push him," she advised. "And don't push yourselves. Use this time to
build up a backlog of intelligence materials so you can double up afterwards."
   My sister Lynn called to ask how things were going.
   "Well, we've stopped the program—"

"*Good!*"

"No, wait. We haven't stopped for keeps! We're just taking a few days to rest up and get organized."

Lynn's disappointment was obvious. I hadn't noticed until now that she disapproved of what we were doing.

"If I can help, let me know," she said before hanging up.

"Thanks. I'll keep that in mind."

Any thrill attached to walking around our immediate neighborhood had faded. Lidwina now said to try for a nonstop *mile*, just to see how long it would take, and for that a new course was definitely in order. Lynn was a marathon runner, and could see a place for herself in this part of our endeavors, if not others. She recommended a high-school track where she trained sometimes. Four laps would equal a mile, so we could dispense with the roller tape.

Joseph accepted this new challenge willingly enough and began pacing off the distance while the three of us walked backwards in front of him, constantly shouting our encouragement. Every few steps I would drop back beside him, and Judy would immediately warn me not to nudge him along in my impatience.

"Let *him* do it," she insisted. "*He can!*"

And he did, keeping up a purposeful, shoulders-back, sternum-first stride, lap after lap.

"I've never seen a little kid with such terrific posture," Lynn observed wonderingly.

We had the overhead ladder to thank for that. I hadn't given the question of posture much thought, but it was true. That ladder had stretched him out and shown him the ideal way to stand. How much more desirable this than learning while holding a parent's fingers or—heaven forbid—hunched over a walker!

The first nonstop mile took 42 minutes. A week later he accomplished the same distance in under 37 minutes.

One of the Institutes' definitions for running was the ability to cover a mile in twenty minutes. We'd be at that stage very soon.

19. VISITORS

Dear Mr. & Mrs. Gallup:

Enclosed you will find a copy of a letter we are sending to a family seeking an initial appointment at the Institutes. We have asked them to contact you because we firmly believe that if they observe and we hope participate in an excellent program in action, their child's chances will improve.

Following their visit, we would greatly appreciate a note from you either recommending this family or not.

Thank you for helping us to help other kids.

Douglas Doman

Here was our opportunity to do for someone else what Silvia and Manuel had done for us. Judy dashed off a note to the family, saying we'd be happy to show them our program. They called, made arrangements to visit, called again to cancel because of illness, and then let the matter hang for several weeks. I was ready to conclude that they weren't interested when they finally set a firm date and then appeared on our doorstep.

Bob and Annette gave the impression of having been an unusually lucky young couple. He was a junior insurance executive with the rugged good looks of a model. She owned a beauty and exercise salon near their home in a resort community. This storybook situation had just one kink. Their toddler had fallen into the backyard swimming pool when no one was looking. Now his crossed eyes, slack mouth, and fisted hands all proclaimed brain injury. They had him in a specially designed wheelchair, with straps and brackets to hold his rigid body in place.

Judy and I watched as his parents began the process of unbuckling him. Then they removed a pair of special foam shoes that kept his feet in a normal position. When the little guy was finally free and lying on the floor, his feet resembled those of a ballet dancer on pointe. His gaze moved across the room, registering each of us. Judy and I spoke gently to him, hoping he wasn't frightened.

His parents declined refreshments. They just wanted to learn what they could expect from the program. "As you must know by now," I began, "the Institutes do things differently." They nodded expectantly. I hesitated. Other parents of hurt kids had taught Judy and me to keep recommendations to ourselves, but these people had just driven two hours to hear us.

"Well, for starters, they'll tell you that that wheelchair has to go." I paused again to see how they took this. They raised their eyebrows but not their defenses. "And another thing. These shoes of his are doing the opposite of what you hope to accomplish. His foot wants to straighten out, and when you force it into a normal position, you just strengthen the wrong muscles. You're making it want to straighten even more. It's like an isometric exercise."

"That makes sense," Annette said thoughtfully.

"It sure does," her husband echoed. "I hadn't stopped to think about that. But everything I hear about this approach just—*sounds right!*"

"That was my initial reaction as well," I said.

Within a few minutes, Judy and I had decided that these people were Institutes material. They didn't complain about the magnitude of the task we were describing. They didn't argue that their therapist had told them something else. As we spoke, I could see them making mental adjustments. Build an inclined plane to encourage mobility? OK. They could do that. In fact, they already had the materials, they said eagerly. Keep him prone on the floor all the time, using an antiroll device if necessary? No big deal. Disassemble his crib and have him *sleep* on the floor, or even on the inclined plane? OK. If it would help—why not!

The story of their accident came out as we got to know one another. Bob had been out of town on business when a neighbor reached him by phone to say Jimmy had drowned. "I just couldn't believe it," he said, staring at the floor and reliving the nightmare. Jimmy's nanny was supposed to be caring for him, but was doing laundry instead. Annette had felt a sudden foreboding and had hurried to investigate, but not soon enough.

While Bob's employer made arrangements to fly him home, he'd wandered outside to sit in a car. "I was praying, *Whatever it takes, we'll do, God. Just spare us our little boy.*" Then someone came running out of the building.

"He told me there'd been a miracle and they'd gotten a pulse."

Now they had something to do.

We showed them our videos that documented Joseph's progress. They saw his early faltering movements with an antiroll device strapped on his back. They saw the parade of patterners coming through the house. They saw him standing under the ladder.

"I cringe every time I see our footage of that ladder," I told them. "We spent so much time marching him back and forth under the thing. Five, six hundred trips a day. It felt brutal."

"But it worked!"

"Oh, yes. It sure worked. It just took longer than I'd anticipated."

"How long was that?"

"He was under the ladder a year and a month."

From the present perspective, a year and a month seemed trivial. The videos continued. In the last one—the recent Thanksgiving news segment—Judy was smiling and holding out her arms as a laughing little boy walked into them. Annette wiped a tear from her eye.

It was great to think about the payoff, but I still wanted to make sure they understood how demanding their program would be, and how unyielding the staff at the Institutes could be regarding their assignment. We'd acquired certain survival skills along the way that helped keep the relationship smooth, and we stressed the importance of these. "You don't confront them," I warned. "Some staff people in particular you *never* want to get crosswise with."

Judy laughed. "Dawn, for example."

They looked back and forth between us. "Yeah," I smiled. "Dawn would be an example. And if your assignment is to mask your son a hundred times a day, and somehow you only manage to do it sixty times? Well, *I'm not saying you should lie about that*, but—."

"I think I get the picture," Bob said.

"Mind you, a hundred times a day is probably what he *needs*," I persisted. "This isn't to say you shouldn't try your very best to accomplish that. It's just that if you don't—."

"Understood," he said again.

We showed them how to pattern, we mentioned a few books that would add to their knowledge, and we gave them a stack of used word cards. In parting, I shook Bob's hand and said, "You're in for some good times and some bad times."

He just grinned. In recent months it had been *all* bad times.

The visit encouraged Judy and me as well. In the daily grind, we continually lost sight of the big picture. We critiqued our performance and Joseph's status, returning every day to the same worries and conversations the way a musical composition returns to its motif. It was reassuring to see ourselves through the eyes of these newcomers. They'd gazed in wonder at the intelligence materials we were currently teaching. Such variety! Annette had begun trying to teach her son to read, but had made the beginner's mistake of showing him the same few words over and over again. Our mountain of *retired* word cards, which now included phrases in three languages, had rendered them speechless.

With the ladder gone, our household looked much more normal, but evidence of our ongoing program was always within reach. Rebreathing masks hung conveniently from doorknobs throughout the house. Even today, when we'd tidied up, it was still a mess, with reference books, rollertape, and all the other stuff shoved hastily into the corners. As if we had reason to doubt it, we were definitely a full-fledged Institutes family. Of course, Joseph was walking proof that we'd been doing something right.

AS YET ANOTHER REVISIT DATE approached, we realized that he had become more *curious*. He stretched to pull items off the kitchen counter. He pulled stuff out of drawers, examined the workings of the dishwasher, occasionally got into things that he shouldn't. Back in the early, chaotic days, Judy had bought safety latches for the doors of our kitchen and bathroom cabinets. It didn't matter that Joseph was completely immobile then. The house had to be child-proofed, and there was no peace between us until I'd installed at least some of the latches. Now, years later, we needed them.

At long, long last, we said, our boy was demonstrably on track to become the healthy, normal child he'd always been meant to be.

20. BLACK-AND-WHITE REALITY

All these years later, I still remember the kids we met through the Institutes. The memory of them haunts me, because, in most cases, I don't know how things turned out for them.

Some were poster children. Jeffrey, a slender, fair-haired boy from Pittsburgh, was near the top of the heap when our paths crossed. Although undersized, he could not only walk but run, talk, and brachiate, and he no doubt excited the envy of every parent there. His own parents were far from complacent, however, and assured us that his small stature was misleading. He still lagged a couple of years behind his age group.

On the other hand, on this next trip back to Philadelphia we could see that Sean's respiratory capabilities hadn't kept pace with his increasing size and demand for oxygen. He was now even more rigid than we remembered from previous visits. His legs had scissored to the point that they were actually becoming dislocated from the hips.

Paul, his dad, seemed to be taking it all in remarkably good spirits. Every time I saw the man, he maintained the same jolly, winsome personality, frequently offering racy jokes at the expense of his tolerant wife. Just a faintly quizzical expression around his eyes hinted at perplexity over the direction life had taken.

He and Laura had long since recognized that Sean needed more than manual respiratory patterning. They believed he needed an actual mechanical respirator. In fact, they'd already purchased one, he said, without waiting for the Institutes to prescribe it, and were pushing for a further measure called CO_2 therapy.

How many more twists like that lay in store for all of us? *How much longer was all this going to take?* Speaking to a small group of fathers in the waiting area, I referred to the drive across town from the Philadelphia airport that Judy and I had managed two nights before. We'd lost our map, but somehow had negotiated the dark streets without a single wrong turn.

"Glenn Doman says the slowest learner is an adult," I recalled. "Well adults are supposed to need up to thirty repetitions of something before they learn it. I just hope we won't have to make thirty trips here before Joseph graduates."

"We've come twenty-six times now," a man from Belgium offered.

My heart sank. "No. Twenty-six?"

"Well, in the early days, families came every two months."

They had crossed the Atlantic with a severely brain-injured—indeed, he said, in the early days a *paralyzed*—child, as often as every two months, for the last ten years.

Of course, by now their son was no longer paralyzed. In fact, he was expected to graduate from the Institutes on his next visit.

"We thought he would be graduating now," the father said. "But in the past year his handwriting has become really poor. The staff decided that meant he had a problem with mixed dominance, and now we're in the process of changing him from being right-handed to left-handed. *Then* he'll be finished!"

Toon, the child in question, was one of the best advertisements for a neurological program that I ever saw. During the week, he made a point of getting acquainted with the different families. We found him a proper little gentleman, very much interested in the younger children and their programs.

And then there was Bobby!

I met his mother, Cindy, when we were both running up to Clarke

Hall for coffee. We stood in the empty dining room there discussing our kids, and she revealed that she too had been making the trip for many years.

"We've been on program longer than any other American family," she sighed. "I wish it weren't so, but what else can we do? Obviously, we wouldn't stay with something like this if we didn't think it was doing some good. But on the other hand, I never expected it to take so long. It was *three* years before Bobby even had a crawling victory! And he's still got light-years to go."

She was a lively, upbeat lady. I couldn't imagine how she'd preserved such a bright and attractive demeanor over a decade of grueling work and almost imperceptible progress. But admiration for an Institutes family is a cheap emotion, worth no more than the simple pity commonly spent on those without a plan for recovery. I knew that well, but I was beginning to admire this parent nonetheless. Then she mentioned that Bobby wasn't even her natural child.

She'd found him in a state institution, where he had been placed at one year of age after being profoundly brain-injured by abusive parents. Although unmarried at the time, she had assumed the responsibility of caring for and hopefully salvaging this pathetic throwaway. She had exhausted the medical resources of her native Chicago within six months, and before his second birthday Bobby had arrived at the Institutes.

"They use a lot of techniques here now that they didn't have back in those early days," she went on. "CO_2 therapy, the respirator—. When *we* started, people just patterned their kids and put them on the floor, and the kids were supposed to start crawling. Maybe if we'd had all this other stuff then, he might be further along now."

At some point, Cindy had married, and now she had several children of her own, fine, healthy boys, each presenting a beautiful reminder of our shared objective for Jeffrey, Sean, Bobby, Joseph, and all the rest. Their raucous play added several decibels to life in the Clinic throughout the week.

AFTER VARIOUS STAFF MEMBERS had evaluated Joseph, we found ourselves Lidwina's office. Joseph seemed thrilled to be meeting with her once again. At home, we invoked her name daily to encourage his cooperation, so there was no danger of his having forgotten who she was. He bounded into her room making lots of high-pitched, playful noises.

Lidwina said, "Joseph, do you want to climb up in your own chair?"

Joseph excitedly said, "Yeah!"

"Well, bring your chair over here, and sit next to us—. You'll have to *pull* the chair. There! You're a mighty big fellow now!"

He giggled and clambered into the seat.

Lidwina then got down to business, and we discussed the good and bad aspects of the previous few months of program, Joseph's strongest and weakest areas, and the areas that had changed the most.

Under the heading of auditory competence, I complained that it was still hard to say how much he understood, since he gave us so little verbal feedback.

Lidwina said, "You've got to become experts at looking at him without the language. Some of the things you mentioned in the report are beautiful indications of understanding. And practically, he gives me the impression that he's taking in a thousand things."

Joseph let out a cheer at this, or seemed to, anyway, and she paused to smile at him for a long moment. Almost regretfully, she returned to the questions at hand. We talked at great length about intelligence, language, and running, and his impediments to faster progress in all these areas. He'd made progress since our last visit, she said, although there were no victories to celebrate. "Statistically," she said, "brain-injured kids have head sizes that are below the 50th percentile for their ages." But Joseph's head had grown at *four times* the normal rate, bringing it within one-tenth of a centimeter of the average.

"I thought Elaine was getting something unusual," I recalled. "Because she went back and measured him a second time."

"This rate of increase is *very* unusual. I think we can attribute it to brain growth."

Judy remained stuck on one subject. "How soon can we expect to see more language?"

Lidwina couldn't predict that. "I think we have to look at whether we go all-out with respiratory patterning to get it," she said, "or whether we mix that with gymnastics, or running, or more creeping. There are various combinations in there that will all affect his language, but which is going to accomplish it faster? I want to discuss it with the staff. But we should definitely push more respiratory development."

We said we liked the results we were achieving with respiratory patterning, in terms of Joseph's improved disposition and better general alertness, but there was a practical problem in accomplishing it manually. What we really wanted—especially if longer hours might hasten acquisition of language—was one of the Institutes' patterning *machines*. We tried to convey this request as clearly as possible, without appearing to dictate anything. (Judy had already broached the subject to Ann Ball, the Institutes' gatekeeper for such devices—a little too forcibly perhaps, judging from Ann's frosty response.)

"I *hate* to see Joseph falling so far behind in speech, as compared to other four-year-olds," she lamented. Then, more brightly, she asked, "How quickly *can* a child pick up language, once he starts?"

Lidwina smiled. "Oh, some of them just blossom! Kids have picked up thousands of words in just six months." But she had a more immediate concern. "How are you both, in terms of health?"

Judy confessed that we'd suffered a series of bad colds. "I guess that's just because we've been pushing so hard. You know, Joseph's program doesn't stop at a certain time in the evening. It stops when we get it all done, and sometimes that's at ten-thirty. And then we stay up later than that, trying to get ready for the next day. So, we haven't taken very good care of ourselves. Maybe you can't expect to stay healthy under those conditions."

Lidwina nodded. No doubt, she'd heard it all before. She reminded us that the Institutes offered alternate plans, and families reaching our level of seniority could choose between continuing with the Intensive Program or switching to another, less strenuous option. "For example, on the Off-campus Program you can decide your level of effort," she said.

I protested, "But on the Off-campus Program we don't have as much access to you folks."

"Right. That decreases. But for any family that has been doing this for two years or more, there's no way I'm going to say *don't call me*. You might think of going off-campus for a year, so you can get yourselves recouped, and work at a pace where you can keep going, instead of winding down. And *then* come back on the Intensive Program."

Judy said, "I've given it a lot of thought, and I would rather be working with Joseph instead of doing anything else. Doing the housework, say—as opposed to late at night, when he's asleep."

"You do that now, during the day?"

This was dangerous territory. "Sometimes I do," she confessed bravely. "When he's eating a meal I'm throwing dishes madly into the dishwasher. But Joseph's time is vital! He'll never have this time again, Lidwina!"

"True. But in the end we've got to have both of you, or we won't have anything at all."

"We'll make it!" Judy insisted stoutly.

"You've got to be able to make it on good health. You may have no choice but to go for a period of time at fifty percent while you make a point of getting enough sleep."

"Do other families have people helping them get it all done?"

"Some do. Some don't."

"Do other families get run down?"

"You both look more ill than most. Now I think you've got to be very realistic. You've got to ask yourselves, if you continue in the state you're in, where are you going to be six months from now? It may even be time to say, 'I have to have another Honeymoon.'"

"I don't want a Honeymoon!" I protested.

"There's no barrier against coming back Intensive when you're ready."

"I'm glad of that. But I remember, when we were on Honeymoon last summer—."

"It was *painful!*" Judy interjected.

I tried to explain our feelings. "Because we had more freedom, we had more exposure to well kids, and the contrast upset us."

"That's not reality," Lidwina said firmly. "At times like that you need to kick yourself in the shin and say, 'Hey, this is unacceptable! My kid has gone from immobility to walking!' I mean, he *could* be sitting in a wheelchair right now. You could be pushing a wheelchair. But on the other hand he's not. He's walking, and he's walking two miles a day."

Lidwina was typically a tough, no-nonsense individual, but I had never heard her speaking so sternly. "That's black-and-white reality," she went on. "You *have* to be able to look at it that way. You've got to be able to see that. Then you can say, 'Great! Why isn't he talking?' The only way we're going to get *that* result is with both of you.

"So, the choice is either: (1) two months of Honeymoon, just going out to the beach and enjoying yourselves with the little guy, and then going Intensive; (2) Off-campus for, say, eight months and then coming back; *or* (3) staying the way we are, but doing so with new energy, new zip, and knowing we're going to survive it."

I scrawled these options on a pad as she spoke. Looking at them, I said, "What this program does is it makes you a problem-solver. Whatever the problem is. If your antiroll device doesn't work, you've got to figure out a way to *make* it work."

"You don't just throw up your hands and say, '*I'll take the problem!*'" Judy laughed somewhat maniacally.

We paused thoughtfully for a moment. Joseph had long since moved off to explore the corners of the office, but now he returned to investigate the abrupt silence. Before I knew it, he was grinning and playing peek-a-boo with me over the edge of Lidwina's desk. We all laughed. "I love you, Joseph!" Lidwina cried. "You're just great!"

"It *is* important to be healthy and full of energy," Judy said at last.

"To get things done, yes! Unless you're healthy you just can't."

"But I couldn't imagine not doing Joseph's respiratory patterning. If it's the answer to getting him fixed, I couldn't go without doing it."

"Right," I agreed. "So let's scratch off that first option, anyway."

"Not so fast," Lidwina protested. "Talk it over. You think about it, and I'll think about it."

THE REMAINDER OF THE WEEK followed the usual format, with two days of stimulating lectures followed by a series of consultations with staff members.

Dr. Wilkinson reviewed general health and diet with us. Joseph applauded when she said we could discontinue the zinc supplement that she'd prescribed on an earlier visit. That was one foul-tasting concoction, as Judy and I well knew, having sampled it ourselves. On the other hand, it may have contributed to the rapid growth he'd recently displayed.

Elaine Lee issued a supply of new masks and told us how to make our own if the need arose.

Maria Lopez demonstrated a basic gymnastics routine that she wanted Joseph to learn and announced that the time had come to start brachiation—swinging hand-over-hand from the overhead ladder. To congratulate him on reaching this milestone, Judy grasped a giggling Joseph by the forearms and spun him around in a wild circle.

Dr. Vasquez looked on nervously, half-expecting Joseph to slip out of her hands and sail through the air. "Hmm, the boomerang program," he commented.

Katie Doman, Glenn's wife, helped us outline a new intelligence program.

She didn't think we had a major problem in the realm of intelligence, even given Joseph's limited feedback. "In the beginning, all parents have to go on trust," she said. "Then, over time, you notice that he's understanding more. It may not seem like much, until you compare it with what you saw a year ago."

We spoke at length about how much Joseph might or might not understand, while he amused himself idly on the floor of her office. Finally, possibly to put an end to all the conjecture, he began digging through the pile of sample reading cards we'd brought from home. He selected one that read *Tengo hambre* and waved it to get our attention.

"Look what Joseph has!" I exclaimed. "That's Spanish for 'I'm hungry!' Are you trying to tell us something, Joseph?"

He laughed at the stir he'd created. Judy had already dashed from the room to find a banana to reward him.

And so it went. There was no further discussion of our doing anything less than the full-blown program, and in fact, we left with an assignment even more strenuous than the last, including as it did *four* hours of manual respiratory patterning every day and a weekly three-hour nonstop marathon walk. Matt Newell predicted, "He's going to be as fit as a buck rat." When he saw our bewilderment he added, "That's an expression you hear in some parts of the country."

I wobbled between being excited over the prospect of seeing Joseph acquire new skills and mystified as to how we would accomplish everything. More manual patterning! Dawn promised that a respiratory machine would be forthcoming if this program did not elicit language, but until then we'd simply have to make it work.

21. PARENTS WHO COULD NOT IMAGINE HOW LITTLE THEY KNEW

I remember once, as a ten-year-old kid from suburbia, taking a short-cut through my grandfather's cornfield on the way to visit a cousin. At some point, the realization sank in that I'd become lost.

At first I couldn't believe I'd gone astray on such a simple errand. But I had stepped abruptly into a different world. The stalks reached far above my head. Overhanging leaves, translucent in the sunlight, trapped a thick layer of moist heat around me. Weird, long-legged bugs jumped from their perches at my approach. Forging ahead between the curved rows, I flailed irritably as cobwebs snagged on my sweaty face. I raised my forearms protectively, and the long, glossy leaves scratched my arms and ears. Coming in here was a bad idea! Stuff was falling down the back of my shirt. I knew I'd begun wandering erratically. I no longer aimed for my cousin's house, but turned in *any* direction that might get me out. But none felt right. How the *heck* was I going to do it? Pushing past the yielding stalks in front of me seemed pointless. There were always more just like them. And more. And then more.

Much, much later, breathing heavily, I crashed desperately through the outermost row alongside the road, barely halfway between my grandfather's house and my cousin's.

Why did that long-dormant memory come back to me at this point? I now think the specter of becoming lost—of choosing a path and then wondering how long to stay with it as doubts accumulate—must have always fascinated me. Since high school, my favorite poem has been the one by Robert Frost about roads diverging in a yellow wood.

After college, I did spend a lot of time in the woods. Throughout my twenties, I loved to hike through wilderness areas, leaving the trails to wander with only a sketchy notion of where I would end up, walking extra miles when I guessed wrong.

Perhaps I sensed that these flirtations with ambiguity were a fore-taste of a less trivial dilemma to come.

Perhaps I sought a formula, some rule to apply when dependable guideposts are absent. I think, subconsciously, I wanted to know: How do you stay more or less on course toward attaining whatever you need, regardless of the inevitable mistakes and surprises? And after wandering into several dead ends, can you backtrack and try again, or does the way close behind you? Can you secure a path of retreat, as Hansel tried to do in leaving a trail of breadcrumbs in the children's story, as Theseus did in unwinding a string in the mythical labyrinth?

Labyrinth? Or maze? There's an important distinction. Strictly speaking, they differ in that a labyrinth leads unfailingly, albeit through seemingly endless twists and turns, to one inevitable destination. But I've operated on the assumption that the struggle of my life occurred in a maze, a network of multiple forking paths, where success depends on making the right choices.

How close to right were our choices now?

Yes, Joseph was greatly improved.

Improved respiration now enabled him to eat his meals without dan-ger of choking, although he wolfed his food down as seriously as ever. "Don't bite your *fingers*," I warned only half-jokingly as he crammed a bran muffin into his mouth. A dismissive glance showed what he thought of that comment.

His daily walks at the track were perfecting a nice, long stride. He never stumbled now. For the first time, he could step up and down off curbs without reaching out nervously for someone's hand. One month after returning from Philadelphia, he'd built up to five thirty-minute walks on marathon days, during which he logged a total of over four miles.

He took shorter naps—or even went all day without needing sleep. His eyes, which hitherto had been shrouded by drooping lids, now took in his surroundings with serious interest. He no longer drooled, and in general he just looked more tuned in. Dawn had suggested that the new alert expression in his face meant that "integrative" areas of his brain were coming into play. But he didn't just *look* more alert; when I bragged to Sally about his performance during the Institutes' evaluation, he broke in with a chuckle from the next room. He'd been eavesdropping. Another time, he handed me a book of Calvin & Hobbes cartoons and deliberately said, "Ha, Ha!" Nancy and Greg had lent it to us to enjoy on the plane. Joseph was letting me know that he'd noticed us giggling over it, that he knew it must be funny.

All this was fabulous. But if we didn't have reservations, Dr. Frymann did.

This time she didn't like our news that Joseph's head size had increased so rapidly.

Judy countered that it was still barely average for his age, but Dr. Frymann insisted that head growth could bode ill and "to be on the safe side" a new CT-scan should be ordered. While we were at it, she went on, we might as well get an EEG and (because he didn't talk) a brainstem hearing test.

One of the great benefits of being on program was the freedom it had granted us from that endless round of appointments and inconclusive tests at clinics all over town. Every day we dedicated to program goals was a day spent constructively. We were in no hurry to resume anything that recalled our unproductive pre-Institutes days.

"This time you might just learn something," Dr. Frymann said patiently. Her manner conveyed a profound, bone-deep weariness with all the parents she saw who could not even imagine how little they knew. She sat at her desk and eyed us silently before saying, "After a hearing test, for example, you *might* change your expectations."

"*Nothing* is going to make me change my expectations!" Judy retorted. "Joseph is going to be perfectly well."

A younger osteopath sitting in on the conference ventured to say that "it's not always easy to understand God's will." I think he regretted doing so, because Judy turned on him.

"I don't agree! I *know* that God's will for Joseph is that he be well and whole. I don't know why it's *taking* so long. But *God* isn't holding up the works. We've asked for it, and we're working for it. The Bible says, 'Whatsoever things you desire, when you pray, believe that you receive them, and you shall have them.' That's a promise. God keeps His promises."

We already knew that Joseph had neurological problems! What would be gained by taking time out and subjecting him to more probing and poking? Still, we wanted to do the right thing, and so relayed the question to Dr. Wilkinson at the Institutes. She responded promptly:

"Joseph's head growth has certainly been phenomenal, but he's shown no signs of increased pressure, so I see nothing to worry about. If we got a CT scan I suspect we would see evidence of brain growth. I see no reason for an EEG. Both the CT and the auditory evoked potentials I would regard as of interest, but would not alter his treatment."

Since the choice was ours to make, we decided to trust our instincts. Joseph had never looked healthier! He was strong and robust, with pink cheeks and bright eyes. He wasn't in danger. We did compromise and got the hearing test. And as we'd expected, it shed no light on the situation. Whatever the obstacle to speech might be, it evidently wasn't his hearing.

"I don't appreciate her raising doubts like that," Judy grumbled. "It's hard enough to stay focused, as it is."

Still, no one denied that his slow language development was discouraging. After we'd sent in two monthly reports documenting little or no progress, Lidwina called to investigate. "The results you're getting are not good enough," she said briskly. "Concentrate on establishing your best respiratory patterning rate, and get in all the brachiation and gymnastics you possibly can. Don't let him hear any music, either, because music stimulates the subdominant hemisphere of the brain. The dominant hemisphere is used for language, and right now that's where the work needs to be done."

No music—. *No music?*

From the "Wee Sing" nursery rhymes to Raffi tapes and foreign-language ditties, to electronic compositions, music had kept us going through rough times over the last few years. This would be an unwelcome adjustment.

We forged ahead with the respiratory patterning. Every day, for as many hours as possible, Judy and I sat across from each other, pulling those dowel rods to squeeze Joseph's chest while the metronome clicked and beeped its stately three-beat guide: Pull-pull, release. Pull-pull, release. Hours of this. Now music was out. We'd grown tired of books on tape. We began talking again, and that old subject of autism began coming up. Janet Doman had commented in the last lecture series that the benighted world outside the Institutes still called non-speaking children "autistic" instead of acknowledging their difficulty with breathing. Autism was just one of that world's many unhelpful terms for brain injury. And yet, we both well remembered the physical therapist at Kaiser who'd suggested Joseph might be autistic.

One day, half an hour into a session, Judy gave words to something that had been gnawing at her for quite a long time.

"Steve, do you remember that woman on the Institutes program who shot her kid?"

"Of course."

"You remember I wanted to write to her?"

"Think so. What about it? Did you?"

"No. I didn't know how to begin."

The metronome ticked and beeped. We pulled and released, pulled and released.

"I—Listen, I don't want you to tell anybody about this, all right? That time you came home and said the therapist thought he was autistic? You remember of course."

Pull-pull, release. Tears were streaming down her cheeks. She didn't wipe them away. Couldn't, without breaking the rhythm of what we were doing.

"Steve, I almost killed Joseph that night."

Pull-pull, release. And again. And again. I couldn't speak.

"You went back to work that night. And I started thinking of what the future was going to be like if Joseph was autistic. I understood there was no real treatment. I understood we've got this society that thinks it's enlightened just because they have stuff like the Special Olympics. I already knew what reality would be like for him, from when I taught. It was worse for the girls, of course. I was *so* disappointed the time Winnie got pregnant in eighth grade, when she still needed someone to wipe her nose. But the way I saw it, all of them ended up neglected, and exploited, and I thought, *Why does he even need to go through that?* And I thought you didn't deserve this. It wasn't your fault. *I* brought this baby into the world! It was because something must have been wrong with me. *Ooh*!" She leaned her head back and howled with misery.

Still, we pulled on the dowels. Fortunately, Joseph appeared to be asleep.

"I thought I'd go to jail, and you could divorce me. You could start over, marry someone else. It seemed like the best option."

"Judy, that's crazy, of course—."

"We don't have a gun or anything like that, but—." She stopped to gulp air. "Well, I took him upstairs on the balcony. I looked over the side. And I saw the concrete down below."

We were both crying now. "And I actually lifted him up. I was going to see what it felt like, before I actually did it. Ooh! And then I cried out, '*Oh God please help us!*'"

Pull-pull, release. Pull-pull, release. Pull-pull, release. It seems odd now that we never stopped the patterning while this was going on, that I didn't go around the table to hold her. Instead, both of us clung to the monotonous task as our anchor.

"And something happened when I said that," she went on. "Right away this enormous peace came down around me, like a blanket. And suddenly I understood that there was no need to do that. I can't explain what happened. But I know—I know God was right there with me. That night changed everything. I really wasn't much of a believer before then, you know."

It was true. Judy had gone out of her way to tell the pastor who married us that she was not a Christian. Had offended him in the process.

"I was brought up in a Catholic family, but that night was when I started believing. And ever since then I've known that God was with us. That's why I don't let people say wrong things, like that person at Dr. Frymann's office. I believe it's important to take a stand when you hear ideas like, like you know, *it's God's will for a little kid to be crippled or disabled*. We need to affirm that His will is always what the Bible says it is. I've tried to learn more about that. Pat helps me."

We continued patterning until the hour was up, and then moved on to the other parts of the program. No more was said about that horrible night. There was plenty else, much more immediate, to occupy us.

JOSEPH'S EYES seemed brighter during gymnastics, an observation that encouraged Judy through the rebellions he staged on the floor of the YMCA. But what would motivate him to care about what they were doing? She cheered, yelled, praised, and even spanked him at times, but none of that inspired much cooperation. He did enjoy trying his luck on a balance beam. So they'd spend five minutes practicing the floor routine Maria had prescribed, and then it was time for a break and a stroll along the balance beam. Then she dragged out a big foam wedge and helped him through a few backward somersaults. She switched tasks in this way, constantly diverting him to head off the rumblings of discontent, until the arrival of an aerobics class indicated that their hour was up.

How do you really reward a kid for all that we were asking him to do? Joseph had a volatile disposition. He'd always had strong opinions. And *there just wasn't time* to allow for them. We tried to keep him amused on the walks by telling stories and periodically popping raisins into his mouth. As he built stamina for longer marathons, we tried some of the more scenic locales around San Diego, such as Balboa Park and Old Town. I started with him early in the day, before the tourists came out in force, and we made our way up and down the sidewalks, across the plazas, and through the gardens, while I pushed the roller tape and tried to keep up a steady patter of encouragement.

Certainly, Joseph *could* be cheerful and cooperative. The first time we completed a nonstop three-hour walk, he seemed as pleased as I was. But pretty scenery meant nothing to him, and other people were just a potential sympathetic audience. He knew Judy and I hated to have him whine in public. We felt self-conscious already, pushing that miserable stick along and enduring the obvious stares of everyone we passed. Probably, our sensitivity came from stress. Whatever the cause, his vocalizing made things unendurable. I've encountered other hurt kids who made noises far louder and more bizarre than Joseph's. Just the same, he could emit a peculiar siren noise that guaranteed no one would miss him.

EVERY FEW MONTHS, Lidwina asked for a videotape that showed us in action, and for that one of our volunteers always graciously stepped in with a camcorder. The requirement was upon us again. For the segment on respiratory patterning, I kidded about splicing in a scene from *Ben-Hur*. I hadn't seen the movie since my childhood, but the incessant drumbeat and the feverish labor of the galley-slaves hauling on their oars came to mind whenever we started that metronome. The parallel was striking. I let that opportunity go by, of course, since we doubted the staff at the Institutes would share our sense of humor. Anyway, securing Joseph's cooperation was the main issue, and that was no joke.

Dear Lidwina,

Hello. We are happy to send the enclosed Interim Report. We have also managed to get a 13-minute video (enclosed) showing Joseph's gymnastics, brachiating, and the respiratory patterning. We think the progress you can see here is encouraging.

Our biggest concern, obviously, is the lack of progress on language development. This is coupled with his reliance on random animal-like noises and whining. (You can hear a dose of that during the brachiating segment of the video.) These noises have a cumulative effect on us. In public, he draws unwelcome attention, even from people who are some distance away. Even little children stare at him, wondering what is wrong. But it's not just a bad-behavior problem. He also makes wild, loud noises when he's happy. For over four years now we have lived with a kid who uses crying and yelling as his primary means of communicating, and we are at the end of our patience.

I don't want to overstate the problem, but on the other hand, sometimes we feel that it couldn't be overstated. Judy is particularly impatient for a breakthrough in this area, but I agree. Something has to be done.

We already knew what Lidwina would say. We needed a new emphasis on the Family Law aspect of the program introduced earlier. The trouble was that timeouts still were no punishment. If we interrupted respiratory patterning to put Joseph into a dull, uninteresting corner—well, that was fine with him! If we stopped a walk to make him sit in the grass, so much the better! We'd gotten nowhere with those tactics.

Lidwina suggested putting more weight on the rewards side of the equation. What evolved was a system in which we paid him with white poker chips, which he could redeem for various rewards, and taxed him chips when he misbehaved. Swimming was by far his favorite activity, so we explained that for every thirty minutes of cheerful cooperation, he'd get a special *blue* chip, fourteen of which were good for a swim.

The "Happy Program," as we dubbed it, served to call the vocalizing to Joseph's attention. He understood the system, knew when he'd lapsed, and reached the point where he'd unzip his bag, reach in, select the required number of chips, and pay them to Judy or me, with minimal prompting.

But whether he protested or not, I could no longer bear to operate in crowded public places. Granted, the bystanders who gaped at us, and even photographed us, and tried to question us were not significant. I knew that, but also knew we'd do better work without them. I tried walking on Fiesta Island, a semi-deserted patch of wasteland in the middle of Mission Bay. The perimeter road was just over four miles long, and Joseph and I managed one lap in our three hours. Along the way, we could watch people out in the water romping with their jet skis. And they were all far too busy to notice us.

By September of 1989 I'd picked an even better spot. My employer operated a park for its employees, and it offered not only a measured track—one less boring than most, and with a handy drinking fountain—but a nearby miniature railroad and a carousel. I gladly put that roller tape into permanent storage and began taking Joseph around the track on weekends. Every time the train chugged by, I reminded him of the reward coming at the end of the walk. "Welcome to the Kearny Mesa and Pacific," the conductor would intone as Joseph handed him our tickets. Joseph would then take his seat with regal satisfaction, and the ride would commence.

BY OCTOBER he was completing his walk in twenty-five minutes. On marathon days he now covered slightly more than five miles in three hours. This being the case, I wondered, how serious could his breathing problem really be? The kid seemed to have enough energy—he just didn't direct it constructively. Without constant supervision throughout the day, his actions immediately degenerated into mere randomness, such as strumming the window blinds or shaking a length of string. Acts like those never grew old to him.

One day, Judy called me at work to say she'd accidentally locked him inside the car. (Yes, she was beginning to slip up that way again.) He could have unlocked the door from the inside, but he showed no awareness of how to do that—and indeed, no awareness even that there was a problem requiring his attention. Possibly he did understand, and *welcomed* the unexpected break from program activities. More likely, we knew, he would have stayed in there until he wet his pants. So I had to come and let him out.

Another afternoon, he fell asleep during the respiratory patterning. Judy and I carefully lifted him from the table at the end of the hour and tip-toed away to confront some long-deferred household projects. I remember gazing at a mountain of laundry in the bedroom that was lofty enough to deserve a name. But then I decided to lie down for just a moment before tackling it. When I opened my eyes the house was completely dark and someone was scraping chairs about in the kitchen. It was—*1:30 a.m.?* Judy was asleep beside me. Making my groggy way downstairs, I found my son sitting at the table, placidly waiting for his dinner to appear.

Why couldn't he understand enough to let himself out of a locked car? And where did he suppose his dinner would come from if we were both asleep? What was he lacking? Initiative? Organization? Clearly, very basic neurological connections of some sort remained undone, even now.

Again, I thought of that cornfield I'd stumbled through many decades earlier. What decision was required of us to get past this? Was our implementation of the program so abysmally poor? Or had the wrong program been assigned? Judy still griped about not having the respirator.

DESPITE OUR GROWING IMPATIENCE, we still felt sure that what the Institutes offered was the only acceptable option. From there, it was a small jump, especially for Judy, to believing it would be right for others.

I suspect that unhappiness with our results prompted her to push for validation via an alternate means. She was, after all, a former teacher, and had always valued the ability to influence others. That was part of the attraction Glenn Doman had in her mind—his talent for inspiring crowds of people to travel every week from all points of the compass to hear him talk. I remember once after a lecture she actually kissed him on the cheek and asked, "What makes you such an effective speaker?" Startled, he sputtered, "Ho ho! It's because I believe what I say."

Believing (or in dark moments at least wanting to believe), she continued to proselytize other parents of disabled children, in places like Dr. Frymann's waiting room. Most were not attempting any sort of program with their kids. Some said they'd been to various "Institutes-style" clinics around the country. We'd heard the Domans angrily dismiss those places as watered-down copycats, and now Judy began to see why.

One day she observed a mother attempting to mask her child, but the woman couldn't do it properly and had no understanding even of what masking was supposed to accomplish. She removed the crumpled thing after thirty seconds and sighed. "It looked so easy when they showed me how to do this," she complained. She *wanted* to complain, Judy realized; she wanted sympathy. Instead, Judy offered to reshape the mask for a snug fit around her child's nose.

"It's important to go for the full sixty seconds," Judy said gently. "I know it can be scary, putting something over his face and seeing him start to breathe heavily. But that's exactly what he needs. When you create this situation he'll receive a surge of oxygen to his brain that can last for several minutes." She hesitated before venturing to ask, "How often did they tell you to do this?"

"Ten times every day!"

It wasn't a contest, but Joseph wore his mask six times in a typical hour. Judy felt a calling to share her knowledge; she owed it to all the hurt kids if not to their parents. But, as before, the parents just felt threatened. Anguish and despair over their children's condition had driven some into a position from which they could scarcely function. They'd made it to the doctor's office. *Wasn't that enough? What were they supposed to hope for, anyway?* Judy talked about intelligence programs, which she thought would help parents view their hurt child in a new light. But as she talked, the eyes before her acquired an opaque glaze. It may have been possible to make the *kids* smart, but you could do nothing about the adults. They backed away defensively, suspiciously. Some indicated that they already knew about us. We were the fanatics they'd been warned about. And anyway, it wasn't as if we could point to our own kid as clear proof that we knew anything at all.

The only mother who showed interest was a young Taiwanese immigrant named Ming. Judy was standing at the counter in Dr. Frymann's waiting room, writing a check, when Ming's two-year-old son Christopher rolled onto her foot. She looked down and recognized an Asian version of what Joseph had once been. The only difference, she learned, was that Christopher had been normal until suffering a choking accident and going into a coma. The rest was familiar. The parents were determined to restore him to his rightful abilities. Ming was so determined, in fact, that the neurologists had labeled her as "difficult" and urged her to seek counseling.

Ming and her husband Kai began visiting us to see Joseph's program in action. Ours was the only approach to brain injury that made sense, they said, and they were especially outspoken on this point the second time they came. They'd just had an appointment with a local developmentalist, whom Dr. Frymann had recommended, and were very disappointed.

"That guy talked for three hours, and he didn't say anything that you hadn't already told us," Kai complained. "In fact, he didn't say as much!"

I said, "Whether you talk to him or us, you're getting these ideas second-hand. The Institutes is where they originate."

"Well, we have a proposition for you," Kai went on. "We can't travel all the way to Philadelphia. But we'll gladly pay *you* to tell us how to help Christopher."

I smiled, flattered. "I wish it were that easy, but anything we tell you is *generic*. It might help. But Christopher has specific problems that are different from Joseph's, and we aren't qualified to design a program for him."

"Look, we mean it. This could be an arrangement that might help us both. We paid that guy three hundred dollars, and I wish we'd paid it to you instead."

"So do I!" I laughed. "But seriously, you need to absorb the philosophy behind this treatment, from the people who can explain it best. It would be a mistake to bypass that." I had already perceived a tendency in these eager souls to select the most appealing parts of the program—using an overhead ladder to get their child walking upright as soon as possible, for example—while ignoring less exciting but fundamental activities such as patterning and creeping. I tried to explain that a cafeteria-style approach would be doomed to failure. "Besides, we wouldn't have time to advise you on an ongoing basis, even if we knew how."

Our visitors looked down at their laps glumly.

Judy said, "You'll find that getting to the Institutes isn't as difficult as you think. I couldn't imagine going when we first heard about it. I thought that sort of thing was for *other* people; not us. And then when we managed to go the first time, deep down I still didn't really expect to go *again*. Now our seventh trip is coming up. We've lasted *this* long!"

There've been sacrifices, of course. We always feel broke. But just because there are problems is no reason to stop."

Ming and Kai obligingly praised Joseph for his accomplishments and departed with a big decision to make.

MY AVAILABILITY for that seventh trip was suddenly in question, as my father had entered the hospital once again, with congestive heart failure. His condition was deteriorating rapidly.

Then it stabilized, and he returned home. However, this second assault on his body appeared to have claimed his mind more conclusively. He stopped walking, evidently having forgotten how. He needed round-the-clock care. My attempts to speak with him on the phone bore out the discouraging reports from my sister Angie. He'd lost contact with reality, and interest in it as well.

There was disagreement back East as to whether what Dad had was Alzheimer's, but in any event no one expected him to improve.

The confusion about his diagnosis again led me to see similarities with Joseph, who also had never been diagnosed by mainstream doctors. But regardless of the label, Dad was suffering grave neurological dysfunction. I felt sure that, like Joseph, he needed stimulation. He needed it with *enormous* intensity, frequency, and duration. He also needed opportunity. Instead, he was spending his days parked in a wheelchair doing nothing.

"He could still be helped," I said wistfully.

Judy said, "Go to him, if you think you should."

But that was out of the question. Any attention I gave to my father would be taken away from my son. I knew a campaign to slow his inevitable deterioration would require enormous effort—far more than I could give at this point. I turned Dad over to God, who had ultimate control in any event, and grimly set to work on Joseph's Revisit Report.

22. AN INTRODUCTION TO THE MACHINE

The Revisit provided another opportunity to go over all the obvious issues with the Institutes' staff. An attractive junior staff member named Claudia sat with us and praised the care we'd put into organizing our Report. Then the familiar evaluation began. She unfolded the familiar Institutes Profile, with its columns defining the six areas where they measured neurological competence. Joseph's earlier attainments were marked from all the previous times this had been done.

This time, I really hoped he would somehow score lots of Victories. He needed them to push up his neurological age. And I needed to see higher numbers there to keep our growing unease at arms' length.

The tactility test ought to be one he could finally pass. When Claudia mentioned it, I eagerly produced a cloth bag with an assortment of little wooden shapes that we'd practiced with in recent months. Several times we showed Joseph two pieces—a little donut shape and a pyramid—and then dropped them into the bag. "Get the pyramid!" we'd say. But the results were disappointing. When he withdrew his hand, he held either the wrong piece, or both pieces.

"Oh well, it looks like he is still not consistent," Claudia said pleasantly.

"He could do it at home," Judy complained.

Claudia smiled. "Children always do what they want. We can't force them."

I was quite let down.

Claudia moved on to discuss mobility, and then language. These areas had seen no change—no measurable change, at least—in the last several months, and we had little to report. Joseph was not running, nor was he saying much, although he sometimes seemed close to doing both.

"Now then, manual competence," she said. "Can he use both hands now? Has his manual competence improved?"

"We have not seen him unscrew a jar," I said slowly, knowing that this was a key test for bimanual function. "But I *have* seen him hold a box of raisins with one hand and reach in with the other."

"Uh-huh. So he's *starting* to use both hands. Have you given him opportunity to screw and unscrew things?"

"Sure. During respiratory patterning we let him play with some big plastic bolts and nuts. We've tried to get him to twist those."

It was another frustrating area. Judy described her repeated efforts to have Joseph pour water from one container into another. "He understands," she said. "He can watch me do it all day. I can hold his hands and go through the motions, but he won't do it on his own."

I suggested that it was a matter of overall neurological organization, and Claudia seemed to agree. She asked about his behavior in general and his ability to interact with others.

Here was yet another troublesome topic! Joseph typically made no response when spoken to by visitors and other children. On the other hand, he had a distressing tendency to approach total strangers in public and to hug them as if they were family members. "Aside from just not being a good thing," I said, "That shows a lack of social understanding."

"Of course, most of the people who've come into our house have encouraged him to hug them," Judy pointed out.

"That's true. He's had hundreds of patterners come in and put their hands on him."

"Strangers to him! And so—what have we taught him? That everybody's your friend!"

"That behavior is characteristic of a certain neurological age," Claudia mused. But she made a note for later discussion with other staff members.

MORE THAN THIRTY FAMILIES were spread across the waiting area around disorderly heaps of coats, blankets, and luggage. A few restless children were throwing a ball back and forth. I wondered if these were nearly-well clients of the Institutes or just well siblings.

Judy scanned the big room and located Jerry and Dora, a lively pair from Colorado whom we remembered from earlier visits. She ran to them eagerly. As Joseph and I caught up she was already saying, "I think we'll finally get the respiratory machine this time."

"Oh, you'll love the machine," Dora said. "It's great. It's the best thing that's happened to Jay." She beamed at their son, a very healthy-looking child poised on hands and knees beside her.

"Is Jay talking yet?"

"Not so far, but he's functioning better. It's going to take more time, but the machine is just pushing him up. He's very close to a *lot* of big milestones."

"Of course," Judy said, "we have no idea how we're going to monitor the thing all night."

Dora smiled encouragingly. "I sort of doze off and on. It's not really sleeping, but I nap for five or ten minutes at a stretch. That's OK. The main thing is just making sure the machine keeps operating at the same rate and pressure. You get to where you can tell if it's changing, just from the sound it makes."

"I've heard that they keep breaking down," I said worriedly.

"You end up replacing motors and parts all the time. The Institutes supposedly has an improved version now, though; one that's far superior."

Jerry interrupted. "We don't use their model anymore. The one they gave us burned out, and we bought a different kind."

"How much do they cost?"

"Almost two thousand dollars. But we were lucky. Our health insurance paid for it."

"Really!"

"Believe me, they didn't want to, but we brought in a lawyer. Before Jay got on program here, insurance was paying for speech therapy, which wasn't doing him any good at all. Since the machine is supposed to take care of the same problem, we said it should be covered, too."

THE HOURS PASSED SLOWLY. Somebody had fallen asleep on top of the bench that contained our belongings. Joseph dozed too, then roused himself, picked out a severely brain-injured boy sitting with his family, and began interacting in the only way he could—by taking the kid's toy. I sprang to the rescue.

"Your son is almost ready to graduate from the program, isn't he?" asked the mother.

"Oh, no. I wish." I wasn't sure how to respond to her obvious admiration. Joseph had a long way to go, but in terms of mobility, at least, he was in better shape than the child before us.

"How long have you been coming here?" I asked.

"Four years. When we started, Toby was cortically blind, and deaf, and everybody said he couldn't be reached. Now he can see and hear. He understands at a three-year-old level, and he reads in four languages."

I nodded, hoping my reaction to her first sentence hadn't shown. *Four years!* I'd immediately wondered how people could keep going in the face of such discouraging results. But recovering from blindness was a very big deal.

Judy and I wanted to compare notes, but at that moment Elaine Lee called them into her office. Shortly thereafter Teruki came to collect us for the Summary.

"What is the single area of *least* change on Joseph's Profile since you began the program?" he asked us.

Judy and I considered for a moment before agreeing that it was language.

"And what is the single area of greatest change?"

This time we didn't hesitate. "Mobility!" That was obvious. "It was our biggest priority in the beginning," I added.

"Yes," he replied. "That's one reason Lidwina asked me to do your Summary tonight, because now the Number One goal is language.

"What prevents Joseph from speaking, or speaking better?" he asked us. "Is it poor hearing? Lack of information? Poor breathing? Poor co-ordination? Poor organization? Poor laterality?"

Judy said, "I suppose it's two things, breathing and organization."

"The question of his hearing has been raised more than once," I remarked.

"Hearing could have something to do with it," Teruki said. "I don't know how much. But obviously if you don't hear well or if you hear incorrectly, then output is affected. So that's a possibility. What's your feeling about his hearing?"

"Joseph understands what I tell him," I said firmly. "The thing is, I think vision and hearing and manual competence and all these things—they're *all* not perfect. That's why we keep coming back to the question of organization."

Teruki said, "That's my opinion, too. And that's why the respiratory machine deserves a good try now. If there *is* a problem with his hearing, better respiration may improve it further.

"We're still trying to decide which is more important in improving respiration," he went on. "We don't know if it's masking and the machine, or physical activity such as gymnastics. But now it's definitely time to think seriously about a machine for Joseph."

He reviewed the newly revised Profile with us, noting the changes. Claudia had seen fit to grant Joseph a Victory in "understanding" this time, largely on the strength of his success with the Law program. But we wanted so much more! I showed Teruki a graph I'd drawn up before we left home. It depicted a normal growth curve, with neurological age advancing steadily with chronological age. Below that I had plotted the growth Joseph had achieved while on the Institutes' program.

"It's a jagged line," I said. "Sometimes it's flat, and then the next time you evaluate him it jumps up again. But the slope is never steep enough to look like it might ever intersect with the curve for normal kids. So I'm looking at that and wondering, is he *ever* going to catch up with where he should be?"

Teruki pointed out that Joseph was now relatively high on their Profile. "From now on, any change he makes from one level to another will have more value in terms of neurological age. The reason he went up six months this time, you see, is simply that from here to here on the Profile is three months, and from here to here is also three months. But if he changes from here to *here*, that alone will represent six months. These changes usually don't come quickly, but from now on, as I say, they'll be worth more. Now, your question is, when does he catch up with this curve—."

"I'm not asking you to give me a date for when it's going to happen. I just want to be reassured that it's a reasonable objective."

Teruki smiled. "I think the question has to be, 'If Joseph goes out into the world, can he survive?' And the answer to that has to be, 'Not yet.' That's what we have to worry about. Why not? Well, his understanding is good, but he still has to learn more."

Judy said, "So he can deal with anybody. A child in school has to deal with the teacher and every situation that comes up."

"Exactly. And again, he needs to improve his speech. So, the question of neurological age is fascinating, but the more important thing is how close he is to living in the world by himself. Three years ago when you first came here, you were concerned because his mobility development was very slow. And you said, if only he could walk. Now he walks, and obviously the next question is when can he go out in the world, and go to school. It's natural that you should be concerned about that. Your concerns and ours are the same.

"In reality, if a child can walk and if his understanding is up to it, then we may say to go ahead and let him start school, even though he may not be running yet. In Joseph's case, most likely what will happen next is this." He tapped the square on the Profile representing that elusive ability to recognize shapes and textures by touch. "And then you can expect this." He pointed to running. "Speech takes more time, and then writing."

"Writing comes last, I guess," I said.

"That, and sophisticated understanding. As far as manual ability goes, Joseph could write now. The reason he isn't writing is his understanding. It doesn't always follow this course." He mentioned one of the older children we'd seen on the floor that day. "Jason can still barely walk, but he could go to school at any time. The parents of course want to see him improve some more first, and we agree with them. We want him to be a walker and a runner so he can do everything the other kids do. But on the other hand, with some kids it's easy for us to create walking and running while speech and understanding and writing come more slowly. I haven't really answered your question. I'm sorry, but it's not neurological age we're concerned about. It's function that's most important."

AS ALWAYS, Tuesday and Wednesday were devoted to formal presentations. This time we had to share the auditorium with a film crew, who were in the process of recording all the lectures. The men moved their equipment discreetly around the room while staff members took turns speaking on a variety of topics: how to teach advanced problem solving skills, and foreign languages, and music, and even swimming.

On Thursday morning we returned to begin assimilating our new program instructions. Inevitably, there were hours of waiting, and Judy and I found ourselves talking with a good-natured little British kid named Wayne. Like so many others in the room, he still had a long way to go in terms of mobility. On the other hand, he spoke quite easily and had no problems expressing the lively intelligence that is the birthright of every child. I saw a rare opportunity to get a brain-injured kid's impressions of life on program. "What's your favorite part of the program?" I asked.

"The overhead ladder!" This was a surprise, since my memories of Joseph's ladder were not pleasant. But Wayne was logging 160 trips a day, and enjoying it. He confided that his least favorite activity was rolling.

"But that's easy!" I protested stupidly.

He looked at me skeptically, fighting back a shy smile. "Easy for *you* to say."

Then we were summoned downstairs along with five other families to begin learning the arcane science of operating a respirator. Ann Ball assembled everyone in a rather small room there and ensured that each child had all the necessary equipment. In addition to the machine itself, which resembled a canister vacuum cleaner, there was a two-piece "cage" that enclosed the child's torso, rather like a turtle shell, and a vinyl "poncho" to create a sealed air-space within the cage. The poncho was connected to the machine by a length of flexible hose.

Two of the families in the room spoke only Spanish and two others were French. Ann's remarks were therefore punctuated by frequent pauses for their respective translations. She reminded us of the ratio we'd used in manual respiratory patterning: two beats for each expiration and one beat for the inspiration. "The same thing is going to happen with this," she said. "That ratio doesn't change. Inspiration occurs when the plunger on the machine goes up. At that point, air in the cage around your child's chest is being pulled out, causing his chest to expand." She showed us the on/off switch and the pressure-adjustment knob. "This is the main thing that needs to be regulated," she said. "A lot of things can change the pressure. For example, as the seal gets better after the child has been in the machine a few minutes, the pressure can go up. Or if there is a leak someplace the pressure will go down. Either way, if the pressure goes up or down, the machine will then be working harder or more easily, and the rate will change.

"Now, how do we adjust the rate and ratio?" She referred us to a pair of knobs on top of the machine, one marked TIME EXH and the other TIME INH. "You'll have to work both of these until it's just right," she warned. "Get this straight, because this is the most confusing thing about the machine: If you want to make the rate faster, you *decrease* the time."

Virtually all that day and the next were spent in this room, with the oppressive droning and thumping of six respirators and the continual beeping of metronomes, which everyone used to calibrate their machines. I found that it took intense concentration to block out all the distractions while trying to stabilize Joseph's machine at the desired rate.

Periodically, different staff members stopped in to see how we were faring. No doubt they knew that learning the machine was a stressful business, and they wanted to offer encouragement.

Phyllis crouched beside Joseph at one point and stroked his hair.

"This is such an amazing kid," she said. "It makes me happy every time I see him."

"How so?"

"Because I remember he was such a mess when he first came here, and now he's taking off!"

I shrugged modestly and gave my standard reply. "We always want more."

"Sure! But don't forget that he's come a long way already!"

JERRY AND DORA were finished with their last conference and heading out the door. "See you next time!" They called.

"Jay's got a really heavy physical program. *Lots* of creeping and clambering." Dora rolled her eyes dramatically. "Plus twelve hours a day on the machine. They also told us to take one hour off every day for ourselves, but I don't know where we're going to find it!"

We wished them well and returned to the respiratory room. I would be flying home on Sunday, but Judy and Joseph needed to stay an extra week to become thoroughly accustomed to the new program. Judy had made friends with a couple from Illinois whose equipment was arranged alongside ours. She showed Joseph's toys to their son, Nicholas, hoping to encourage some interplay between the children while they lay there, and I fastened the poncho around Joseph's legs once again and started the machine. Ann materialized at my shoulder to watch. I carefully twisted the dials for several minutes. After a number of false starts, the steady thumping of the plunger finally appeared to be synchronized with our metronome.

"There! I'd say it's right on the money," I said triumphantly.

"You need to give it at least ten cycles before you know."

She was right. As I watched, a very small error became magnified until the respirator was perceptibly out of sync. I sighed and crouched over it again, and Ann moved on to another family.

Fortunately, Joseph had adapted to the new situation without much protest. Judy and I took turns, with one of us talking to him and the other fiddling with the controls. I became convinced that the rate drifted, which meant we had to make adjustments constantly.

AFTER I'D GONE, Ann took Judy aside to discuss the details of our respiratory program.

She referred to Lidwina's notes in the file. "I see you're also going to have a two-hour running program."

Judy said, "Good. I was starting to worry that Joseph might decrease his activity level too much."

"No. No. We don't let that happen. So—the time *out* of the machine is going to be those two hours, and—. It also says there are vestibular techniques here. I'm sure it's going to take you more than two hours to get all that in; you mark my words. Let's allow three hours to do the physical program. Now then, how much time do you need to feed and bathe him?"

They finally arrived at a goal of at least eighteen hours per day on the machine and six hours for doing everything else. Ann wanted to know who would be monitoring the machine at night.

Judy wasn't sure. She said, "Some of our old volunteers have offered—"

"Really!"

"—for a couple hours at a time."

"At *night*, you mean?"

"Well, none of them said *that*. But there's a college near us, and perhaps if we advertise exactly what we need, we can find somebody whose schedule fits. Students tend to stay up late and study, so—"

"You've obviously got to teach people how to do it. There's *that* route, and if it works, great. If you do have to stay up, you need to make sure you don't wear yourselves out. By the way, I happen to think that family members are more responsible at night than *non*family members. So we're always in favor of the family staying up, although we don't want to ruin you."

"Possibly volunteers could do gymnastics with Joseph in the day, and I could sleep a little then," Judy suggested hopefully.

"No."

"No?"

"No. You have to make yourself available for *all* of that. But for two hours you could probably have somebody reading to him, or something like that, in the machine while you're getting a little extra rest."

"How long do people usually stay on the machine?" Judy asked, clearly dreading the answer.

"Some people here get it twenty-four hours—all day, except for eating. And others just at night—"

"I don't mean day hours, but—six months?"

"No! Two or three or four *years*."

"When a child graduates from the machine, how do you know that time has come? His breathing is adequate to support his activity?"

"It's *that*, as well as just having him go up the Profile and finish, like any normal kid would do."

"So you graduate from the machine when all your functions are normal."

"Yes. That's right," Ann said brightly.

I HEARD THE ABOVE DISCUSSION on tape after Judy and Joseph had rejoined me in San Diego. Listening, I thought Judy's anxiety was so obvious. Ann seemed deaf to it. I knew Judy could not imagine spending the next few years without sleeping at night. But after begging for a machine, she couldn't protest the prescription for how to use it. I had plenty of misgivings, too. Teruki's distinction between neurological age and function seemed like no distinction at all. If you had one, by definition you had the other, did you not? But we sensed that these doubts were not going to be resolved until more time proved whether these people were right.

Now that we were away from all the other families, and the din of multiple respirators, I expected the task of monitoring our own to be much easier. However, the continuing noise of even one machine amounted to a frontal attack on our sensibilities. The thing made a dreary whining and thumping noise that inhibited conversation and invaded our very consciousnesses, until seemingly every thought and movement was in waltz time at a ponderous sixty-three beats per minute.

As a matter of survival, Judy threw herself into the task of building a plywood box around the machine to muffle its noise. A plexiglass lid enabled us to see the pressure gage and access the controls, and strategically placed vent holes and a small fan inside kept it from overheating.

Not content with that, she then put the box on wheels. She also added wheels to the sofa upon which Joseph lay while connected to the respirator. To ensure he remained comfortable at night, she made a little blanket with a hole in the middle to fit around the hose. Next, she turned to the problem of optimizing the arrangement of the room itself, adding dimmer switches to the lights and setting up a drawing board for late-night assembly of intelligence materials.

For the most part, I was a bemused spectator of these projects. She conceived an idea and rushed to carry it out the same day, before I even came home from work. Some of the changes addressed problems I had not even recognized. With the sofa on wheels, and Joseph sleeping on the sofa, she explained, we could easily turn it in such a way that he would be shielded from lights in the next room. Then we could assemble Bits while he simultaneously learned to breathe better.

That was the plan.

23. ESCALATION

A stint of several hours on the respirator would mean improved oxygen delivery and better overall performance, or so we expected. As it turned out, however, he showed no signs of being particularly invigorated. We studied him closely each time we unsuited him and had to conclude that he might even look worse for the wear. *Now* what was going on? Fortunately, yet another appointment with Dr. Frymann was coming up. We took the apparatus along, and demonstrated it in her office.

The concept of putting a brain-injured child on a respirator was new to her. She confessed that she couldn't speak about it authoritatively, but nevertheless she didn't approve. "Physiologically, it doesn't look sound," she said. "You're superimposing something from the outside on your child's own rhythm. It's in conflict with what his body's trying to do." She shook her head and scowled. "I believe that this is assaulting the body's whole mechanism."

Recalling the philosophical underpinnings of osteopathy that she'd explained years earlier, I saw that this reaction could have been predicted. However, it was more than just a question of theory. The child before us had already spent two weeks on the machine. Was he any better?

Preliminary indications were that he was worse. Dr. Frymann reported that the very subtle movement of his skull bones, which corresponded with respiration on a cellular level, had slowed to half the prior rate. His face had become swollen, due, she thought, to prolonged inactivity while lying in a face-down position. And it was suddenly clear that he was ill. But there was more.

"This child is nearly five years old," Dr. Frymann said sternly. "It's high time we got to the bottom of his difficulty with speech. Now, as I've told you before, *I'm* not at all sure he can hear. He may need a hearing aid. He may need to learn sign language."

"*We* think he can hear us," Judy protested. "And the Institutes has just given him an Understanding Victory. That means he understands speech at a three-year-old level."

Dr. Frymann looked at her skeptically. "I'm not that much interested in what the Institutes says. I *am* interested in the child before us. Does he get to see other children in the course of his day?"

She already knew the answer to that, of course. "It would be great if he *could* play with other kids," I said. "The trouble is that he doesn't know how. We haven't observed that he even takes much notice of them."

"What else would you expect, if he never has the opportunity!"

We really didn't want to argue with Dr. Frymann, whose intentions were obviously good. But as important as play no doubt was, in the order of Joseph's priorities it remained pretty far down the list. No doubt, plenty of brain-injured kids *did* have social opportunities. But as far as I knew, none of them ever got well as a result. Judy said, "Dr. Frymann, other families aren't especially interested in putting their well kids together with Joseph. He has adult friends, but people in general don't accept him yet."

"I think you might be surprised by the acceptance he'd receive."

"That may be so, Dr. Frymann, but just out there in your waiting room one time an older boy said that he was a *monster*."

Dr. Frymann looked distressed. "That child should have been *corrected!*"

JUDY HAD BEEN STANDING at the receptionist's counter that day, scheduling the next appointment, when the word *monster* brought everything in her world to a halt.

Over her shoulder, she heard the boy's mother voice a mild objection. "Honey, why would you say a thing like that?"

"Well, look!" the child retorted. "He's just sitting on the floor making noises. He can't even do as much as my little sister!"

Judy turned and crouched beside Joseph, stroking his hair, and explained that he was the way he was because he'd been hurt. "But he's learning. He's still learning, and he's getting better," she promised. "He works hard, so he can be like you. See? Let me show you what he does." She fished some snapshots from her pocketbook, noticing that her hands were beginning to shake, and showed the boy some of the things Joseph had been doing every day to get better. Then, taking Joseph by the hand, she fled. As she crossed the sidewalk to her car, great heaving sobs began wracking her, with such force that she couldn't breathe. She leaned against the fender, fighting to regain control. This was exactly what she'd always dreaded: ridicule and rejection. All Joseph's life she'd taken pains to dress him in the cutest possible clothes, combed cotton turtlenecks, corduroy overalls, and the like. And he *was* cute, more than cute. But also still disabled, a monster as far as some were concerned.

Joseph giggled nervously at her tears, which was his way of relieving the tension when grownup emotions became too overpowering. He'd encountered more than his share of those.

"ANYWAY, surely you can see why we want to speed up his development," Judy went on.

"There are more reasonable programs for doing that." Dr. Frymann named a colleague, the one who'd recently seen Ming's son, and also mentioned Carl Delacato, a former partner with Glenn Doman who had split from the Institutes to form an independent clinic.

"We know families who've been to both of them," Judy said. "And they don't have a lot to show for their trouble."

"Well, *I* know families who have been to the *Institutes* and don't have anything to show for it, either!" Was she talking about us? "A *lot* of families I know have been made very unhappy trying to do that program."

There was no agreement in sight. As we stood to go Judy said, "We know you mean well, Dr. Frymann, and we do value everything you've done for Joseph. But Steve and I have to decide what he needs most."

We left with a homeopathic remedy and instructions to hold an ice pack against Joseph's face to reduce the swelling. As it turned out, during the next three days we did this and little more. His cold worsened. I held him in my lap, with his head resting miserably against my chest, and gave up on daily program goals for the time being.

No one at the Institutes had given us guidelines on when to suspend use of the respirator, but we assumed they would be the same as for manual respiratory patterning. Joseph had become very congested, and so we concentrated on masking and let other parts of the program slip.

Ann Ball confirmed that this move was correct, when Judy reached her by phone. It was the first of many anxious conversations with different staff members and other Institutes families over the next several days. Ann strongly resented the suggestion that the respirator might be connected in any way with Joseph's illness. "We've had seven thousand children on respirators at the Institutes," she said, "and none of them has gotten sick because of it."

"No, I'm not saying that it *made* him sick. I don't know enough to say that."

"If you don't want to use the respirator you can just send it back."

This was not the exchange Judy had anticipated. She hastened to assure Ann that we did want to make the new program work. However, getting started with it was difficult, and we merely wanted to do the right thing. Ann accepted the apology, but let it be known that she expected no further challenges to her machine.

The next time Judy called she reached Dawn, who conceded that some children didn't respond well to it and that Joseph might be one of these. It was too early to tell, and among other things she wanted us to reconsider the rate we had chosen. We'd reported a rate of breathing that was suspiciously slow, she said. Had we counted accurately? If so, perhaps the rate on the machine should be turned back somewhat.

A few days later I found myself on the phone with Lidwina, to whom these breathing rates were just further evidence of Joseph's need for respiratory patterning. "Fifteen breaths per minute is an unusual low, low rate, especially for a walker," she said. "Most of our kids are in the twenties or thirties."

This was astonishing news. I asked if well children breathed that rapidly.

"Maybe towards twenty-one, twenty-two probably. But when you watch Joseph walk, he walks as if he's breathing very, very slowly. So it doesn't surprise me that you've counted such a slow rate."

"OK. So we need to use the machine to increase it."

"Right. You may need to come down a little bit, initially, until you find what he's comfortable with. But you've got to put in something that's better, in order to get him to a point where he will come out with language."

Incredibly, that was our final conversation with Lidwina. Just one week later a note arrived saying she'd resigned from the staff and was going home to Australia. She didn't share her reasons. "I will always be Joseph's advocate," she promised.

We fervently wished that could be true on a practical level, because it was hard to imagine anyone else filling her place. Others on the staff had their various areas of special expertise, but none of them knew Joseph as Lidwina had. We didn't realize until now how heavily we'd relied on her advice.

Almost every family we knew who had been using a respirator for any length of time had invested in an alternate model, which was manufactured and sold by a man in Pennsylvania. He sent us literature promising that it required no complicated adjustments. The rate and ratio were digitally set and remained accurate within one breath per day. "It's worth its weight in gold!" Cindy assured us in a letter. "It saved my sanity!"

On the other hand, it was very expensive, and it might even involve rewiring the house and making other major alterations. Apparently, certain costly accessories were going to be necessary, whether we switched to the new machine or kept the present one.

To begin with, Judy ordered a new poncho—a vinyl suit, actually—and a smaller cage that she hoped would fit Joseph's chest more snugly. The bill for these two items exceeded five hundred dollars.

"Why would you want to do that, when we still aren't sure a machine is right for us?" I asked.

"How can we know whether it's right until we give it a fair trial?"

"I would like to go on record as saying that I'm not made of money."

"I know that. But I see this as our last chance to speed up Joseph's development so he can go to First Grade with the other kids."

What other option was there? We could go back to manually patterning him. But the rate of progress using that route did not point toward a timely entry into school. On the other hand, how long could we keep this up?

About this time, Ming phoned with a suggestion. They'd decided against taking Christopher to the Institutes. But they appreciated the time we'd given them when they felt so directionless. At the moment, they had an acupuncturist from China actually living at their house and treating their son. We were welcome to bring Joseph for treatments, too.

Judy thanked her but declined immediately. And when she told me, I agreed that we shouldn't run off on tangents. We had no reason to think acupuncture could help at all. And more importantly, no time to explore it.

For several months now I had been operating in a survival mode. All I hoped to achieve each day was the task immediately before me—the current monthly report to the Institutes, the next marathon walk, preparing the next day's Bit cards. I couldn't imagine handling any further challenges. And now even *this* much seemed excessive. I was faltering, and so was Judy, who dropped further and further behind in the race to complete each day's program goals. As always, I relieved her when I could, but even on weekends, with both of us available, we fell short.

"Dr. Frymann has a point," she sighed. "The Institutes gives people impossible assignments, and then parents become miserable trying to do them. I do think our program is what Joseph needs. But there's no way the two of us are going to get it all done!"

As for our veteran volunteers, they were out of the picture. Sally had a new baby now. Nancy and Greg had new careers. Probably everyone was dismayed by how long this was taking. They were all still our friends, but they had their own lives. And no one new materialized to take their place. Evelyn agreed to monitor the machine on Tuesday afternoons, which enabled Judy to get an extra hour or two of sleep, but aside from that we were on our own.

Following Nell's last visit to our house, I walked her to her car with an umbrella, since it had begun raining. Before driving away, she had some final words for me.

"What you two are up against is too much," she said. "I worry about Judy. She's so wrapped up in this. Something is driving her. I wish you would stop and think about whether the time has come to call it quits. Be satisfied! You've done a lot with that little guy."

"I've done nothing if I let my only kid perish."

"*Perish?* Oh, for crying out loud. Who's 'perishing?' Huh? Think about that. It's not Joseph."

During the time we'd known her, Nell had come to dislike me because of my unbending insistence on following the Institutes' directions. At least, that's what I sensed. I accepted the fact regretfully, feeling that I had no choice. The prospect of contributing to Joseph's recovery meant everything to me. Of course I wanted him well, needed him well, because he was my son, but it went beyond even that. In the first part of my life, I'd expected to become a doctor. Even though that dream had not materialized, even though I'd then made hasty and immature decisions that negated all my preparations for a career in the healing arts, even though it seemed nothing I'd touched since then had gone particularly well, fixing up this helpless little boy would make everything right. Life would then move in an uncharted but wholly acceptable direction. Joseph would merge into society on an equal footing with his contemporaries, and I would have overcome the doubts that had beset me these many years. I did not consciously think this, in so many words, but I can see now the importance I attached to participating in the recovery of a child who'd been dismissed and ignored by the professionals. The achievement would mean nothing to them, but it would validate everything for me.

But on the other hand if this campaign were to fail—No, it *couldn't* fail! I refused to contemplate what that would mean, for myself as well as for Joseph. I avoided comparing the energy and passion I spent on his behalf with what I displayed at my day job. The managers there had faith in my ability to support tight deadlines with high-quality work, but I had no remaining bandwidth to offer much creativity or leadership. They rewarded my steady presence with steady employment, but no promotions. Like Nell's contempt, that too was ok. I could not excel in my career because I had this program to do! Therefore, the program must not fall short of what I needed as badly as Joseph, because then neither of us had a way out.

JOSEPH RECOVERED his usual good health and seemed to demonstrate a new curiosity about life in our household. He wanted to help load the dishwasher. When reminded, he put his dirty clothes into the laundry hamper. Judy wrote up a recipe for cookies, and he helped her follow it through all the steps of measuring and mixing ingredients.

I shared the results with coworkers at the office, and then prepared a homemade book for him describing everyone's delighted reaction to "Joseph's cookies." He seemed gratified.

Life with the respirator began to look possible. Either the machine had passed an initial break-in period or we had finally learned how to set the controls, because now it operated reliably for as much as fifteen minutes with no need for adjustment.

And so our fortunes ebbed and flowed. The utility company gave us a discount on our hefty electric bill to offset the use of the respirator. We did our best with the daily goals, and somehow didn't go bankrupt.

Sleeping in shifts remained the big hurdle.

Judy insisted on taking the graveyard shift, which meant that my own sleeping schedule was scarcely affected. On days when all went well, I'd arrive home from work by five o'clock to find Joseph in the respirator and Judy just finishing dinner preparations. The plan was for her to go to bed at that point. I monitored the machine, kept Joseph company if he was awake, and did the chores until midnight, at which point I was supposed to rouse Judy and go to bed myself. Then she was on duty until five p.m. the next day.

That was the idea, anyway. Often, I'd find Judy in the wrong frame of mind for sleep. Against my advice, she'd stay up until seven or even eight o'clock, discussing the day's events with me or winding down with a long phone conversation, a magazine, a bath—whatever. Could she get by on four hours' sleep? Experience soon proved otherwise, because I noted a sharp decrease in the morale around our house. She complained about our situation in general, our shortage of helpers, and not infrequently, about me. I no longer showed her love and support, she said. What did she mean? "You don't know," she responded bitterly. "Of course you don't know. Why would anybody expect *you* to understand showing love and support for your own wife?"

When she did get more rest, all this abated, and she reverted to her usual, more sunny disposition. Accordingly, I began to postpone the changing of the guard until one or two a.m.

"*Why didn't you wake me?*" She'd protest irritably. "Now how are *you* going to function tomorrow? You're undermining our whole arrangement!"

Downstairs, Joseph would be sound asleep in the respirator, breathing audibly—sometimes even with a flute-like whistle—as the machine repeatedly forced his chest open and sucked air into his lungs. Sleepily, and not too happily, Judy made her way to his side to doze and check the rate every few minutes, and I'd collapse on the bed.

I didn't always wake up to the same sound. Many times, Judy became dissatisfied with the machine at some point in the night. It would begin overheating, she thought. Or the pressure would gradually tighten Joseph's poncho until the circulation to his hands and feet was being restricted. Unable to make further adjustments, she just shut the thing down and went back to sleep herself.

So he didn't get the requisite eighteen hours. He got fourteen hours. Or twelve. Or nine.

Like Dr. Frymann, Judy still harbored inner misgivings about this machine. It appeared to put a lot of stress on his little body, bouncing him around almost violently inside the cage. She fretted over what it might be doing to his bone structure.

DISTANCE WALKING remained part of the schedule, too. Desperately, we redoubled our efforts, *shouting* encouragement to him on the walks, really oblivious now of curious bystanders. He still had not progressed from walking to running, the next step up on the Profile. Running would help his respiration still more, in addition to buying him a big boost in neurological age.

On weekends, Joseph and I still did our marathons at the park near my office. We'd used that track all winter without drawing attention, but with the coming of spring a softball team began playing in the infield. Before long, the players indicated, in not-so-subtle ways, that they disapproved of us. I gave little thought to this until partway through a marathon walk one Sunday, when a beefy guy standing in right field bellowed, "Hey, man, give the kid a rest!"

It was easy to imagine the picture we made—Joseph doggedly measuring off lap after lap with his little steps while I bent over him, glancing at my watch and barking encouragement like some self-appointed drill instructor.

People commonly mistook him for a younger child—three or even two years old (actually, he was now turning five), and no doubt perceived me as an overzealous parent trying to rush a baby into world-class competition.

"Did you explain that you were doing physical therapy?" Judy asked later.

"Couldn't. That guy was playing ball, and we were in the middle of a timed walk. We don't owe explanations to everybody we see."

"Well, you might find that people would be more understanding if they knew why you're doing it."

The very next day, however, Judy had a story of her own. She and Joseph were on their customary morning walk around the university track when a young woman jogging past them began to take an unwelcome interest. She looked at Joseph very closely as she came by and asked if they were doing some kind of therapy. Thereafter, each time she passed she'd offered an opinion.

"You have him dressed too warmly!" she snapped. "Children get overheated faster than adults."

Then she was away on another lap, before Judy could point out that Joseph was only walking, and therefore not generating as much heat as a runner. The track was situated on a hilltop about a mile from the ocean, from which a cool wind was blowing, and she felt that Joseph's long sleeves were appropriate.

"He should be drinking water when he exercises!"

An interesting observation. Judy might have discussed liquid balance if the other had lingered. But she had not, and now these peculiar attacks *en passant* were taking on a hostile tone.

Next lap: "Do you think he's *enjoying* this?" Clearly, this woman thought he did not, although thus far Joseph had been forging ahead with no complaint.

The runner came up behind them once again, and this time she just muttered, "You idiot!"

"Wait a minute," Judy called after her departing back. "You can't say that! I've been trained to handle his program, and I know what I'm doing."

"Well, *I'm* certified," the other flung back. Whatever that meant. Certified creep, maybe. Or certified something else. Judy shied away from the more satisfying words even in her thinking.

Out loud, she yelled, "Just because you've taken a few classes doesn't give you any insight into my son's medical condition!"

Picking up on the strife, Joseph began crying as he walked.

Matters escalated rapidly. The woman had slowed and was jogging backwards in front of them as she shouted a rebuttal. Apparently, she'd been unwilling to sacrifice her lap times to discuss things rationally but was quite ready to take time out for a fight. However, at this point they happened to be alongside a grey-haired man whom Judy saw at the track every day. He was always there, it seemed, pacing silently around the outside perimeter, always wearing earphones and apparently always deep in thought. They'd exchanged nods once or twice, but each respected the other's privacy. Now he switched off his tape player and said, "What's all this?" He looked at the runner and said, "Why don't you leave these people alone?"

Outnumbered, she turned abruptly and left the track.

The man looked back at Judy and said, "I've been watching you folks for the last year. *I* think you're doing a great job." That much said, he replaced the earphones and resumed his pacing.

The runner had vanished, but her effect lingered in Joseph's tears and Judy's elevated blood pressure. They managed to complete their mile with Judy singing a lighthearted song for him, but now the day was off to a rocky start.

"I wish I hadn't yelled back at her the way I did," Judy said to me that evening. "Maybe she had good intentions. Initially, she was making some intelligent comments. But she ended up hurting us. Mainly, I'm sorry Joseph saw me get upset."

I argued that her response had been more than justified.

"No. I shouldn't have let it turn into a shouting match. That was destructive. We've got to prepare ourselves in advance for run-ins with people, so that we can defuse them."

A tall order. In truth, we both lived on the edge of conflict, every day. Once, as Judy was unlocking the car in front of Dr. Frymann's office, a young guy bounced his motorcycle up over the curb, en route to a sidewalk café next door. He came very close to colliding with Joseph, whereupon Judy came very close to attacking him physically.

"Your kid didn't even try to get out of my way!" The biker protested feebly.

"What? So you can drive down the *sidewalk*, at fifty miles a hour, and it's people's responsibility to get out of *your* way? You asshole! You could've killed my son. I'm calling the police."

The biker changed his mind about stopping at the café. He was gone.

Back home, Joseph protested as they climbed the stairs from the garage. Another hours-long session in the respirator loomed ahead and perhaps he felt unhappy about that. At the top of the stairs, he abruptly flung about in a temper, lost his balance, and fell backward. Judy told me all about it that night.

"I short-circuited," she confessed. "I didn't know what I was doing. Joseph was tumbling down the stairs and I just reached to turn on the light switch. Except it was already on, so I turned it off. Then I turned it on again. And the light went on and off and on and off, and Joseph was somersaulting—he was actually doing backward somersaults, just like we taught him, all the way down the stairs! And at the bottom he landed on his feet, with his arms out, even! Not even bruised, can you believe it? But with the light going on and off, I was seeing this strobe effect. It was like an old newsreel. It was like I was watching a tragedy in the news." She paused to regain control of her breathing. "Anyway, that's why I didn't put him in the machine this afternoon. After the motorcycle and then the steps, neither of us could face it."

Thus went the days, until yet another Revisit was upon us. We didn't have a perfect record of meeting our daily goals (far from it!), and I had to fudge some figures on the report. But we'd survived. At this point, that alone felt significant.

24. A BIT GENERIC

"Are the changes you've seen during this last period worth the effort you've put into your program?"

That old familiar question! This time, Glenn Doman's daughter Janet was asking it. And for once, a ready answer didn't spring to our lips.

Joseph's eighth evaluation at the Institutes had been less than inspiring. Language, running, tactility, manual competence—all had been targeted for growth but showed indifferent improvement, at best.

Now it was Monday night. The last six months were painful history. Judy was depressed, but she answered bravely.

"I just have to say a program is better than no program."

"And how do you vote, Mr. Gallup?"

I didn't want to answer. "There's a temptation to be short-sighted, when you just see problems and no change over a period of weeks and weeks. It helps to take the long view. Compared to where we were when we began, it's been worth every minute. But going back just from December to now—*I don't know!*"

"Joseph *has* made *some* changes this period," Judy pointed out. "He just recently got to where he can catch a ball, for example."

"That's the result of better visual convergence," Janet said. "It shows you that *something* clicked in a big way. *I* think you've gotten good results. He's not where we want him to be—but that's the purpose of your week here."

Janet felt that there was "some key element" that hadn't been addressed sufficiently. As Lidwina and Teruki had done before, she listed the most likely issues and Judy and I tried to rank them. General neurological organization remained a prime suspect.

I recalled that creeping was said to be a treatment for midbrain organization. "Joseph hasn't crept since he began walking, two years ago," I commented. "I wonder if he should do more."

Janet smiled. "That's very interesting, because when I picked up this chart I started asking the same question."

The Institutes did indeed sometimes prescribe what was called a Primary Human Development treatment (coyly dubbed their "PHD" program), which involved long-distance creeping and crawling for children already able to walk. The purpose was to clear up any weak areas that persisted in the lower brain levels, which might then facilitate faster progress overall.

"We've *got* to accelerate his neurological growth rate," she said. "His overall rate now is only 39.3%. What I'd like to see is sixty percent, or above. Because if a kid is sustaining sixty percent over a long period of time, he's ultimately going to win. And he's going to win in a time frame when you and I will be here to see it."

IT WAS TURNING OUT to be a hard trip. Among other issues, Judy was sick again, with frequent violent coughing spells. At one point during the week, Ann Ball even asked in alarm if she was all right.

"She's gotten a little run-down," I confessed. The coughing subsided and Judy leaned weakly against the wall behind me, dabbing at her eyes with a tissue.

Ann gave us a knowing smile. "Maybe it's Honeymoon time again."

What I remember most about that last week was the final conference, again with Janet. "How was your week?" she asked.

"It got better," I said. "Your lecture on problem solving was especially interesting. Of course, your focus was on how we train our *kids* to be problem-solvers, but we adults are wrestling with questions, too. A big question in our minds these days is the relationship Joseph's going to have with the school system back home. He's fast approaching the age when kids normally start school. We've operated on the assumption that he'd be well when that time came. Now it looks like that'll take a while longer. Obviously, we aren't keen on putting him into a special-ed class—."

"Of course not!" Janet scoffed. "But the trouble is that the *whole world* is special ed. And when they take a curriculum that's already slow, and slow it down even more for special ed, how would the kids have any hope of catching up? If you took well kids and put them in special ed, *they* wouldn't progress normally, so how could anybody expect it of hurt kids? Special education is not the answer for *our* kids, that's for sure."

There was an alternative course of action. "It's legally possible for a mother to home-school her child from birth to age eighteen," Janet reminded us. "All you have to do is agree to have him tested once a year, and that's perfectly reasonable. He takes the Stanford Achievement Test. To a home-schooled child, this is fine. It's no problem for him at all."

"We were trying to gage Joseph's reading level," Judy explained. "Is he at the First Grade level yet, or—."

"We can help you with that. As soon as he's reading smaller print, *we* will give you the Stanford Achievement Test, along with the booklets on how to administer it. It's very easy. Then you just give the test at home, send it in, and we'll mark it.

"The Institutes is fully accredited," she continued. "When Joseph's ready to enter school—at whatever point you feel comfortable letting him do that—we can issue a certificate that will get him in at the right grade level. We've found that to be totally effective, worldwide."

I said, "One argument for putting him in school is the benefit of social interaction with other kids."

She laughed. I'd stumbled into one of her favorite topics. "This is something that our parents get a lot of harassment about. *'Oh! How's he going to become socialized?'* But here again, experience has shown that our kids are profoundly affected by being home longer than the average kid. And the effect is a profoundly *good* effect. When you incarcerate a child at age six—because, let's face it, a well child is incarcerated, he's institutionalized, at six—he goes in as a sweet, sensitive, civilized little guy, with a pretty good idea of right and wrong. But after just a year or two, already the parents are beginning to be uneasy, because they are less and less the opinion leaders for the child. By the time he's in Third Grade, it's the other third graders. Then the fourth graders, and so on. And they see that school, rather than being an environment for socialization, is actually an environment for *de*-socialization.

"All the things the kid learns about sharing, about caring, about being fair, being just, he learns at home from Mother and Father. And the more time he spends with Mother and Father, the more sane his environment will be. When he goes to school, he learns that the world is a world of injustice, that the biggest kid calls the shots, that the noisiest kid always gets the attention. *And on the bus!* Well, he might get rough-housed by kids four or five years older than he is."

I nodded. There was truth in all this, although it felt a bit generic.

"What he gets in school is a dog-eat-dog viewpoint. So we've learned that when we put a kid in, say, Fourth Grade, who's never been to school a day in his life—and the world is saying, *'How's he going to cope?'*—It turns out that he is much stronger than all the other fourth graders, because he comes in much more like an adult. We often hear of report cards where the teacher is saying, 'Well, yes, intellectually he's strong, and physically—*but socially!* He's incredible. He's like an assistant teacher!' And this has happened so many times. Again, I'm talking about kids who'd never been to school before.

"Maybe the epitome is Feruccio Liguidi, who graduated from the Institutes' program two years ago. Now Feruccio started on program at age four; we graduated him at seventeen and a half. He's got the world's record for time on program. He never spent a day in school. He missed grammar school. He missed junior high. He missed high school. He went from the Institutes directly into the University of Padua. How did he get there? He got the top math scores in all of Italy. And I'm sure he was the most mature college student Padua ever got, because he's lived the life of an adult—all his life. *He* had no problem with socialization. At all."

"Everybody's job is to grow up and be an adult," Judy offered, dutifully quoting one of Glenn's lectures.

"Yes! And to compare the standards in your household to those in even the best classroom—! Even the best Third Grade teacher in the world is no match for thirty youngsters. *She's* not setting the pace or the standard! The most outrageous kid in the class does that. It's a terrible thing that our school systems are falling apart. But it's good that parents are able to take responsibility and write their own ticket if they choose."

It helped to hear all this. Unfortunately, it was just philosophy, with no immediate reference to Joseph himself. I wondered if Janet understood *how far* he was from being able to take a standardized test. We wouldn't feel good about the situation until events at home began to reflect her scenario. I just didn't know if they ever could.

25. COURSE CORRECTIONS

For months, Judy and I had been putting one foot in front of another, sustained by habit and little else. Now Janet had allowed us another Honeymoon. Even if she hadn't, I doubted that Judy or I could have geared up to carry on as before. Elaine Lee had mentioned that West Coast families generally got their new programs sorted out on the plane going home. We did not. Back in San Diego we just wanted to sleep, and no amount of sleep was enough.

"Has Joseph made *any* progress?" Judy's father asked by phone. His tone of voice betrayed his opinion. "Maybe you should just put him in some kind of *school*," he said. "Don't they have schools he could go to?"

A former volunteer was blunter. "He hasn't really changed in two years, you know." She slipped this observation in smoothly between innocuous comments, but she meant for Judy to notice it. As she saw things, this was simply a conclusion that we needed to accept.

Joseph *had* changed, of course! But most of our evidence for believing that was anecdotal. No one could pretend he didn't still had a long, long way to go. Honeymoons had a way of bringing that out.

"A little boy can get by only so long on cuteness," Judy said one night. "After a certain number of years, the world expects to see real performance." It made little difference that Joseph did perform well compared to his own past. He still did not begin to measure up to the world's standards. The same playgroup moms who'd accepted him unquestioningly two years earlier now appeared just a little reserved. Since our previous Honeymoon, some of them had had second or third children, and even these toddlers were leaving him behind in some areas.

We *couldn't* give up. But what else would it take? Judy was hearing messages at church to the effect that God never gives one a greater burden than he can handle, but experience didn't necessarily bear that out. "This past spring I was working as hard as I possibly could, and it still wasn't good enough," she said glumly. "Getting up at midnight to monitor the machine. I never had a good night's sleep. And I *hated* taking him through that gymnastics routine! Time after time he'd do a somersault and then just lie there. I had to *pull* him up and tell him to *do* it again. I'd get dirty looks from the other people at the Y. I know they thought me terribly mean. It got to be a hair-pulling experience for me, every day."

And so I said, "Listen, Judy. You don't have to do it any longer if you don't want to. I can quit my job and take over the program full time. We could still get by."

Exactly how we'd get by without my income was not clear. We might sell the condo and live on our equity for a year or two. We could move back East and stay with my mother.

"I've been over that already, and it's not the answer," Judy sighed. "I have to fix my own attitude. That's what we've both got to do. Then we can fix Joseph. Don't you worry. We'll see this thing through to the end, whatever it takes."

And with that much settled, we began our Honeymoon—now known however as the "Motor Opportunity Program." (Time away from the full program was never meant to be *empty* time, and to counter what appeared to be a misguided enthusiasm among parents for taking breaks, Janet said the term "Honeymoon" had been replaced.) In addition to staying physically active, we needed to use this time to learn the rules of a complicated new diet. Plus, Ann had asked us to start right away with the CO_2 therapy we'd heard other families mention. This "oxygen enrichment program" involved giving him thirty-second doses of a special blend of oxygen and carbon dioxide. It relied on the same principle used in masking. By creating an imbalance in the levels of these gases, we stimulated the brain to call for a surge of blood, resulting in a net increase in available oxygen.

Any spare time we discovered *still* had to be spent in the respirator. Even now.

In the three months that followed, Joseph enjoyed frequent long walks on the beach. Judy told him about tidal action as they went, or they stopped and she demonstrated how to draw pictures in the sand.

In the evenings, I took him into the neighborhood pool. Swimming had always been one of our joys, and no well kid of our acquaintance swam nearly as well as Joseph—even those who'd had lessons. At the Institutes we'd heard that swimming was good from the standpoint of brain growth and development. Obviously, it was also closely tied with respiration. When you hold your breath under water, you're doing a form of masking. This leads to chest growth, better language, and all the benefits of good respiration. Joseph had no trouble going under for ten seconds or more, and he brought himself up laughing and ready to repeat the trick. Before I knew it he was crossing the pool without assistance.

"Joseph, if I painted you black and white you'd look just like Shamu," I said, referring to the well-known mascot at SeaWorld, a killer whale. He emitted an exasperated snort at the comparison, but then smiled.

He attended Sunday school and even a week-long vacation Bible school, always with Judy close by to help with the unfamiliar tasks of cutting and pasting and painting—and to ensure he ate none of the Oreos and similar garbage routinely handed out in these settings.

"Why doesn't he talk?" the children asked Judy. It was interesting that little kids seldom spoke to him directly. Something about him signaled that he wouldn't reply.

"When Joseph was a baby, he was hurt," Judy explained patiently. "He's still catching up from that, but he'll be all right soon."

The children were troubled to find someone like themselves so unfairly limited. But what impressed them more was the level of adult attention this kid received. Taking their cue from Judy, most kids were affectionate toward Joseph—even protective of him. For his part, Joseph allowed himself to be babied. In fact, he *enjoyed* it. This was not a relationship with the world that we wanted to encourage.

The highlight of our summer was a weekend trip to Palm Springs, where we visited Jimmy's family and helped out with *his* program. Familiar tasks in a new environment, and with somebody else's kid, did not feel like work. On the contrary! Between patterning sessions we joined our hosts in frequent short dips in their infamous backyard pool (now belatedly enclosed by a sturdy fence). The dry desert air enabled us to run between pool and house almost without toweling off.

At the moment, Jimmy's biggest challenge was logging 130 meters of crawling per day, and his parents' living room was taken up with a smooth track for that purpose. He didn't enjoy it very much—but he did it, just as Joseph had done so many things we'd asked of him. Judy and I added our voices to the cheering section, and Joseph watched Jimmy's dogged efforts with interest. *So other kids had to do this stuff, too!*

Judy and I observed his parents as well, and with great respect, because unlike us they were handling the program without going crazy. Granted, they had a live-in Mexican housekeeper who helped with respiratory patterning. That was a stroke in their favor. But whatever the reason, they'd preserved something from their former lives. Annette even managed to keep up her own business. Bob and Annette had admired our program once, but now the tables were turned.

We drove home with the conviction that we needed more balance, or more accurately, a bigger picture. I felt that obsession with meeting each day's program goals might have narrowed our vision to the point where we could be missing something. This seemed more likely when, a few days later, I found myself holding a hospital newsletter that promised:

The idea of illness or injury to our neurological system can be a frightening prospect. But today, diagnosis, treatment and rehabilitation of neurological disorders have moved light-years ahead of where we were even five years ago. And thanks to these ongoing advances, surviving and thriving after a brain illness or injury is the rule rather than the exception.

In the article, a local neurologist extolled his new high-tech methods for studying an injured brain's electrical activity, blood flow, and metabolism. He said it was now possible to locate a problem area in the brain with great precision, opening the way to effective treatment.

This was too much to ignore. I knew we'd been out of touch with current events, but it was hard to believe that we could have missed the kind of medical breakthroughs this article suggested. I sent the doctor what I hoped was a thought-provoking letter about Joseph's history and current status and asked for his recommendations.

He had none. To his credit, he did respond, but only to confess, "We are still in our infancy in understanding the growth capability of the brain, and I am afraid we are a long way from applying these processes effectively in the case of someone like your son." The article had been written only to generate buzz over the launch of a new clinic.

Although it was a long shot, he said an esteemed colleague at the University of California might be able to help. I drafted a new query to this learned individual, and included copies of Joseph's medical records, but received no reply. I made several phone calls that were not returned. Apparently, without high-powered names from NIH to drop, I wasn't going to get anyone's attention.

I fired off more inquiries to various meccas for brain study such as the nearby Scripps Research Clinic and the Salk Institute. Perhaps someone there would have professional interest or compassion as well as the expertise necessary to reach Joseph, to open doors of expression for him as Annie Sullivan had once done for Helen Keller.

No one took time to reply, except for one well-known doctor who returned my letter with a note scrawled at the bottom: "I regret I know of no useful therapy for your son's unfortunate developmental struggles. I work only on experimental animals and know of no appropriate other physician to recommend. So sorry."

Despite the Institutes' bold claims about being years ahead of the times, and despite encouraging reports that still appeared from time to time in the papers, nobody had a handle on the problem. One article on neurosciences began with the dismal prediction, "At the current rate of progress, if you were to ask me when we will have some real understanding of complex vertebrate neural systems, I would answer perhaps in one thousand years, maybe 500, but certainly not 20."

I even wondered whether I should be involved in furthering that work. Admittedly, my pre-med background was rudimentary and outdated. Still, I could have thrown myself into the cause with religious zeal, if only one of these labs would consider having me as some kind of lowly technician. If possible, that proposal met with even less enthusiasm.

GAMELY, I revised our daily checkoff sheet to reflect the various program tasks that had been assigned to us. That alone was a project! I was hard-pressed to fit everything on one piece of paper. When I did, Judy couldn't bear to look at it.

The new Primary Human Development program included a resumption of old-fashioned cross-patterning, which meant we were going to need volunteers once again. Also, Joseph would be crawling and creeping greater distances each week, until by Interim Report time he would be covering a mile every day on his hands and knees and another two hundred meters flat on his belly.

There would have to be thirty trips under the brachiating ladder every day, regardless of the fact that blisters had always prevented him from achieving even half that number.

At least, the CO_2 treatments were easy. We'd rented a huge tank of compressed gas, formulated per the Institutes' prescription, and all we had to do was give him short doses of it throughout the day.

And of course we still had the Institutes' respirator.

"We've *got* to buy the improved model," Judy decided. "If we don't have the money, I'll take some out of my IRA." She'd tapped that resource once already. I started to protest that the tax penalty made it a rotten deal, but she said, "Listen, if we don't make life easier now, I won't be around at age sixty-five to *need* a retirement fund! I can't stay up any more nights twisting dials back and forth and listening to that stupid metronome! *I can't!* Not and do the rest of the program during the day!"

Well, OK—. But a bank loan made more sense.

We resumed the full program on a weekend in mid-September, 1990, four years to the day after our original mass mailing to call for volunteers. I concentrated on getting off to a good start. The first day, Joseph achieved eight trips of brachiating before his hands became sore, after which point he refused to hold the rungs of the ladder. He crept and crawled the requisite distances and submitted willingly enough to some cross-patterning.

Then, late Sunday night, my father died. For months, Dad had been virtually unreachable. He'd examined his fingers endlessly or just stared into space, seldom speaking or even acknowledging his frustrated visitors. What he *had* said was mostly nonsense, although my sister told me he occasionally called out to anyone who happened to be near, "Always keep a positive attitude!" Evidently, he'd held onto that last piece of wisdom until the very end.

Judy and I sure needed that advice.

For several days she bore the full responsibility of doing the program. But she attempted very little of it. "I'm *tired* of this!" she said angrily when I returned from the funeral. "I'm *tired* of rushing from one task to another all day and falling further and further behind as I go. The last three programs they've written for us have been *absurdly* difficult! There was a time when this was all I wanted to do. But it's meaningless now. And I can't shake the feeling that the staff hasn't been listening to what we tell them. They just recite the party line and send us back for more. They've taken all the joy out of our lives. They even took away music. You know what? I'm *not* doing this anymore."

There was no point in arguing with a statement like that. As Lidwina would have said, our "dynamics" were not good. Matt might have nodded and observed, as he'd done before, that Americans were lazy. Presumably, *that* explained why most of the senior families were from overseas. Whatever the cause, "dynamics" explained the effect. As Glenn Doman's latest book put it, a successful program had to be "mutually joyful and fulfilling for both parent and child."

In any such equation the joy has to precede the success. But there comes a point at which it must be reinforced with results. "I'm *tired* of always having these one-sided conversations with Joseph," Judy went on. "Why won't he make choices? Why is he so passive?"

I said, "He's learned to let us do things for him because we're always racing to move on. We have only so many hours in a day. How long should we wait for him to uncap his toothpaste tube, for example? How long do we sit around waiting for him to answer a question? We *can't* wait! We're always charging ahead to the next thing."

I think we could have carried on if we had a better sense that Joseph was truly on board with us. He gave less indication of that than ever, and now spoke even less than before. He could be extremely *vocal*, but most noises he made bore no semblance to words. We could assign meanings to them if we wanted. That was Doman's tactic. The child says *Guh* and the parent takes that to mean *Good*. Thenceforth, when the child says *Guh* he's using a word of the family's accepted vocabulary. Joseph gave no indication of caring, and the exercise led nowhere.

In the early days, Joseph *had* wanted to creep and walk; and he did his part. But we'd all been increasingly drawn to more normal pursuits since the wonderful day when he took his first steps. At the same time, the respiratory aspects of the program had made our lives increasingly *less* normal, and had also produced less obvious results. By now Joseph had perfected his own compensatory mechanisms, his own ways of dealing with people and getting what he wanted. He gave us less reason to feel confident about things that we'd always had to take pretty much on faith—that he enjoyed and benefitted from his intelligence program, for example. He *wasn't* benefitting from it if he wasn't attending. It might have helped to discuss the situation with Lidwina, but alas she was gone. Teruki, our new advocate, had been out of the country for several weeks, and conversations with other staff members were not productive. Judy actually avoided talking with them.

Living means dealing with problems. I knew better than to look for a time when we'd have no challenges at all. But we wanted to move on to some *new* ones. When could we realistically hope to do that? *How much longer would this take before I even knew how long it would be?*

Paul wrote to concede defeat. "We believe the Institutes' program helped Sean's intelligence and more importantly our ability to know how intelligent he is, but physically they did not help at all." Sean was due for surgery on his hips, after which he would be entering the public school system in Canada. His parents were thinking about their careers and about each other again, because "Without us, Sean will not survive."

Judy had several conversations with Silvia, the mother in Mexico who'd described her daughter's program for us back in those early, heady days. Angie was now well into her seventh year with the Institutes, and the outlook was no longer so bright. "I've seen it time and time again," Silvia said. "Families start the program and get good results. Then the changes stop coming so rapidly. Finally, they reach a plateau. Their kids stop improving, and eventually they get discouraged and quit." In their own case, she said, they'd just kept plodding along, hoping things would improve again. Instead, during the last couple of years, Angie had regressed. She now suffered from scoliosis—and may even have had typhoid, they weren't sure. She was so run-down that they'd canceled some Revisits. Now the Institutes was questioning their dedication and threatening to kick them off the program.

She and Angie had even been summoned back to Philly for a reme-
dial on-campus encounter. It hadn't been fun. Their advocate would
not believe Angie could fail to improve with the regimen she'd been
assigned—at least, not until after Silvia had worked very hard for two
weeks under the staff members' unremitting and almost hostile scru-
tiny.

Cindy wrote, saying that Bobby had reached his fourteenth birthday.
"He has been working real hard on using his hands in a functional
way—holding a spoon, hitting a switch, etc. Nothing for him comes
easy. We're back to crawling, plus the machine, some balance development, and lots of reflex masks! *Ugh.*" They were looking forward to the
encouraging influence of another week in Philly.

We felt increasingly certain that *we* were not. Asymptotically smaller
and less quantifiable changes were not getting us where we needed to
be. I mourned Joseph's blighted childhood and Judy's chronic anxiety. I mourned the fact that domestic preoccupations had long since
brought my career advancement to a halt, stunting my ability to provide for them.

Sure, we admired Janet's story about the Italian boy who graduated
to wellness after thirteen years on program. On the other hand, how
confident could we be that his condition had ever been comparable to
Joseph's, or that any number of years on program would bring us the
same result?

I thought yet again of the time I'd been lost in the cornfield, the way
it had seemed that going in one direction was about as promising as
heading off in any other. I thought of Dad's sudden perspective in the
hospital, when he announced that endeavor was pointless.

And again, was our life a labyrinth or a maze?

If my basic assumption had been wrong, and all this time we'd been
in a labyrinth instead of a maze, then there never was much question
regarding the outcome.

The many advisors we used to see who recommended acceptance
of Joseph's disability must have believed that we were in a labyrinth.

When we sought to prove them wrong, and achieved interim victories, their answer was that "It would have happened anyway," without intervention. Since, in their view, a disabled child always becomes a disabled adult, the destination was given. So the path of least resistance would have been the healthiest choice.

But what to do with my conviction that fatalism was wrong? That wellness was still his birthright?

OFF AND ON—since the very beginning, in fact—we'd grappled with the idea of a spiritual response to all this. Obviously, Judy and I couldn't heal Joseph by ourselves. And it was useless to blame the rest of the world for not helping more. That left God. However one defines it, the Ultimate Creator had to be brought into the picture in a way that would make a difference.

I, too, had become a churchgoer now. Actually, as I learned more about the congregation that had helped fund our trips, I gathered that they'd been humoring us in a way, believing that a more direct solution would be available once we were prepared to receive it. The church Judy had selected was different from others in my experience, in that it emphasized the divinity of each person. It didn't burden its people with an inventory of their sinful nature, nor did it pressure them for money. It taught that those who sowed would also reap, and it left matters there. And so I joined the Unity movement, eager to repay Joseph's benefactors in any way possible, and more than eager to redefine our problem.

Wellness was *still* Joseph's birthright. A normal life was his birthright—and ours! To achieve it, I heard, we had to learn something called *scientific prayer*, so named because it could produce demonstrable results, time after time. We had to control our thinking. Blair, the minister, put it quite simply. "What you think about, you bring about." This was perhaps too simple. I took him to mean, *What you can believe, you will experience.* We did believe that all the potential of a well boy was in there, behind the barrier of brain injury. To honor that belief, presumably, we needed to affirm wellness in prayer, to bless the abilities he already had, and to align our thinking with a full recovery as if it were an accomplished fact.

Judy and I tried using our imaginations to visualize a well Joseph. What would he be like? My experience with well kids was so limited that I hardly knew what to expect. Back East for Dad's funeral, I'd seen the son of an old high-school friend. Now *that* kid had been riding a bicycle, climbing trees, and teasing his mother by bringing frogs into the house. I thought he must be advanced for five years, but that was his age—the same as Joseph's.

Judy said, "I can picture Joseph coming up to me and asking for a glass of water."

"That still has him in a dependent role," I argued. "*I* want to see him running outdoors to play with his friends, yelling goodbye to us over his shoulder." I had to stop speaking. Just putting this in words made my eyes sting with tears.

What you think about, you bring about. (Catchy phrases like that abounded in our new circle. *Name it and claim it*. Have *an attitude of gratitude*.) Yes, Judy and I were game, but what was *Joseph* thinking about?

He didn't tell us, although frequently he did sing or chant a phrase that, with some imagination, sounded like "Good enough." That's what Judy heard, anyway.

Was he saying that the progress he'd made thus far was *good enough*? Our objective was no secret. We had explained it to him many times, but that did not mean he'd accepted wellness as something real for himself. I thought ruefully of all those hours we'd spent around the patterning table with his volunteers. It wasn't the time I regretted but the *conversation* that Joseph had been forced to hear. To satisfy the more or less idle curiosity of our helpers, Judy and I had repeatedly talked about *why* he couldn't do all the things regular kids did. We were working to improve his coordination and his breathing and so on—but meanwhile *he'd* been learning that he was imperfect! He had probably absorbed that lesson at a deeper level than anything in his intelligence program. He now *hated* to hear about his shortcomings, by the way. That much was obvious. Whenever a conversation started to move in that direction, he yelled in protest. We respected his feelings about this, of course, but also didn't want him to ignore the problem.

Our studies revealed that deep-seated beliefs were most subject to revision when one was in an "altered" state of consciousness, such as that induced by beautiful music or when falling asleep. Accordingly, we developed a series of affirmative statements, which we recorded on a three-minute loop. For several weeks, Joseph went to sleep at night listening to constant repetitions of messages that promised:

> "Past events no longer detract from your abilities. Talking is easy for you! You think about something, and right away you can open your mouth and say it. Every day you have *more* exciting things to talk about, and every day you talk more. You *like* to talk. It makes you happy to talk, and it makes Mommy and Daddy so very happy to hear you talk. We're all happy, and we're all winning. You are clever. You are intelligent. You are smart. It feels very good to know that you can do anything for yourself. All the cells of your body are bathed in the perfection of your being, because you are a child of God. God is perfect, and God made you in His image and likeness."

Another part of establishing a normal life—for us all—meant getting rid of the consciousness of *lack*. I vowed to ask for no more financial help. We didn't need to seek out benefactors. *We were prospering!* That statement was *true*. We would *make* it true with an attitude that attracted abundance, and by donating to the church and other worthy causes, starting now.

We pursued this question with the same determination, the same sense of being hot on the trail of something, that had first taken us to

Glenn Doman. We attended workshops at the church, and pored over metaphysical interpretations of the Bible.

I'd always thought it improbable that the followers of Moses could have made some ridiculous statue and worshipped it in his absence— but according to a book I found (in Dr. Frymann's library, of all places) Judy and I had done the same thing. Like the golden calf, brain injury was a false god. We didn't worship it in the usual sense. We certainly didn't love it! But we'd allowed it to dominate our lives. Everything we'd done, every waking thought, had conformed to this obstacle. Scripture became startlingly relevant and even exciting when viewed this way. Hungry for more, we sought out counselors.

A visiting minister played a tape of an infant giggling and invited the participants in her workshop to imagine we were holding that baby. Then, "Imagine that *you* are that baby," she said. "The baby you are holding is yourself! Love it." The recorded burbling and cooing went on while everyone adjusted to this idea. "And now, what would you say to this baby, knowing what you know about life? What would you say to yourself?"

A voice in my head promptly shouted *Don't kill yourself*, and I winced, reluctant to admit that a nerve had been touched. The idea of ending my life had been occurring to me lately. I knew I'd never be able to live with myself if I abandoned my family, so I would never just leave. But life itself didn't mean much if I could not help them.

People often tried to tell Judy and me that we were strong. We never believed it. Or if we were—well, I was tired of being strong. No, that wasn't right; I had no desire to be weak. I just wanted out from under all these accumulating burdens that had no resolution. Deserting my family was no option. I loved them all, and that was why I could not bear to see so many knotty problems besetting them—first Joseph and then my dad, and my mother no longer seemed quite right, either now, although I simply had no remaining capacity to deal with that. How could it be that *nothing* yielded to all our positive thinking and determination?

I asked the visiting minister for individual counseling.

She felt that something about me must be attracting all these insoluble problems. Perhaps I harbored a deep-seated belief—inspired by events in a previous life, even—that I needed or somehow deserved to be in this position.

"My own position is secondary," I insisted, falling back on the argument I'd used with Joseph's first doctors. "Yes, it's a big problem for me, but how could anything *I* might believe deep down inside have an effect on my son's development or on family members who live far away?"

"Your souls are all connected, and they go back many, many lifetimes," she assured me. Exploration of previous lifetimes was her specialty, it turned out, and she thought Judy and I might both benefit from the exercise.

She spoke very gently, for a long time, like someone coaxing a desperate person in off the ledge of a building. Judy and I both had to relax, she said. We had to be patient and keep visualizing Joseph in a perfect body. "Look past outer appearances and see the beautiful, whole, and radiant being that he really is," she said. "The process is like putting water in a tea kettle and putting it on the stove. You're going to wait for the steam. And you're going to visualize steam, spurting out of that spout, knowing that at that point it is ready. Then your purpose will have been served.

"But in the mean time, as you look at the tea kettle, nothing is happening. Even though the heat is applied and the water is getting hotter and hotter. At 180 degrees nothing is happening. At 200 degrees nothing is happening. And then, at 212 degrees, steam bursts forth, and there it is. But all along, something *was* happening, although you didn't see it. That's the way faith is. You keep asking, you keep expecting, you keep knowing that it *is* happening. With every positive thought that you have, and every time you visualize wellness, you're adding another degree to the water. Then one day, when you have added enough energy to that image, and when Joseph is in agreement with it, the steam will manifest."

But you can *visualize* steam all day, my literal mind insisted, and water on the stove won't boil unless there's heat. That, ultimately, was the question. Was the right burner turned on? And didn't I have to be actively involved in some way to find out?

So far, nothing in particular was going on with Joseph. He'd developed some disturbing new habits, such as continually flexing his fingers in front of his face. This was some kind of game he played with his vision, but it was one more obstacle between him and normal social interaction. He still loved to strum on the window blinds and he dragged my shoes around the house as if they were toys.

Operating on habit, I continued making new reading materials and Bits whenever I hit upon an interesting idea, but there was no reward in trying to present them to him. Usually he just pushed them away. He was tired of that stuff.

"What's the point, anyway?" Judy wondered, quite seriously. "If he hasn't established basic things—like what's his, and where the boundaries are, and how to behave accordingly—then how is it going to help him to learn about state capitals or the life cycle of a butterfly?"

She still hoped that Sunday school, exposure to life in a structured group, could make a difference. Her skills with children were a big hit there, and before long she'd been put in charge of whole classrooms full of well kids. However, when her back was turned, anybody left with Joseph packed him off to the nursery, *with the babies!* This was totally unacceptable, and we protested. Joseph's behavior may have been unusual, but it was no more disruptive than that of any other youngster in the bunch. He did need occasional reminders to stay in his chair. The trouble was that since he said nothing, people assumed that he *understood* nothing. We couldn't convince them otherwise, and finally just took him to Sunday school at a different church. To make sure this one worked out, Judy or I was always present with him, making sure he participated and behaved appropriately. Whichever one of us was "off duty" went back to Blair's services and continued to pursue answers.

Judy sought further counseling and heard some disturbing opinions, to the effect that she was in no position to say what Joseph's purpose in life might be.

"I'm sure his purpose is *not* to live out his days with subnormal abilities," she retorted.

The kindly old gentleman who said this had been a guiding light for her, ever since he delivered an inspirational lesson on the radio back during the early days of our program. But his advice now was not helpful. He seemed to feel that Judy and I wanted Joseph well in order to satisfy our own egos, that we were imposing something unnatural on him. As if it weren't natural to be well.

After that, our steps led away from the church where we'd begun to find a spiritual bearing. Their exercises had showed us a diverting new side of religious experience, but hadn't changed our life. Who could do that?

Judy's sister Pat had long since introduced us to the television ministry of Kenneth and Gloria Copeland, and we now began tuning in their daily broadcasts for another perspective. We found Kenneth staring earnestly from the screen. The answer was clear-cut for this guy. Every problem should be viewed with reference to very explicit promises in the Bible, which he cited as if they provided a legal basis for making claims. Contradictory evidence from other sources was worthless.

His wife Gloria specialized in explaining the promises for healing. "'Bless the Lord, and forget not *ALL* His benefits,'" she proclaimed, quoting from Psalm 103. "'Who forgiveth *all* thine iniquities; who healeth *all* thy diseases.' The benefit of spiritual redemption is certainly the most important one, because it's eternal. But you don't have to choose! God is offering *all* of His benefits to you."

The first time I'd heard one of Kenneth Copeland's energetic deliveries on tape, much earlier, I'd wondered how an intelligent, educated person could seriously listen to that stuff. But now that I *was* listening, I realized that this message resembled Blair's in its focus on a better life on earth, as opposed to patient suffering. "I thank God for the sweet by-and-by," as he put it, "but what does He say to do about the rotten here-and-now?" He had at least one key point in common with Glenn Doman's philosophy: that winners *expect* to win, that it's better to plan to win than to plan to fail and then succeed at that.

Copeland was surely speaking to us when he said, "You must never let a problem become the biggest thing in your life. If you dwell only on The Problem, then all you're doing is moving on toward more disaster and further away from what God has already provided for you. Refuse to speak any words contrary to your victory. Answer every doubt out loud with the Word of God. 'He *is* my fortress! He *is* my refuge! And in Him I trust!'"

The big difference here was in recognizing evil as an active force that had to be defeated, and in doing so with something more than constructive thoughts. "Stand up to whatever it is that's trying to destroy you, the same way that shepherd boy stood up to Goliath," he commanded. "David said, 'This day will the Lord deliver thee into mine hands.' He's calling things that be not as though they are. He said *This day* it'll come to pass—Aw, now, David, you're just a *young boy*! Let's use some *wisdom* about this, Sonny-boy. It might not happen *today*. Maybe you should say, '*One day*, if it's God's will—.'" Kenneth Copeland loved to parody conventional wisdom with these little asides, which he delivered in a comical whining voice.

"But David said, '*I'm not only going to take YOU, Shorty, I'm going to take the whole Philistine army, and feed 'em to the fowls of the air and the beasts of the field.*' Where's that little whippersnapper come off talking that way? He's talking according to his covenant. And I'll tell you the Bible says God called him a man after His own heart. When you're standing up there and telling the devil where to get off, when you're saying, 'In the Name of Jesus, by His stripes I am healed, I'm well and I'm whole. I'm going to be a witness unto His glory, and I'm going to walk in power!' God's not going to put you down for that! He's going to help you just like He did David. He's saying right now, 'I put the armor on you. I paid the price for the power that's in the Name. I told you to take my Name and lay hands on the sick and they'd recover. I told you whatever you bind is bound and whatever you loose is loosed. Now bind and loose, and have some fun at it, because I'm with you. I'll never leave you nor forsake you.' Hallelujah!"

26. THE EVIDENCE OF THINGS NOT SEEN

Our new focus on help from Above cost me the friendship of a fellow I'd known many years. He sneered, not exactly at Christianity, but rather at our reliance on promises from sketchy sources. In countless late-night college discussions, he and I had agreed that even though one might pursue science or medicine or *any* discipline and in the end know only one's own limitations—nevertheless, the greater tragedy would be to hand over the power of decision and pin one's hopes on someone else for the illusion of settling doubts and satisfying mere needs.

That shared belief had formed the basis of our ongoing connection over the years and miles. Now suddenly my old friend would have nothing to do with me. I told myself that for him the question was still theory. On the other hand, as Shakespeare put it, "There was never yet philosopher that could endure the toothache patiently." Life had handed us a challenge for which no conventional response was available. The alternative response I'd selected, and into which we had poured so much of ourselves, had not been a complete solution. No other alternative looked as good, either on its own terms or in view of our remaining capabilities. The Institutes had primarily been *my* choice. Judy had gamely followed. She was in the driver's seat now, and I saw no reason to doubt her chosen course.

On November 2, 1990, Kenneth Hagin, one of the grand old men of the full-gospel movement, came to speak before an immense crowd in Los Angeles. Such events had never held the slightest attraction for me before. If I encountered one when spinning the TV dial, I kept right on going. However, being there, awash in the energy of thousands of believers, was a different matter.

We listened to a very ordinary-looking man with a rustic country-preacher's delivery tell stories of miraculous healings he'd witnessed during a career in the ministry that spanned more than half a century. He strolled among the first few rows of his expectant audience while he spoke. Wheelchairs crowded the aisles. A few very sick people lay motionless on stretchers. Here and there in the crowd I saw anxious-looking parents holding children who had floppy limbs and vacant expressions.

Of course, Hagin didn't claim to heal people himself. But sometimes, unexpectedly, an anointing came upon him, and spectacular things happened when it did. Now, these supernatural interventions were the exception. God performed them for reasons of His own. But even without them, Hagin went on, listening to the Word of God was medicine enough. *Informed* believers did not need miracles! They already knew what belonged to them and how to claim it. The Word was so powerful that no evil thing could withstand it, unless reinforced with our own fears. "*Terminal cancer!*" he snorted derisively. "*Ha!*" He emitted peals of raucous laughter to show what such threats were really worth. Whenever he cited a piece of scripture, a gentle, airy rustling filled the auditorium, like the sighing of wind among leaves in a forest: the sound of fingers scrambling through the tissue-thin pages of innumerable Bibles. Matthew 21:22. Romans 4:20–21. Isaiah 53:4–5.

We took Joseph through a healing line. Hands were laid upon him. And that night, after months of pressure from Judy to do so, I took the step of becoming born again. "God has not given us the spirit of fear," the crowd sang jubilantly, in a driving, strangely compelling amalgam of scriptural affirmations that resonated within me for a long time thereafter. "He has given unto us a spirit of power, a spirit of love, and a sound mind."

Outwardly, the weeks that followed were no different, although I felt considerably happier. We took comfort in believing that the healing anointing *had* been administered to Joseph. An instantaneous change in him would have suited us, but when that did not occur we said new things had been set in motion. Supernatural help might yet come via apparently natural means. Our trust was now in divine intervention, but we saw no reason to shy away from new avenues that suggested themselves.

So when we read about a woman offering treatments using an electronic "digital audio-visual integration device," which reportedly had improved the communication skills of autistic children, we called her. Joseph enjoyed the sessions, but instead of evolving into words, his random vocalizing just became louder.

Likewise, there was a new diet of "regenerative" herbal foods, said to be derived from ancient Chinese formulas. We had no doubt that these foods promoted health. Joseph's hair became glossier. Performance-wise, however, he made no progress.

There were about thirty-five sessions with an elderly Chinese acupuncturist. We felt that we couldn't neglect this possibility, because Ming and Kai had seen amazing results with their son Christopher after trying it. The kid had recovered the ability to walk and run, which he'd lost after his injury, and could now talk as well! Aside from minor problems with his vision, he seemed perfect. They hadn't even patterned him! Another huge regret: We should have seized the opportunity when they invited us over to share their acupuncturist. Now that guy had gone back to China. Christopher's parents didn't necessarily credit acupuncture for his turnaround, but since they'd done nothing else it was the only explanation. However, the local acupuncturist we used did not produce any changes.

We tried various new techniques that, we later learned, were part of a protocol called "sensory integration therapy." The promise here was that Joseph's use of language would be enhanced—and certain bizarre, self-stimulatory movements that he was making more and more frequently with his arms would diminish—in response to activities that challenged his vision and sense of balance, such as standing barefoot on a wooden swing and riding prone on a scooterboard.

At the end of 1991, we actually journeyed to Taiwan to learn about this latter approach. By then, Ming and Kai had returned to her hometown on the southern end of that island and, having formed a very close attachment to us, insisted that we visit them there. They wanted us to have a vacation (and a vacation was all we expected from the trip). But they also believed Taiwanese therapists and educators had more to offer than those in the U.S.

By this point, we'd grown accustomed to taking extraordinary steps that would have violated any rational person's budget. Still, traveling across the ocean to that very exotic place turned into one of our greatest adventures. I can't say that sensory integration accomplished more for Joseph than any of the other measures we were attempting. However, the exposure to Taiwan became a watershed event in my own life. Perhaps what impressed me most was the universal acceptance of Joseph—no, the outright admiration for him—that we encountered there every day. Granted, the people were reacting to the novelty of his blonde hair and blue eyes, and even if that were all they saw, I would have loved them for it. But it was more than that. Uncritical acceptance of children is one of many aspects of Chinese culture that I learned to appreciate. When we returned home, I belatedly began trying to learn their language. Just why, or how I might use it, I did not then know.

Still the campaign went on. When nothing else looked good, we led Joseph on a few more timed walks around the track—and even resorted to some old-fashioned masking, although we no longer worried about respiration.

We tried all this, and more, telling ourselves that each new treatment might yet be the solution we'd been seeking. Anecdotal reports indicated that each had indeed been the solution for someone. But for Joseph, *nothing worked!* At least, we had the meager satisfaction of establishing that first-hand. I always felt grateful for our freedom to explore all these avenues. I found it hard to believe that they consistently led nowhere.

It's easy to dismiss such measures as desperation. It's easy to be "realistic" and say there are no magic bullets for solving complex problems. Doing so would have saved us considerable effort, but each time a new idea came before us, we couldn't escape the thought that perhaps we had been led to this point. If that were true, if the new venture were the one to clinch that long-sought breakthrough, then neglecting to give it a chance would be the worst of tragedies.

Prayer, home study, and many more huge believers' conventions provided our only defense against an undercurrent of frustration that still threatened our future. No local church adequately reinforced the message we wanted to understand, so every time Hagin or the Copelands or any of their associates appeared in Southern California, we were present. At their gatherings, we heard gentle disapproval of the weak faith displayed by mainstream churches—not unlike Glenn Doman's dismissal of mainstream medicine. I noted the similarity and acknowledged that we'd transitioned from one set of mavericks to another. Still, all we were doing was taking God at His Word. Isaiah 55:10 promises, "My Word shall not return to me void." By confessing it, we were returning it. We were making our move. And as if the process were some metaphysical game of checkers, God's move was supposed to come next.

Judy and I sought to absorb the lessons on an emotional level, reminding ourselves daily that we had to eliminate strife and resentment from our lives if we wanted blessing. We couldn't find fault with each other, or blame the people who thought our cause was misguided. We absolutely had to be careful of the words we used, particularly avoiding expressions of discouragement, because we weren't just hoping for Joseph to be healed *someday*. We needed to affirm, along with 1 Peter 2:24, that he *WAS* healed! In order to see it, we had to believe it, utterly. Out of the abundance of the heart the mouth speaks, and our words would mean little if our hearts weren't right.

Was this indeed all we needed? If so, were we wrong to want some kind of outward manifestation?

Much has been written about the human tendency to be drawn to charismatic personalities. I think the attraction increases with the degree to which people feel a loss of control over their situations. The scriptural promises provided the basis of our hope, and gave it legitimacy, but it was the man standing on the dais, in the middle of the convention center, who gave it shape. Otherwise, we could have simply stayed home and read our Bible. In our case, however, the need was too acute to slip over into revering the messenger, as I suppose some did. The ultimate point of all this, for us, was not to feel mere encouragement, but to see results. It was to come away with something that changed our lives in a fundamental way.

Brother Hagin and Brother Copeland could pack a coliseum, but without that change, the exercise was pointless.

So I buttonholed Kenneth Hagin one morning, as he descended from the speaker's platform, to ask *what else* I needed to do. I began to elaborate on our situation, but he cut me off. "Praise God," he said, and turned away.

This pat answer hurt my feelings. But I decided he was right. The Bible says God inhabits our praises. So that night, sprawled backward across my bed, I prayed, "Lord, I do want to praise you and give you the glory—. *But I want my boy healed, too!*"

"Yes."

I thought about that, mildly surprised. Somebody other than me had just said, "Yes"! OK, it wasn't necessarily audible, but I heard it plainly enough. I heard a voice that was gentle and yet strong, fatherly, freighted with authority.

Hagin had spoken of direct communication from God. He said

that once God had even begun by directing him to get paper and pencil in order to take notes. If that kind of situation were the next step, I was ready and willing. Yes.

Yes, what? Excuse me, but yes what?

THE LATEST NEWS from Chicago was that Bobby had broken a leg—not for any clear reason, other than the fact that he was still immobile and his bones had become porous and brittle. Cindy had therefore canceled an appointment in Philly, getting in return a surprisingly caustic letter from their advocate. She wasn't quite certain yet, but it appeared that their many years on program were finally ending.

Annette and Bob knew for sure. They had returned with Jimmy for a scheduled Revisit, only to learn on arrival that they'd been terminated for sending inadequate monthly reports. "You can stick around for the lectures, or you can leave now," they were told indifferently. "But we aren't assigning you a new program." This blow was delivered, apparently without warning, after they'd mounted a major fund-raising effort just to get there. They returned home reeling with disappointment, outrage, and self-recrimination. And now they were talking divorce.

Judy and I couldn't regret our years with the Institutes. With their help we'd learned to keep an expectant attitude and had cleared some big hurdles. Families with newly brain-injured children still approached us for advice sometimes, and we still told them about the Philadelphia option. At last we handed on Lucas's old patterning board, which showed little wear after many thousands of hours of use.

We liked the mother who took it. No question, her baby's choking accident just a few weeks earlier had turned the family upside-down, but she was resolved not to be a victim of circumstances. She said, "People try to say that it's so terrible, that I'll be looking after Mary for the rest of my life. I don't need to hear that. My girl is getting better every day." Judy and I talked to her about the nuts and bolts of providing neurological stimulation and opportunity, and also shared our evolving beliefs that, we felt, complemented the practical side.

AT AGE SEVEN, Joseph had become a good-natured, cooperative, and healthy kid. It was hard to imagine that he had once cried almost incessantly, or that he'd complained so bitterly about doing the program. A speech therapist from the school system came to visit and praised his ability to follow complex directions. "He has excellent behavior, considering how frustrated he must be with his communication disability," she noted. Several of her colleagues passed through our house. They all expressed admiration for Joseph's library of Bits and homemade books, while voicing the usual reservations. They especially weren't convinced that he could read. To get credit for that, he'd have to read aloud. Just asking him to make selections did *not* constitute an adequate test, they said. One protested, "A child who couldn't read might still recognize the letter *D* and then be able to guess which word was 'duck,' for example."

"Well, then," Judy said, "We could show him two words that both start with *D* — 'duck' and 'dog,' say. If you want to test his comprehension you could even ask him which animal flies. Let's try that."

"No. No. No." The other smiled patiently and chuckled. "That's not reading. That's science."

It was not the introduction to school that we'd planned, but we weren't prepared for any other. We had never established the kind of sustained attention to the task at hand that educators call "instructional control." We knew our claims about his intellectual prowess sounded hollow.

As far as the school system was concerned, parents did not have the last word on what their kids needed. Some educators expressed this point more tactfully than others, but we got the message loud and clear. If Joseph was going to school—and the time for that *had* come.

He was bored at home, and Judy was increasingly plagued by back pain, and after all our trust, ultimately, was in God—then the school expected free reign. Everyone agreed that he'd fit in quite well, in a special education classroom, that is. And that's where Joseph landed, along with a varied collection of nonverbal, multiply-handicapped kids, kids who'd never had the benefit of any program. They ranged in size from one who looked like a two-year-old to some almost as big as the teacher. Many were in wheelchairs. Because Joseph required less maintenance than the others, he received less attention.

Nevertheless, the school seemed a good interim move, for he picked up skills there that Judy and I had never managed to impart. "He has started pointing with his index finger and using the communication board!" His teacher reported one day. The communication board was an array of small pictures that kids could touch to indicate their needs. Since he'd always been agonizingly slow and inconsistent in making choices, this sounded like an important step forward. Soon he was readily selecting menu items, both at school and at home—pressing the illustrations firmly and deliberately, as if they were buttons on a vending machine. In spite of our misgivings, he seemed pleased with the idea of going to school.

He looked less pleased—in fact, he looked panic-stricken—about his mom. The back pain and the limp she'd lived with for several months were still evident and in fact rapidly growing much worse. A wretched family doctor had suggested that this might be "tendonitis" (or even intestinal gas!) and had let matters rest with that. Two osteopaths and then a chiropractor had failed to provide more than temporary relief. (The chiropractor asked her to please stop screaming during treatments. She was scaring off his other patients.) Now she bought a walker, because suddenly she could no longer get around unaided. That's when I finally insisted that she see someone else.

A friend at my office suggested an orthopedic surgeon. The orthopedist ordered a bone scan. On November 3, 1992, he announced that Judy had tumors scattered throughout the bones of her body. I wasn't with her at the time, but my coworker, who was a personal friend of the doctor's, told me what happened next:

"This doesn't sound like a very good report," Judy had mused.

"Do you want me to call anybody for you?" the doctor asked solicitously.

"No, thank you. I'll handle this."

"So—? You're just going to get into your car and go home?" He apparently worried that she wasn't showing more of a reaction. But neither Judy nor I, when she told me that evening, felt inclined to panic. Perhaps we'd just grown accustomed to bad news, and our capacity for emotional extremes had been seared away. What we said was that God still had an answer. We meant to receive it, in whatever form it might take. And so Judy grew thoughtful but not alarmed. In terms of bedside manner, this particular doctor was really fine. She liked him more than anyone in his profession she'd encountered in years. It seemed a pity that he had to send her on to another specialist.

Joseph's case moved very quickly to the back burner while Judy and I adjusted to her increasing helplessness. We wondered how this added affliction could have come our way. *We should not have been open to it!* Judy in particular had long been a lay authority on matters of diet and health. For years she'd been steering all of us away from fast food and chemical additives. She'd tried to enforce positive talk in the household. In fact, we could think of *nothing* in our family experience that could have led to this.

Except unending stress.

The oncologist speculated that her cancer had begun growing at a time corresponding with our later days at the Institutes, when discouragement had peaked and Judy in particular had felt there was no script for the future. He wasn't sure the events in our lives were the cause. But anyway, the real issue now was treatment. Not that there was a cure. He said there wasn't.

She faced a long, uphill battle—tougher than it might have been, he said, because while the average patient beginning treatment had "millions" of cancer cells, she now had "billions." Incidentally, he wondered mildly, why had she waited so long before coming in?

This was a humbling experience for Judy, to be putting her life in the hands of MDs after having lost respect for them over the years. Humbling, too, to realize how misguided her choices had been. "I sure was foolish about this," she said tearfully. The cancer had begun as a lump in her breast. She'd told herself it had to be a cyst, because a tumor was unthinkable, and had reflexively claimed wellness for herself as well as for Joseph. Having settled that in her mind, she didn't draw a connection as she gradually, progressively lost function and almost unthinkingly accommodated herself to that—finding one month that she couldn't lie on her side without pain, somewhat later discovering that it was no longer possible to pick up a dropped item from the floor, and then reaching the point at which her right hand couldn't even twist a car key in the ignition.

To their credit, the people in this branch of medicine, at least, had a protocol. Better still, they knew how to act decisively. Within weeks, her deterioration stopped and began to reverse itself.

If mental outlook did have anything to do with triggering the disease, it might affect the recovery as well. This was certainly no time for feeling like a failure. It was no time for guilt, but rather for taking authority over the situation. She complemented the chemotherapy with the spiritual device of talking to her body every day, commanding the bones to be normal, in Jesus' Name, forbidding growths and tumors to inhabit her body, and so forth. Such language no longer felt natural in my own mouth, but when the chemotherapy made her feel sick, I offered the encouragement that those lousy cancer cells probably felt worse.

I did not tell her that I was also now reading up on cancer and the mechanism by which tumor cells "cascaded," via the bloodstream, from the original site to take up residence in other parts of the body. The bones were a very common secondary site, I discovered. The brain often came next. Chances of survival after metastasis occurred were drastically lowered.

But of course, understanding what we did, we knew Judy would be in the minority that recovered.

By the end of January 1993 she was mostly out of pain and walking short distances on her own again. The pace of recovery actually surprised her doctor, who asked if I thought she might be "denying her symptoms." He'd warned that cancer patients who lose the ability to walk often don't regain it. She *had* actually lost it for a few weeks, had gone to appointments in a wheelchair—had been more than half-dead: unable to sleep comfortably at night and only semi-consciousness for long hours in the day.

In June she was still weak but confidently promising to be his "star patient." She said, "I want you to be able to brag on me to the other doctors."

"I'm doing that already," he replied agreeably.

"I feel pretty good now," she observed to me. "And that sure makes a difference, let me tell you! In times past, when I noticed that I felt good, or happy, I let it go on for only a little while, because there was so much to do. *Now* I want to get *everything* out of it. I want to savor it with every fiber of my being!"

She laughed and spoke of an old friend back in Virginia, a fellow who had prided himself on being a wine connoisseur. "Remember the time Chip sat in our living room, chattering away while he slurped his wine? And then when he stood up to go he noticed the bottle and said, '*Mumm's!* Why didn't you tell me we were drinking Mumm's, so I could've enjoyed it!' I think life must be like that—more wonderful than we know."

She found herself starting animated conversations on any subject with strangers in line at the grocery store and on elevators, and even going so far as to exchange phone numbers now and then. At home she indulged in multiple viewings of the musical *South Pacific*, which prompted affectionate memories of her father.

She had given herself permission to stop worrying about Joseph, or at least to stop fighting the battle, heart and soul. His unmet needs did remain always before us, it is true, remained a source of recurring grief. But life was nevertheless "interesting," as she put it, regardless of setbacks and injustices.

Even if our fight to help Joseph over the last eight years had led to this, neither of us could bring ourselves to regret the effort. Given that unconventional therapies do help some disabled kids, and given that those therapies are the only course of action offering any hope, the justification for our choices still seemed obvious. We'd seen enough to know that the answer for one kid may be unrelated to what works for another, that very seldom is any answer complete, and that there's no escape from guesswork. The only feature the various success stories shared was a willingness of each family to reject experts who would not help. Where we'd gone wrong, I decided, was in attaching too much negative emotion to that. Instead of letting our energy take the form of stress, and rage at our many obstacles, we should have spent it—and still ought to spend it—in mutual support for each other and demonstrable affection for Joseph. We hadn't given ourselves enough credit for being such a dynamic team; we'd always been in danger of overlooking Joseph's beautiful disposition.

"The kid doesn't have one mean bone in his body," Judy said. "He's really something special that way."

At times now he received no attention from us, and unproductive habits emerged to fill the void. He waggled his fingers, played endlessly with shoelaces. He took delight in pressing his elbows against hard surfaces for the tactile feedback. I knew we were seeing hallmarks of autistic behavior. Dr. Frymann had always insisted that he related with other people too well to fit the stereotype of autism. Nevertheless, when I completed a questionnaire provided by San Diego's well-known Autism Research Institute, his score was on the spectrum. When I took him to a neurologist, he did get that diagnosis. So here we were, belatedly confronting the issue that had been raised long,

long ago by that well-meaning, discredited physical therapist.

But now a profound weariness was taking root. One night I told Judy, "There's this basic assumption, formed while I was growing up, that the passage of time brings, not just change, but *improvement*. As we got older we learned how to do new things. We got promoted to higher grade levels in school. When we were adults, we graduated from living in dinky apartments and driving jalopies, to owning our own place and buying nice cars. And the *world* was improving, too, with break-throughs in science and technology. Yeah, and sometimes there were setbacks—. But the long-term trend was *up*! And especially, with effort you got improvement."

We talked, once again, about the fact that, despite our best efforts to help him, Joseph now spoke and interacted with others less than ever, and was making vocalizations that seemed at times to be beyond his control. We couldn't ignore the fact that, despite tackling her cancer with every known remedy, spiritual as well as medical, nutritional— you name it, Judy still led a very circumscribed life and was again growing weaker. These were not improvements.

She said, "If you believe in God, you also assume that there's some meaning or purpose to it all."

"Well, you have to believe in a God of some description," I returned. "There's no other explanation for the world. I *refuse* to believe that things happen randomly." I paused. "That's why I've always insisted that that there was some cause for Joseph being hurt."

"God didn't cause Joseph to be hurt," Judy pointed out.

"No, I'm not saying that. I'm just saying it's one thing to believe, and an entirely different thing to claim you understand anything at all about that subject. A lot of people who do are lying." I could feel the rage returning. Understanding the danger of one's emo-tions and controlling them were two different matters. "*A lot* of people have sold us bills of goods. These characters who stand up in front of crowds and pretend to have something to say. I should have known better. I *did* know better. We've been vulnerable to them because the people who *should've* helped us didn't."

"If the doctors knew what to do for Joseph, they'd have done it."

"They could've shown a little more interest in trying," I insisted bitterly.

She smiled at me sadly. "I hope you'll marry again after I'm gone," she said. "Move out of this place. Make a new start."

I coughed and cast about for an acceptable answer. "How about we make plans for moving out of this place together?"

She gestured helplessly. "Steve, I wish you'd acknowledge what's happening. It makes it harder for me when you don't."

"But," I said forcefully. "You were getting better. Remember? And I am tired. Of failure. I know you are, too."

"I understand what you mean," she said. "But maybe this isn't failure. I know I'm going to a good place." She paused for a long moment and added thoughtfully, "I promise you *this*: If it's possible for me to do anything on Joseph's behalf when I get there, I will."

I'D DONE ALL I KNEW TO DO for Joseph. Then I'd handed his case to God. And now, in fairly short order, I found myself turning Judy over to Him as well. "I've asked You to heal my son," I prayed. "And now I'm asking You to heal my wife, too. I see clear scriptural basis for asking this. But if I haven't been asking as I should, please show me the right way to ask. If there's something I need to do from this end, please show me what it is and I'll do it. No matter how this is accomplished, the glory for it is all Yours."

As far as I could tell, these pleas met with utter silence.

And that silence continued as Judy's decline steepened. The cancer did spread into her brain, where the doctor said there were now in-numerable "BB-sized mets." We didn't ask to see the films. We never asked for percentages, either, or for projections of how much time she had left.

Then it was in her left eye—an ugly brown shape that started small, and grew. There was one point when we were looking at each other and I gasped involuntarily when I saw how it had completely obscured that lovely blue iris. She nodded grimly, saying nothing. She knew. Her other most attractive physical attribute, her hair, had of course long since been lost to repeated chemotherapy.

Finally, the chemo was discontinued. I drove her to the clinic, with an amusing videotape she could watch while the needle was in her arm, but the results of a preliminary blood test told the doctor that there was no point in proceeding. He seemed rattled when telling us this, perhaps because we didn't respond. I suppose we were habitually numb by that point. He touched the videotape. "*Amos and Andrew!*" He smiled desperately. "A great movie! Go home and watch it. What a hoot!" We nodded and left, and at home Judy just slept.

Sometimes she tried to talk with me about the event that was looming. I didn't refuse to listen, but I never encouraged that line of discussion. Admitting defeat ran counter to everything. Someone might be trying to deliver this "package" to our door, but I didn't intend to sign the receipt for it. So I preferred to talk about daily trivia, about Joseph, and then about the parade of home-hospice nurses coming through our doorway every day. One of them said she had a disabled child, too. I did not willingly talk about what was really happening.

And then something began coming between us. Judy was perceiving things quite differently. One day she informed me with great joy that Joseph had been miraculously healed of his disability. She had already been on the phone sharing the tidings with our old volunteers. She'd even called the TV station. Since Joseph had made the evening news during his home program, she thought they'd want some new footage of what he looked like well. She couldn't understand my reluctance to celebrate or the muted responses of everyone else.

"You understand, don't you, that she's dying?" This was the hospice nurse, handing things off to me when I came from work one Tuesday afternoon.

"Um. But I don't know how close she is."

"She's *close.*" She looked across the room at Judy and called out a goodbye. "I'll see you on Friday, dear," she said. But she said it half-heartedly. She didn't expect to be needed by Friday.

Judy took no notice of the nurse's departure. She lay comfortably in the hospital bed that had been set up in our living room, since the second-floor bedrooms had been inaccessible to her for several months. The catheter bag was tied to the rail on one side, and on the other side a morphine pump made periodic little peeps as it delivered its regular doses. Joseph was upstairs.

For lack of anything better to do, I brought the mail in to her: a church bulletin and a catalog. She placed her palm on the catalog. "Eddie Bauer," she murmured fondly. In recent months, mail-order shopping had become a diversion. She'd been buying things to give people as gestures of affection. She closed her eyes.

"Would you like something to eat?" I asked.

"Something small, maybe."

I cast about cluelessly for something small. "How about some nuts?"

She accepted a pecan and began chewing it methodically. Five minutes later she was still chewing the same nut, and beginning to look tired.

"Barbara's coming tonight," I reminded her. "The plane lands at eleven."

Judy considered her big sister's arrival, or perhaps the hours remaining before then, with an expression of vague anxiety, then closed her eyes again.

I had to prepare for our guest. The bed needed fresh sheets. The towels in the bathroom needed to be changed. I started some laundry. I fed Joseph, who seemed to be staying as far away from that bed in the living room as possible. I got him ready for sleep.

"Hey! Only three more hours until Barbara gets here," I said encouragingly. Judy was paying no attention, although she opened her eyes with a bewildered expression as I hurried past with an armload of bed sheets warm from the dryer.

Then I noticed that the catheter bag was still almost empty. By now, it should have been almost full. And Judy's breathing was becoming more audible. Audible? I could hear it plainly in the next room when I called the nighttime hospice nurse.

"If she is not producing urine," the nurse said, "it means her kidneys are shutting down." She was trying to speak gently, and choosing her words carefully. "This means she's entering into the last part of her life."

"Is there anything I can do? What about her breathing? It's getting really loud!"

"I'm sure you're doing everything you should. This is all perfectly natural."

Judy took no further notice of me, other than to mumble, "I love you," every time I said it to her. I gave a running countdown of the time remaining before Barbara's arrival. I told her when the plane was probably touching down, said that Lynn was probably meeting her in the airport by now, driving her to our house.

Then Barbara was with us. "She's here, Judy!" I announced loudly. We sat on opposite sides of the bed. By now the agonal breathing had subsided. Judy was very quiet. Barbara tried speaking to her, but when there was no response she spoke to me. Inevitably, within minutes we were exchanging family news.

Then something felt different. I looked at Judy. She was still. I listened for her heartbeat, felt for her pulse. Wide-eyed, Barbara and I looked at each other.

I noted the time on the wall clock. I turned off the morphine pump. Judy had held on as long as possible. Now, having heard Barbara's voice one last time, she was done.

Finally I said, "I guess it's fitting that we're both here. Between the two of us, we've been with her practically her whole life. You saw her first twenty years and I've had the last twenty."

Epilogue I

I continue to believe in powers, both spiritual and professional, that can aid and guide us through our challenges. Wonderful results *can* be achieved when we find the right mix of reliance on external support and our own innate strength and wisdom.

There have been times when things I wanted very much fell right into my lap, with no effort at all, or with just enough to make the pursuit and achievement all the more enjoyable.

I don't understand why other goals can be so resistant.

Judy died of unhappiness, I feel sure. She had done absolutely everything in her power to bring about change, exhausting and weakening herself in the process so that she couldn't withstand the disappointment when reality took another course.

I am aware that our story could be used to reinforce the position of those who said that our cause, from the very beginning, was foolish. It also shows the risk people run in succumbing to the attraction of charismatic personalities. But at the same time, our story points to the conclusion that we, as a society, must find better answers for developmental disability. And we need to begin doing that soon. As I write this, one of our favorite patterners has become the mother of a baby with poorly understood problems. She feels cheated. In a moral universe, the natural logic would be that the energy she invested in Joseph should have exempted her child from this fate. She still doesn't realize how common it is in a country that congratulates itself on medical breakthroughs. She is indignant to find the medical establishment deflecting her requests for help. She and her husband are rushing from one appointment to the next in a desperate search for any approved therapy. Clearly, they do *not* want to start down the same road they saw us travel. The road they prefer, however, leads nowhere without a medically approved and insurance-certified "qualifying diagnosis." If then.

I believe our story shows that interventions can help disabled kids. The problem is that it's very hard for an unguided family to know in advance which interventions hold promise in their child's particular case. I didn't presume to tell our old friend what to do—only how to cope. "You must have a plan," I said. "Even a bad plan is better than no plan, because at least you'll feel like you're accomplishing something. And that'll keep you going for a while."

I owed her far more perspective than that, but had nothing else at the moment. The Institutes in Philadelphia certainly helped Joseph in a measurable way. That positive reinforcement created the expectation that *another* alternative treatment would help him further. But now I feel like a laboratory animal in a Skinner box. Something's got to help! In the quest for it, my behavior becomes almost random. I cannot give up this optimism for my Joseph.

Nor, at this point, can I fault anyone who's suspicious of alternative paths.

Throughout this experience, I felt grateful that at least we had the freedom to follow our own judgment—and to choose whom we would believe. I still am not sorry that we did so. Knowing what I know now, I would act somewhat differently today; and quite possibly a different attack would have achieved better results. But everybody could say that. As my father observed during his illness, current actions must be based on current understanding, however limited it may be.

MEANWHILE, what about Joseph?

At first, he had no discernable reaction to his mother's disappearance. I tried to explain what had happened, but he gave no indication of understanding. A month later I took him East to spend Christmas with my mother and younger sister Angela, and on the flight back home I noticed that he appeared much more animated and cheerful than usual. Then we arrived, to a dark house, and he seemed crestfallen.

I didn't realize it right away, but surely he'd thought that she would be waiting for us.

The news finally sank in a few nights later when we were at a restaurant with my older sister Lynn and her husband. Something one of us said in conversation must have made the connection for him. He looked at the three adults sitting in the booth with him, registered that his mother was not among us, and understood that she would never be with us again. He began screaming.

All this is obvious now, but at the time it still escaped me. Nevertheless, in my muddled way, the next morning I did the right thing. I took him to Disneyland. Just inside the front gate, a park employee dressed up in a fuzzy Br'er Fox suit jumped out and greeted Joseph like an old pal. In the photo I snapped, Joseph has one of the sweetest smiles I've ever seen on him, and since then he seems to have accepted the turn life has taken.

He's going to school as before. He has a comfortable routine.

I don't believe he likes the food I cook. One evening when I placed a chicken pot pie in front of him, he started crying again. So I don't think he's really happy. Gotta work on that. The happiness and the food.

January 1995

San Diego

Epilogue II

One very good reason for solving problems with dispatch is that additional problems inevitably come along. If current issues aren't helped off the stage, the place becomes pretty crowded.

By the time I lost Judy in 1994, the post-Cold War recession had essentially wiped out San Diego's aerospace-related industries. The job I'd held for over ten years was unquestionably about to end. My colleagues were making new plans, striking out in new directions, but I felt stumped. I'd given little thought to professional development and knew almost nothing about the job market. So I began 1995 with new and rather urgent objectives.

This time, I was just lucky. When General Dynamics closed its plant, I moved to another, far more stimulating position without missing a day of work. Now, instead of writing about launch vehicles and communication satellites, I found myself working to promote global acceptance of a new cell-phone technology.

The irony of enabling such wonderful new modes of communication, when even basic exchanges with my own son remained problematic, did not escape me.

Joseph was spending his days in a nonpublic special school where Judy and I had moved him after his disappointing placement for first grade. The staff here called him "Jo-Jo," a clownish name Judy would have hated. I didn't mind, because it was used with affection. Perhaps this new school would help. I knew of no better option, but hoped in due course that one would suggest itself. At the end of each day, I drove across town to pick him up. Sometimes, when my day's work was not yet finished, I returned with him to the office. One night he agreeably slept on the floor of a conference room, while I pulled an all-nighter along with my boss and several others.

So much change and so much busy-ness meant I had little time to absorb what had happened. People who knew me assumed that I was in mourning, and surely on some level I was. I recall a phase during which I often literally found myself standing in a room with no recollection of why I'd gone there. Also, I fretted irrationally about the fact that no doctor had ever confirmed Judy's death. I'd called a hospice nurse when she died. The nurse in turn had called the oncologist, and he'd filled out the death certificate. Everybody had taken my word for it.

This was stupid. I knew it. But still, *what if I'd been mistaken?*

But despite the aftershock (or perhaps because of it), I found little time to dwell on recent events. Suddenly, this new thing, the Internet, was beckoning. When I went online, I discovered a realm in which parents of disabled kids and a few involved researchers around the world were sharing what they knew and debating issues close to my heart. Online discussion boards continually introduced young families with newly diagnosed or undiagnosed kids, some of whom sounded startlingly similar to Joseph. These folks were beginning to duplicate my family's experiences. I hoped the information now available would lead them to better outcomes.

To that end, I became a conspicuous presence on several forums. When someone fretted that her child was several months behind schedule, developmentally—and said the pediatrician *still* advised only patience—I insisted that she needed a new doctor. When the child was further said to be vomiting frequently, and arching his back, and crying inconsolably, I offered specific leads. When someone else then stepped in to warn about quacks, I became testy.

Without a doubt, I had enriched alternative providers along the way who *never* expected to help my son. I acknowledged that sorry fact, but put it in context by adding, "Anxious parents who go around and around with their disabled kids in the revolving door of ordinary clinics may conclude that the people they're paying are no different."

I still thought very highly of Dr. Frymann, still believed in much that was espoused by the Institutes. But I knew neither resource had adequate answers for the enormous range of disabilities confronting them. Their philosophies were incomplete, their treatments little better than hit or miss.

I recalled my father's theory regarding the comic futility of endeavor. If there really were no reliable solutions, and if a wholehearted effort to find one could end badly, then—why bother with all the churning?

But then I considered Joseph, who was now cooperating with my efforts to teach him how to roller-skate, and recalled the fundamental gains he had achieved. Was even limited progress not worth the risk? Where would he be had we not demanded more than his doctors wanted to provide?

Recently, I read *Better: A Surgeon's Notes on Performance*, by Atul Gawande, MD. The book jolted me, because here, at last, was a physician saying precisely what I had always expected to hear from that profession. The hardest thing about the practice of medicine, he writes, is "to know what you have power over and what you don't." However, he adds, "Even when we don't know that a patient can be completely normal and healthy, we want doctors to fight. ... We want doctors to push and find a way." He concludes that "the most sensible rule for a doctor to follow is: Always Fight. Always look for what more you could do. I am sympathetic to this rule. It gives us our best chance of avoiding the worst error of all—giving up on someone we could have helped."

I think what Dr. Gawande describes is an ideal that has receded before the business realities of running a profitable practice. But if

WHAT ABOUT THE BOY?   361

a child's doctor doesn't follow this rule, and if the child's parents don't insist on it, what are the implications for the child? Can we call that *abandonment*? Is it all that different from what happens in the story in which Hansel and Gretel are intentionally deserted in the wilderness? What parent would be so heartless as to do that? For that matter, what self-respecting professional would choose to let a patient and his family wander off on a trackless search? We know of course that when the children in that folktale thought they'd found refuge, it turned out to be otherwise.

The online argument that distressed me most was one I encountered quite often. Many people maintained that a special child was a gift not to be tampered with. They promised that disability in your child could "transform your own life to profound awakenings." Every week, somebody posted an intellectually dishonest parable suggesting that having such a child was no worse than planning a vacation to Italy and arriving in Holland instead.

Granted, there are different degrees of disability. I'm sure the above analogy works for milder varieties. It had no bearing on my experience, however, and my reaction offended and angered people every time I saw the thing.

Eventually, having developed some new job-related skills, I created an informational website intended, in part, to address such notions. Here's an excerpt from it:

I realize that there are disabled people who lead active, productive lives and have unique ways of viewing reality that might even be an asset.

But most parents I've met who are looking for answers represent individuals who are incapable of saying anything coherent about any subject. These individuals would not be able even to live without a lot more than mere supervision. Some of them have to be protected from hurting themselves. Some of them have no concept of personal safety and would wander away with any stranger. Year after year goes by and they don't change. These children were born to parents who naturally hoped they would participate in the family and in the world. Any rational person would view their inability to do so as a serious malady.

Years ago, I declared war on my son's disability. Please understand that I did not declare war on my son. I love and accept him, and I admire his good qualities—his sweetness and gentleness and very subtle sense of humor. He is lovable; his affliction is not.

The media are full of "inspirational" stories of how modern medicine saves Siamese twins, children with deformed hearts, kids with rare genetic disorders. Such stories happen to rub me the wrong way because modern medicine has never done anything for my son, but the point is that these victories were possible because the world DID NOT just accept those kids as individuals. They were "forced" to be something they were not: i.e., healthy people. The result was that everybody benefited. When a disabled person recovers, he has a new life ahead of him, and the world has one less life-long dependent.

And finally, what right do we, as parents, have to assume that our children are here to teach us or indeed to do anything for us? It's far easier to defend the assumption that they need our help if they are even to survive in a world that, by and large, does not care a damn about what happens to them. Helping the next generation is our responsibility.

Oh yes, I had an axe to grind.

Joseph, of course, did not benefit from any of that venting. However, my primary use of the Internet was to carry on the search for a way to find help for him. Whenever I read about a researcher anywhere in the world doing work that might be related, I sent an email with a link back to Joseph's medical record, which was available on my website. This practice led to occasional online discussions. Questions were raised about his sulfur metabolism, his ability to break down long-chain fatty acids, and so forth. These inquiries prompted me to persuade bemused local pediatricians to order blood tests and other lab work, none of which led to new insights.

JOSEPH MEANWHILE was ten years old and marking time at his school. The staff provided limited speech therapy and so-called occupational therapy, and they listened politely every time I entreated them to step up the intensity or to introduce something with more promise, such as Applied Behavior Analysis. I'm sure they grew very tired of my assurances that here was a kid who had already accomplished a great deal, and who clearly had the potential to do much more. Over time, I perceived that he was continuing to lose ground. I recalled the classic science fiction story "Flowers for Algernon," which I'd read in high school, about a mentally disabled man named Charlie Gordon whose intelligence dramatically increased following experimental surgery, but then declined. Near the end, Charlie tells people, "I used to be smart," and they laugh in disbelief.

I hired special advocates who coached me on the language to use in presenting my requests to the school, but the other side proved quite adept at keeping control. For all my emotional involvement, I no longer had the capacity to take charge of providing daily therapy myself, so this time, if the professionals weren't going to help, there would be no help.

Aside from the need to earn a living, I found myself bone-tired. I also needed to establish more balance in my life.

INCREDIBLY, my personal life did begin to improve. My new job had put me in daily contact with friendly Chinese engineers who smiled indulgently on my stumbling attempts to use their language. Thus encouraged, and still inspired by that 1991 trip to Taiwan, I set forth on a solo vacation in mainland China. While there, I made a new friend. Our lives up to that point had been completely different, unless one wants to compare her frustrations during the Cultural Revolution with mine in the disability wars. She liked the fact that I'd seen hardship, said we had more in common because of it. The friendship deepened. Her mother suggested fate must have brought our paths together.

In 1996, before joining me in America, Song Yi insisted that I allow Joseph to stay with her at a clinic in Beijing, because she thought he could be helped via traditional Chinese medicine (primarily acupuncture). Amazed by her willingness to take on that responsibility, I pulled him out of school and left him with her there for six months, which indicates the degree of trust I had already placed in this stubborn young woman.

Halfway through his stay with her, I was roused from bed in the middle of the night by a phone call, which my answering machine captured:

Steve: Hello?

Song Yi: Hey! Somebody wants to talk to you.

Joseph: [Explosive exhalation in my ear] Ai!

Steve: Joe, are you doing ok?

Joseph: Yeah.

Steve: Do you miss me?

Joseph: Yeah? [His tone suggested that he found this a dumb question.]

Steve: Do you want to come back to San Diego?

Joseph: Yeah! [This time his tone of voice was indignant, challenging: What do you think, Dad? Of course I want to come home! I reflected that, if Joseph were significantly improved, my relationship with him might change. Imagine getting back-talk from my kid! It was almost scary.]

Song Yi: [Laughing] Can you hear him? He's smiling.

Steve: He was talking to me! This is great.

Song Yi: You should come back. You can see Joseph change every day. Every day.

Steve: [Awed] That's exciting.

Song Yi: Sure! Very interesting. [Laughing] Yeah. Everyday! If you come to China you will see. At first, when you go home to America, in treatment Joseph is afraid. And fighting me. He doesn't like acupuncture. But today was a holiday. We went shopping. Walking, walking, maybe three hours with me, take bus, no problem. He's very happy [Laughing] because no treatment today! I tell him to do something. He understands fine.

Steve: Do you talk to him in Chinese?

Song Yi: No! I want him to speak English. Also, Dr. Liu said you should make some tapes and send them. So he can hear more English.

Steve: That sounds like a good idea. I'll do it. But tell me, how are you?

Song Yi: [Laughing uncomfortably] So-so. I take care of Joseph. Just very busy.

Steve: You're tired, right?

Song Yi: Sure. [Pouting tone] Too bad.

Steve: Let me know if you want to stop.

Song Yi: Not now. Maybe June. And I have new—You know, China, so many people, the population? So many disabled children. So we have many, many hospitals to treat the disabled children, just like Joseph. I mailed you information about another one, in Guilin. You know Guilin? Very beautiful place. Many foreigners go there.

Steve: [Surprised] Well, I'm always interested in learning about treatments.

Song Yi: Joseph becomes more and more smart, but he's too old. Eleven years old! *Two years old* may be better for this.

Steve: Can't change his age.

Song Yi: This treatment is more slow because he's old. And it's very conservative. Just acupuncture, traditional medicine. Maybe he needs more. I want to promote his speaking ability. I talked to the doctor in Guilin. If you want to go there after this, I need to extend his visa and change his airplane ticket.

Steve: Yeah, well, Song Yi, I suggest that we do not plan on another therapy right now. I hesitate to rush straight from one treatment to another. I need to evaluate how Joseph has benefited from acupuncture. And also, I don't want *you* rushing from one thing to another, because it can be bad for you. I've seen this before. It's dangerous—for you—to put too much of yourself into this.

Song Yi: [Misunderstanding me] It's not a dangerous operation.

Steve: Maybe what they have in Guilin is a good thing. But if so that's something for the future, not now. Because I think you are already doing too much.

Song Yi: I just try my best, to find the best information!

Steve: I know you're trying your best! And I appreciate—.

Song Yi: OK! You decide. Also, my friend mentioned a hospital in America.

Steve: What? You mean for Joseph?

Song Yi: Yes. Best hospital in America [Pausing while she unfolded a paper to read it]: Institute for Human Potential.

Steve: Oh! In Philadelphia?

Song Yi: [Surprised] You already know about this place?

Steve: Sure! We went there. Joseph learned to walk because of what we did with the Institutes. Your friend is very smart, but we've already done that.

Song Yi: [Not wanting to give up] The address is Stenton Avenue? The phone number—.

Steve: I assure you, it's the same place. Thank you for the information, though.

There was no more sleep for me that night. First, I felt absolutely delighted to have had the short conversation with Joseph. Granted, he'd used only one word, but he had used it very appropriately. I knew he must have been in rare form indeed to inspire Song Yi to call me, because normally she waited for me to phone at a set time, once per week.

But this renewed search for new therapies suggested that the acupuncture was not fulfilling all our hopes.

WHEN I RETURNED to China, the boy I found was essentially unchanged. I guess he'd just been having a good day when she called me.

Song Yi has since acknowledged the reality that he is beyond the reach of any help available, and forgoing her earlier single-minded determination to solve the problem, accepted him as-is with admirable patience and equanimity. I continued pursuing answers, at a rate of about one new serious endeavor per year, and she accepted that as well.

At one point I found my way into a "Defeat Autism Now!" conference, where I spent two days in a huge room with many hundreds of other parents who scribbled notes while scientists took turns discussing arcane lines of inquiry. Autism had a genetic component, they agreed, but genes only conferred a susceptibility to the disorder; they didn't cause it. Environmental factors were the trigger, and there was much discussion as to what these might be. The evidence seemed to point to some immune disturbance, perhaps caused by yeast colonization of the digestive tract or misuse of vaccines. Or something else. Different speakers presented the case for exploring various possible remedies—using vitamin A to reverse a protein defect, using chelating agents to clear mercury from the body, eliminating dairy products and wheat.

I dutifully took notes, wondering all the while whether any of this had bearing on our own situation. Yes, Joseph now had a diagnosis of autism, but his problems had been apparent from the outset. If, for example, vaccines had hurt him, which I was prepared to believe, that injury would have been secondary to an already-serious condition that I still did not understand. I did grasp much of the material presented, but some of it went well over my head. Most was entirely too theoretical to take home and use. I wondered at the dedication of all those around me who continued to sit there, straining to understand. When one lecture concluded, the first parent with a question said (to appreciative laughter and applause), "Dr. Gupta, I'm flattered that you would go through all that for us. I just wish I could *get it*. I want to take what I learn here back to my doctor, but I don't know how to speak this language!"

I wanted to know why the lady—why *anyone* who didn't speak this language—found it necessary to be here taking notes for her doctor.

So guided, I continued to chase leads. Among the multitude of online parents who had no answers, I found a few who could not say enough good things about one intervention or another: injections of fetal cells, hyperbaric oxygen therapy, and off-label use of a hormone called secretin. I think I gave each of these a fair trial.

I *hope* each trial was fair.

None were easy, or cheap.

None worked.

The problem, of course, outrageous though it sounds, is that I still did not truly understand his problem. And without an understanding, I could not target it with anything specific. I continued taking him to doctors, and again heard what Dr. Frymann had always maintained. This young man is *not* autistic, they assured me. He may display certain behaviors that go with that condition. And for the purpose of getting services it may be convenient to say he's on the spectrum. But he represents something else.

Joseph was now eighteen. He had stopped growing at five feet, because his legs never lengthened in proportion to the rest of his body. Other traits had become more obvious. His fingers are unusually short, and the fifth fingers have a slight inward curve. The pads of his fingertips are "elevated." These, I now learned, are clues indicating that some unknown genetic error occurred early in his development. Quite likely the heart murmur is part of the same picture. In any event, that picture had no name. "He has something, but we don't know what," was the best diagnosis offered by San Diego's leading geneticist. No diagnosis. No treatment.

If I knew how this unnamed condition hurt him—for example, if I knew that it suppressed some neurotransmitter—then conceivably there might be rationale for a medication. No one shares my interest in exploring that. Oh, I'm sure I could find someone willing to prescribe a drug, but at this point I want more than the typical indifference.

As he enters adulthood, I find Joseph to be a good companion, rather like a quiet fishing buddy. We take comfort in each other's presence. I miss him when we're apart.

His reaction to music is pleasant to behold. I've seen him

transported by "The Ode to Joy." The building intensity of "Kashmir," by Led Zeppelin, is almost too exciting for him to bear. For a time, he concocted his own little tunes, which he liked to hum or whistle. But now that has stopped.

I spent some time just watching this guy the other day. He sat on the tile floor in the entryway of our house. One of my shoes was at his side, and he held the lace in his right hand, flopping it back and forth, a very intent expression on his face. With his left hand, meanwhile, he repeatedly thrummed the flexible doorstop. After a few minutes of this, he abruptly threw down the shoelace, as if that task were completed, and stood. He strode directly and purposefully to an easy chair in the living room, where he perched. Leaning forward, he lightly rubbed the back of his hand against the edge of the coffee table, experimenting with different degrees of pressure, while he stared in the general direction of the ceiling, again with an expression of serious concentration. Completing that, he found a sheet of paper, which he held by a corner and moved so that its weight fell first to one side of his hand and then the other. I don't know whether he is systematically progressing through a hierarchy of tactile needs or simply groping for an activity to help him make sense of the world. He seems content in these activities until one of us prompts him to attempt something more constructive.

Song Yi and I eventually added a new child to the household, a delightful little girl I named Susannah, who effortlessly hit all the developmental milestones ahead of schedule. Language in particular came to Susie early, and from the beginning she displayed an unusual alertness to the value of words, and how they can be exploited. Early in her second year of life I intervened once when I thought Song Yi was scolding her a bit excessively. "Lighten up. She's just a little girl," I said soothingly. A week later it was my turn to speak sharply, and those words came back in the form of a carefully preserved get-out-of-jail card: "I'm just a little girl," Susie reminded me sweetly. I began predicting a brilliant future for her in the law.

Susie has always loved her big brother. As a toddler, she dogged "Puffoo," as she called him, like a shadow whenever he was in the house. He, meanwhile, alternated between signs of annoyance at having a pesky little sister underfoot and (I think) pride in her. In recent years she has become touchingly protective, nurturing—almost like a parent to him.

I should mention that I approached the risk of parenthood again with enormous misgivings, since I did not feel at all capable of raising another kid with developmental problems. But my fear was no match for Song Yi's confidence and formidable determination.

Ren bie ren, qi su ren is a Chinese expression that can be translated as: "If you compare your lot to that of someone else, it'll make you crazy." There's no justice in remembering that Judy would have given anything under the sun to raise a child like Susannah. This girl is precisely what she hoped for when she spoke of trying again, a couple years before her illness. I don't feel deserving of the good fortune given me so late in life. But neither does Joseph deserve his fate.

More recently, we've added one last child, a son named Braxton, after my father. Braxton was delivered by C-section, seven weeks ahead of his due date, so I got a repeat of that experience of visiting my baby in a neonatal ICU. This time we were in one of the elite hospitals—the same one in fact that had the illustrious Dr. Merritt on its staff back in Joseph's infancy. An astonishing array of medical resources was deployed for our new baby's benefit, and he responded admirably. In due course, he was discharged with no reported issues.

As a preemie, Braxton was considered to be at risk, and so the hospital referred us to familiar resources, including CCS and the Regional Center. We said thanks but no thanks when they called, and instead I applied various Institutes principles, such as keeping him prone on the floor. I even tracked down Lidwina, whom I found living in Australia. She was only too happy to offer suggestions for optimizing his chances. And he thrived.

Parents often observe that their children are very different from each other, and that's the case with us as well. Braxton has yet to display his sister's gift for words, but he is the toughest, most physically active kid I've ever encountered. As he becomes mobile, this means continually going from one misadventure to another, all day long. I once secretly believed that parents whose children were injured should have been more careful, but nobody could shield Braxton from all the bumps and tumbles he suffers in the course of an average day. Thankfully, thus far, none has even slowed him down.

WE'VE MOVED from the old neighborhood, of course, away from the familiar places where Joseph and I logged so many miles on hands and knees in the grass. Sometimes I wonder if we really did all that stuff. But when an errand brings me back, as it did today, and I see the settings again, the memory is strong.

What we did then, we did well. I can take pride in that. We launched Joseph in a new direction, on a course that has not yet concluded. I step from one flagstone to the next under olive trees near the steep grassy hillside in Presidio Park. We were creeping on that slope one Independence Day years ago when a Mexican family walked past us, carrying the fixings for their picnic. Just as they passed, the father dropped a watermelon, which broke into large pieces. Laughing, he jumped sideways, scrambling to intercept them as they spun down the hill.

The people here today are quiet, mostly reading in the sunshine, as people did then as well. Perhaps I know some of them, or more likely perhaps some of them remember Joseph. Many times, in the first year or so after Song Yi arrived from China, she told me people stopped their cars as she walked through the neighborhood with Joseph. "It's Joseph!" They shouted. "How's he doing? Do he and his parents still live over there?" She was too shy, still too uncertain with her English, to introduce herself or get their names.

I turn back. Song Yi and the kids are a couple blocks away in Old Town, buying flower pots, I think. She'll be impatient to move along to the next item on today's list. I look once more up at that long hillside, recalling all that expended energy. Joseph's mobility was worth the cost, but further reward would have been nice. Oh, to have a real conversation with him. Even one. His last word to me was at least five years ago, now. We were walking together when he stopped and frowned at the sound of distant barking. "Dog," he announced seriously, like a toddler.

I can still hope for more. Is there even such a thing as *false* hope? I always said no to that.

I will *never* give up on him.

How can I, when every year brings promise of new untried avenues? There remains the possibility of a scientific breakthrough. For example, recently I read of a project to develop targeted treatments for the very symptoms Joseph displays. I contacted the principal researcher, as I always do when these things come along. She assured me that, because she has a grown son like Joseph, she is highly motivated to find something useful in our own lifetime, as opposed to doing basic science. There is also genetic engineering and synthetic biology. There is even talk of thought-to-speech technology. If the research is more promising, there may yet be a bridge to clinical experience.

In addition, we have the option of simply holding on to the vision.

It's not too late. On days like this, I think something new for him may not be so far away. It could even be today. There is no better place for it to come forth. Maybe when I turn once again I'll see them. Susannah will be running ahead, ecstatic, shouting to me, like the kid I hear right now, who's still too far away for me to understand more than "Daddy!"

I'll see them straggling up Mason Street, Song Yi laden with her package and a squirming Braxton who insists as always on getting down. You can never hold onto that little rascal for long when he's awake. Joseph hangs back beside them, but as we draw closer I see that little smile of his, shy and proud at the same time. *Don't be shy, boy. Don't hide your light under a bushel.* No, I should be quiet. I've said too much to him.

We have eye contact, even across this distance. He has his mother's eyes, and I see in them a fading recollection of the pain he suffered as a baby, his fury at not being understood so many times, the fatigue of the program, the confusion and boredom of being moved along by other people's agendas. Could he now be at a new threshold?

"He's talking, Daddy!" Susannah is beside me, breathless, her up-turned freckled face wide open with excitement. "You are not going to believe this. Joseph just started talking!"

And this is one of those moments in life, like when he was born, like when my father recognized me again. Lord, they don't come along very often. Maybe they're never deserved. All we can do is welcome them and give thanks.

"Don't tell me any more," I'll breathe. "Let me hear for myself what he has to say."

May 2008
San Diego

ACKNOWLEDGMENTS

I WISH IT WERE POSSIBLE to express adequately my profound appreciation to the many wonderful people who did everything they possibly could to help Joseph. Two professionals deserve special mention: Viola Frymann, DO, FAAO, FCA, founder of the Osteopathic Center for Children and Families in San Diego, and Lidwina van Dÿk, a developmentalist now based in Victoria, Australia. There were also a great many individuals who stepped forward to help simply because it was in their nature to do so. I cannot name them all, but special mention is owed to Sally Arguilez Smith, Marzi Atwood Gerard, Greg and Nancy Eberhardt, Jackie Glascock, Andy and Donna Guevara, Marge Hawtree, Elaine Heffernan, Pat Jenni, Frank and Evelyn Kleber, Shirley and Cara McKevitt, Ric and Carolyn Nelson, Nan O'Hara, Isabel Sapien Gallick, Becky Rodenbush, Will Shelton, Ruth Wenger, and Carolyn Wilson.

Writing this book contributed to my mental health during some difficult years, but several individuals subsequently played a major role in helping me refine that work into the product you now hold. I wish to thank participants on the authonomy website who offered feedback, including Paul Clayton, Kate Kasserman, Juliet O'Callaghan, Sue Parker, and Jenny Ruhl. Thomas Larson, author of *The Memoir and the Memoirist*, chaired a critique group composed of several writers, notably Linda Hutchison, Joan Mangan, Patrick McMahon, Ollie

McNamara, Steve Montgomery, Sue Norberg, and Kay Sanger. We met regularly to pick apart one another's work, and I thank all of them for convincing me that this story needed to reveal more of my own emotional journey. Previously, I had thought it sufficient merely to document the events. Peggy Lang, editorial director of Silver Threads, led a series of insightful workshops at a writers' conference that I attended and later advised me on the structure of the narrative. Jeanette Green, a very accomplished editor who also has a professional background in mental health issues, read the entire thing and offered salient advice. I am indebted to Deborah Bell for providing the cover illustration. Finally, even the best of books have little value if they never see the light of day, and Jared Kuritz played a vital role in shepherding this one through production and into the market.